POSTURAL FITNESS

Significance and Variances

Charles LeRoy Lowman, M.D., Sc.D., F.A.C.S.

*Chief of Staff, Orthopedic Hospital, Emeritus; Director School, Physical Therapy,
University of Southern California; Consultant, Rehabilitation and Director
of Education, Orthopedic Hospital*

Carl Haven Young, Ed.D., C.C.T., F.A.A.P.M.R.

Professor Physical Education, University of California, Los Angeles

61 Illustrations

Lea & Febiger
PHILADELPHIA

Library of Congress Card Catalog Number 60:7370
Printed in the United States of America

To the memory of Claire Colestock, teacher and student of corrective physical education in the Pasadena City Schools; and to the many inspired leaders and capable individuals who through the years have continued to extend the orbit and liaison of physical education, orthopedics and movement, this text is respectfully dedicated.

Foreword

THE authors of this book have avoided the conventional cliche that good posture may result from vigorous living, and, concerned with far more than the physical mechanics of posture, have encompassed the relationships between posture and personality.

It has remained for these writers to go beyond the exposition of the evolution of the subject of human posture and its philosophical emergences, into the organization of a practical method providing available sources for the proper identification of faulty posture and a regimen of treatment, training and rehabilitation in which the modalities of physical education play an important and effective role. This in itself is a difficult, complex task, but, fully cognizant of the need for a reevaluation of existing methods, the authors point out that the conventional regimens of holding and overcontraction of the muscles as primary methods in postural reeducation are being restudied from the standpoint of their promotion of necessary body awareness.

Scientific data available in this and many other contributions point to an extensive, indeed alarming prevalence of postural defect and deficiency. From 30 to 40 per cent of all individuals examined for induction into the armed services since the Korean War were rejected. Conservative statistics would seem to indicate that approximately 70 per cent of this group had postural divergency. It has been noted in statistical studies that even physical education and drama students, who might be expected to have good posture, show an alarming high incidence of postural deformity.

One has only to observe people in any community to be impressed with the array of incongruities of gait, walking, standing and sitting. The characteristically lowered heads of the regressed schizophrenics and the haughty elevated heads of the paranoids, examples which can be repeated many fold, demonstrate the prevalence of postural disorder in pathological cases. A noted pediatrician avers that adults have not overgrown the period of childhood when the important thing was to walk, not how to walk, and as a result we have well nigh universal poor walking posture. To this can well be added the tensions and hurry of our highly socialized and industrialized lives, which occupy one's attention to an extent that purposive concentration on such natural activities, as are associated with locomotion and rest, for example, becomes increasingly difficult. Ensuing chronic fatigue becomes a recognizable factor and as the authors aver, "Segmental troubles can strike catastrophically."

Further, there is confirmation of the need for more precise instruments in the organization of methods for health training with its many implications for postural education. The new science of labor, itself being physical performance and to a large degree dependent upon efficient posture, is taking cognizance of the prevalence of faulty body mechanics as a factor affecting economic production.

Now that the need for such a contribution as this is evident, the next problem pertains to the provision of scientific means. What is required in specific method? The authors take a broad and intensive look at this problem and gain a perspective which is able to relate such progressive concepts of habilitation, rehabilitation, education and reeducation to the treatment aims prescribed by the physican. Concern is expressed for the quality and extent of teachers' training which equips them to serve in this newly developing paramedical area. They find that exercise modalities must be far more specific than sports and games for recreation. They naturally look to the physician for the criteria and standards for such specialized training required. Paramedical disciplines represented by occupational therapists and physical therapists and nurses are being augmented by new professional groups, such as the corrective therapists, who in addition to a physical education and education background have specialized instruction in medical subjects and a rich clinical experience gained in a hospital setting.

Since most of these paramedical personnel work in hospitals rather than schools, however, there is a great dearth of the individuals trained in the necessary technical skills for schools, where need for postural training in both its preventive and corrective aspects is so evident. There is equally a very great need for the provision of specific and highly specialized subject matter for such instruction which, as the authors point out, must go far beyond the principles of adapted physical education, oriented primarily to social aims and values. To insure the educational application of anatomical principles it is necessary for the educator to gain more than didactic instruction, he needs to secure experience in a clinical setting. A general introduction to anatomy, in relationship to weight bearing and the movement function of the muscles and neural mechanism associated with posture, needs to be complemented by clinical experience to avoid the errors which can so easily creep into the situation when the physical educator overstresses uncritical physical conditioning as a primary approach to postural training. Such procedures must take into consideration the variations in type, skeletal, physiological, neurological and mental, and must be fitted into a concept of postural fitness which includes, in addition to physical health, neurological functions, physiological health and emotional well being. It is this spectrum of an all determinant of health that will give a rational outlook for a professional approach to the dual problem of therapy and education.

According to social scientists, any progressive innovation in the forward march of health services depends to a great extent upon its understanding acceptance by the man on the street. An effective medical regimen is not enough without public education. Happily, the authors have put into practice this fundamental principle. They have provided not only medically validated, specific procedures through formal therapeutic exercises and modifications of informal sport activities, but have also made an attempt to persuade individuals concerned, including parents and school administrators, to take the required remedial action. A well-organized scientific study of physiological actions and anatomical structures with graduated exercise is elevated to the perspective of a philosophical presentation in a broad yet intensive approach which extends far beyond the mechanics of the problem.

In a style, lively, interesting and richly personalized by the deep interest and dedication of the authors, the reader will find real substance which will stimulate him to do something about a problem which contains both a promise and a threat. The aim is to motivate the individual to attain this enrichment not only of his organic functioning, but of the democratic way of life. This "development leads to larger plans of action and understanding" as the community through various approaches attains greater segmental consciousness with its strengthening associations of dignity and pride. The citizen must realize that good posture is everybody's business and there is even more to the problem than its esthetic aspects. The concept of a significant relationship of segmental alignment to social stability and behavior orderliness, while still at the level of theory, is well within the imagination of the man on the street and the progressive outlook of the social scientist.

The visualization of the approach to this problem as a communal attack seems well taken. One must give recognition and respect to the dominant role of the physician in all medical matters. Just, however, as one accepts a totalistic concept of exercise in the sense that no single movement is considered isolated but a member of the motor community interacting with others, one accepts the concept of a team composed of medical, paramedical, educational and community personnel working together, with the strongest cohesive force of this union being the patient conceived as a doer as well as a receiver. This principle though well accepted requires a realistic viewpoint for its execution. Clear guide lines have been presented for the role of various team members to insure that the job will be done when and where it is needed, and that these people in the various categories are properly trained with both medical and educational equipment for the task. The importance of giving not only responsibility, but a sense of importance to the individual team member and fostering his feeling of individuality and sense of personal accomplishment is recognized as an essential of successful human engineering as applied to medicine and education as well as industry.

This contribution is vitalized, further, by progressive concepts of rehabilitation which conceive the problem as a social movement, in which the potentials of the well become active factors in the restoration of the unwell, postural fitness being a segment of this relationship. Sensitive to the motivational needs of a people in an industrialized culture, ways are sought to motivate the individual to do something about his postural divergency. The broad suggestion is to work *with* not *on* or *for* the person being treated, so as to build up the constructive elements of independence. The word "with" looms large in this perspective. One must work with not only the patient, but also his fellow workers and the community. It seems that only in this way can the dynamics of education enthuse the procedures of medicine, stimulate the participation of citizens and motivate the individual being treated. Thus he is motivated by these multilateral forces to follow the fundamental principle of helping himself. The upright posture as a reality and an aim dignifies the individual and the efforts to attain it.

JOHN EISELE DAVIS, SC.D.

REHOBETH, DELAWARE

Executive Director, Association
Physical and Mental Rehabilitation
Former Chief, Corrective Therapy,
Veterans Administration Central Office,
Washington, D. C.

Preface

POSTURAL fitness may be defined as that fitness which each individual should seek to achieve, whereby he may assume and maintain proper segmental relationship in all movements of the body. Such a state of fitness provides functional efficiency in handling the body in all postural positions undertaken in work, play or everyday living. The significance and variances of postural fitness, as they appear here, are limited chiefly to the observable conditions and deviations affecting health, appearance, psychological attitudes and social characteristics. No definite standard of postural fitness for all is proposed, other than the suggestion of urgency for individual effort in striving toward the ultimate in body build and in efficiency of movement.

This text has been prepared to provide, with a modicum of scientific details, practical guide lines pertaining to:

(a) Prevention of potential growth faults,
(b) Discovery of divergencies in structure and function among people of all ages,
(c) Significance in the relationship of proper segmental alignment to the systems of the body,
(d) Various procedures for the development of necessary musculature.

Such information is of special significance to the students majoring in physical education, to teachers in the area of corrective or adaptive physical education, and to those working in clinical situations, such as physicians, therapists and nurses.

It is hoped, further, that this book will serve to inform classroom instructors, school nurses, and parents of the importance of early observation and referral of irregularities in structural and functional patterns to those on whom the responsibility rests for arranging the developmental, maintenance and therapeutic phases of programs concerned with the afore-mentioned problems.

Throughout this book attention has been directed to those leaders and administrators who have opportunities, while conducting their services, for inspiring special reliance and confidence in people. Such persons are school principals, counsellors, specialists in health, physical education, recreation and rehabilitation, and orthopedic physicians. No one of this group has a priority in caring for the need and treatment of those individuals burdened

(9)

with divergencies or weaknesses. On the other hand it is this leadership through a team approach which bears the responsibility to recognize, refer, prevent, or correct such conditions as may be discovered, and to maintain at a high level the postural health of those persons within their area of jurisdiction.

In addition, there is a belief that this book will arouse many lay persons and individuals in the professional and business world to an appreciation of the necessity for improving or maintaining their own postural fitness, and for guarding against possible postural relapse in later adult years.

Much of the content material and many of the techniques outlined have been tested in practical situations throughout the nation. Effort has been made to point out:

  (a) The prevalence of irregularities in structural and functional patterns,
  (b) Transitional stages in growth, development, maturity, and adjustment,
  (c) Interrelationships of body segments and their importance to efficiency,
  (d) Dissimilarities which exist among people,
  (e) Procedural techniques for determining variations,
  (f) Fundamentals of exercise beliefs,
  (g) Individual group planning in terms of needs,
  (h) Clarification of group procedures and individual measures,
  (i) Specific exercise precepts and recommendations to follow.

Due to many requests, for the convenience of students and teachers there has been included in the Appendixes A and B, a series of exercise plans modified from the texts on *Corrective Physical Education for Groups* and *Fundamental Exercises for Physical Fitness*. This material is centered chiefly on the adaptation, progression, arrangement and application of exercises to suit major group needs.

Since the class in physical education is usually the focal point in reaching early young people with postural difficulties, greater emphasis has been directed to the school situation. There is no intention of neglecting other approaches in the solution of these problems, for all have a part in the team endeavor to promote postural fitness for the members of society.

C. L. L.
C. H. Y.

Los Angeles, California

Acknowledgments

GRATEFUL thanks is expressed to the many young people in universities, colleges and public schools and to those hospital patients whose lives have furnished a constant challenge and a demand for pioneering research and application in an effort to make their future more meaningful. Their faith and hope have hastened the productive search for better ways and means of meeting individual needs and capacities. Personal interest in their welfare has likewise offered a steadying influence which has fostered caution in practices as the most beneficial procedure.

Friendly understanding of colleagues through the years and their personal examples of dedication have furnished considerable encouragement and motivation. Of particular significance has been the inspiration derived from fellow members of the faculty of the Department of Physical Education, University of California, Los Angeles, as well as those at the University of Southern California, Los Angeles, and from San Diego State College, San Diego, California.

Special appreciation is due many administrators and teachers of the Los Angeles City and County Schools, Pasadena and Alameda Public Schools for the many opportunities for service, as well as all other educational institutions whose personnel and students have given of their time, assistance and cooperation. Particular mention should be made of the outstanding contributions for many years by physicians and staff members of the Los Angeles Orthopedic Hospital, Los Angeles, California.

Worthy of recognition was the outstanding work of the officers and enlisted men of the United States Navy Pre-Flight Schools, who through their diligent efforts and sincerity of purpose made possible the development and maintenance of physical fitness. Expecially valuable in the conducting of beneficial programs and the collating of data were all those members of the Mass Exercise Department at St. Marys Pre-Flight School, Moraga, California during World War II.

Sincere tribute is offered to Dr. John Eisele Davis, formerly Chief, Corrective Therapy, Veterans Administration, Central Office, Washington, D. C. for his writing of the foreword; and Dr. Elwood C. Davis, Professor, University of Southern California, as well as the former authority, for their critical review of the manuscript and helpful suggestions for implementation. The advice and counsel of Arthur Steindler, M.D., Professor, University of Iowa, Iowa City, Iowa in respect to requests as to questionable procedures have been of particular assistance and guidance.

To our wives, Elizabeth Lowman and Florence Blood Young, our love and gratitude for their continuous help and encouragement during the span of our careers in the conjoined professional fields of Physical Education and Orthopedic Surgery which has resulted in this collaboration. Outstanding credit and appreciation are due Florence for her sensitive editing of the text and diligent pursuit of reference source materials applicable to the subject field.

The vital encouragement and patience of the editorial members of Lea & Febiger, our publisher, are worthy of note and have inspired our devoted energies in an attempt to justify their confidence and trust.

C. L. L.
C. H. Y.

Los Angeles, California

Contents

Contents

18　　　　　　　　　　List of Figures

Postural Fitness

CHAPTER 1

The Broadening Concept for Opportunity and Service

TODAY, more than ever, this nation is vitally concerned with the potential growth, development and maintenance of *all* its citizenry, which is due in large measure to the high standards of living available to the majority of people. Emphasis in the past has been centered, largely, upon those best able to adapt their capabilities to the demands of society. Yet the wealth of resources inherent in those individuals needing attention has often lain dormant for lack of adequate assistance.

Evidence of such concern is apparent in the recent national conferences and research investigations by prominent leaders in the fields of health, physical and recreation education, and medicine. Justification for the many criticisms as to the fitness of young people may be contested on the basis of methods for determining fitness as well as for the comparisons with the youth of foreign countries where the study originated. However, it is recognized that there is need for an expansion of efforts by those qualified to better organize the nation's forces, and that attention and direction must be given to all during the growing years in order that the maturing period of life may be meaningful.[1]

An expanding democratic philosophy has contributed to a broadening concept of the possibilities for opportunity and service in the desired achievement of a more inclusive national fitness. Such a concept has evolved through:

1. Changing perspectives as to:
   (*a*) the necessity for integrated effort for *all* age groups;
   (*b*) the shifting of educational method from a specialist to a team approach;
   (*c*) the urgency for educating and treating the individual as a functional unity;
   (*d*) the importance of the experienced instructor in detecting early variance in individual performance;

      (*e*) the increasing significance of required attention to adult needs.
2. Recognition of the necessity for well-established, adequate fitness programs which will function equally well in the normalcy of peace or during the exigency of war.
3. The scrutiny as to the prevalence of variance in postural conditions in various decades and situations.
4. A comprehension of the increasing responsibility of the school and the administrator in providing services for meeting therapeutic needs arising in achievement of all phases of postural fitness.

Education in our democratic society is faced with tremendous responsibilities, many of which have been delegated to the teaching profession. Public and private agencies as well as schools and commercial enterprises have been established to provide services necessary for all-round mental, social, and physical development, maintenance and rehabilitation. The import of the physical, mental and social welfare of all individuals, irrespective of race, color or creed, challenges all the resources of the schools and society. As the White House Conference, 1930–1931, declared:[2]

> If we want civilization to march forward, it will march, not only on the feet of healthy children, but beside them, shoulder to shoulder, must go those others—those children we have called 'handicapped'—the lame ones, the blind, the deaf, and those sick in body and mind. All these children are ready to make their contribution to human progress; to bring what they have of intelligence, of capacity, of spiritual beauty. American civilization cannot spare them.

The task confronting the educator, physician, parents and community today is not only to habilitate and rehabilitate this group, but to assist in the prevention of potential growth faults, and to aid in the maximum development and maintenance of all the citizenry in order that they may function through life to their optimum efficiency.[3]

The tremendous importance of this need has been attested to by the medical profession, educators, social workers, therapists, and many others. Efforts must now be centered upon the collating of pertinent information for ready reference and the liaison of all resources for best results. There is a rapidly growing recognition of the necessity for continuous evaluation of individuals' needs, and the implications physiologically, psychologically and sociologically inherent in these experiences. Only when the worker utilizes all avenues of value in contributing to the desired goal, not only *to* and *for*, but *with* the individual, will the eagerly sought outcomes accrue.

Physical education programs in this nation, when conducted by competently prepared instructors, offer one of the best means for carrying out many of these precepts under the direction of and in conjunction with physicians. Physical education must surely assume the major responsibility for the development and efficient use of the antigravity muscles, which are essential for the adequate maintenance of skeletal function throughout life. Performance is contingent upon the efficacy in alignment of body structures and physical fitness in accordance with physiological laws.

The concept of opportunity and service is consistently broadening in keeping with the possibilities for reaching a higher degree of national fitness through the extension of the ever widening orbit of educational facilites and programs. The dedicated efforts of all concerned must be earnestly solicited if America's greatest resource, human beings, is to be fully conserved and utilized.

CHANGING PERSPECTIVES

The importance of the individual in society has resulted from the changing concepts of an enlightened people in this nation, who have chosen as their philosophy the latter of two diametrically opposed ideas. The autocratic or totalitarian state requires for its continued existence blind obedience to the will of its self appointed rulers, and calls for an unquestioning group discipline with no freedom of thought or expression. In the democratic state there is dependence upon the freeing of the individual through education, with a greater understanding of and a more intelligent participation in social and political problems related to personal welfare.

Without this type of thinking it is impossible to consider the well-being of the individual, his rights or privileges and the educational objectives for society. This is what Democracy stands for, and only when we seek to discover and advance the potentialities of our fellow man are we true to our ideals.

In terms of the demands which are being made on people in the present social order, and the belief in the worth of each person, it is necessary for a better understanding of the basic needs of those with whom we are dealing and of possible ameliorative procedures for their benefit. The crying demand for an *integration of effort for all age groups* rather than an isolated segment of the population is a growing trend. It is evident upon reflection, that each subject field or resource, in its own small sphere, is striving valiantly to supply the necessary understanding and equipment essential in this race called life. The collating of energies would make more productive and lasting the effect, for age is but a circumstance and the years are like a piece of string which slips quickly through the cat's paw.

There has likewise been a shifting in the methods of teaching and treatment of individuals from specialists in education and medicine, directing their efforts separately within a narrow field or subject area, to that of *the coordinated team approach.* This significant change has taken place through the realization of the important influence of every cohesive contact, which multiplies many fold the benefits possible through this fanning out process and thus supplies the concerted rather than uncoordinated experiences and motivational influences. Such an approach permits the leader to utilize all available resources and to visualize the importance of his efforts and implications in terms of the life span, as well as the teachable moments, opportunities and influence upon present and future generations.

Through the belief advanced in the organismal approach may be found a means for further clarification of interrelationships, in which the mind and body are considered so closely related as to be one, so close in union that the condition of one has a corresponding effect upon the other. On terms of this holistic approach, all parts of man are tied or woven together as in a web. The human organism is considered as a highly complex ensemble of intricate mental and physical traits that are intertwined and interdependent upon each other.

As one part functions, all other parts are affected. They exert reciprocal influence upon one another and are mutually influenced by environmental and hereditary forces. Therefore, the physical and mental are two aspects of the same organism, and any program or treatment must give due consideration to all of the factors affecting the growth, development and maintenance of the human organism as a whole or as a *functional unity.*

It is difficult to understand the encompassing interdependence of the organism without appreciating the radiating influence which those who deal with children and youth may have upon the present and future well-being. An ever extending peripheral horizon of thinking, which visualizes goals of activity directed toward continued attention during adult and senior years, has been perceived and realized. The underlying purpose is so directed that the cumulative investments in people may result in greater accrued profits of physical vigor and happiness as well as in productive ability.

There is general acceptance in a Democracy of the principle that attention to growth factors is essentially the prerogative of the parents and family physician because of their personal interest, concern and knowledge of proper procedures. Yet these persons

accept the fact that much of the obligation for physical development is delegated in the growing years to the role of the physical
education departments in schools.

Education offers a vehicle, by means of a wide range of activities,
for the motivation of the individual through participatory experiences conducive to maturing development.   In the controlling
hands of competent and experienced instructors are the following
possibilities:

1. Innumerable opportunities for early recognition of potential
   growth divergencies and for referral to the orthopedist who
   collaborates, integrates all resources, and makes provision
   for preventive measures to avoid possible difficulties from
   arising through procedures which may be harmful to some.
2. Opportune moments when pertinent health practices may be
   caught rather than taught in the medium of the game.
3. Favorable circumstances wherein the greatest good may be
   derived unknowingly in respect to physical development
   through participation.
4. Adjustable hours in providing for adapted programs for
   those with physical limitations who may take part in certain
   prescribed activities, and in establishing developmental
   classes for those needing knowledge as to habilitation and
   rehabilitation, or for the underpar individual.

The connotation inherent in the term *developmental* implies a
postiveness rather than a negativism so often connected with such
titles as remedial, corrective, adapted and others.   In certain
instances there is a place for the use of such terms, yet they are
more specific to certain types of treatment of various conditions
rather than of general meaning.   It should be pointed out here
that conditions of a divergent nature are often due to the functional or structural failure of unilateral balance in antagonistic
muscle groups.   More often there is a complete lack of proper
development or a weakness of specific antigravity muscles as a
contributing cause.

The term *developmental* came into common use during World
War II, when it was applied to special classes needing to receive
postural attention or to overcome certain physical weaknesses
found among cadets in the United States Naval Aviation Pre-
Flight School training program.   A description of its application
may be found in the text, *Mass Exercise, Games, Tests*,[4] or revisions
entitled, *Conditioning Exercises, Games, Tests*.[5]   Necessity for a
phrase which implied positive motivation to cadets and officers
was apparent.   Therefore, the term *developmental* was adopted
serving to encourage correction of divergencies or weakness, and,
hence, to make for more capable flyers.   Through this service

there was a considerable lessening of the effect of injuries from the strenuous athletic program, and a noticeable interest created in the maintenance of condition gained in this type of classes.

A comparable situation exists today in civilian life wherever there is a need for personal attention of a like nature. Such cases require development of the individual in certain specific areas in order to reach a peak potential, while others, to attain best results, call for habilitation or rehabilitation of a therapeutic form.

Education is a public enterprise with its tools of the trade, facilities and trained technicians readily available, with no time limits prescribed as to the length of the educative process. What better conveyance is more suitable whereby programs similar to those for young people may be offered in adapted form for the *adult and senior citizen*? Physicians, perhaps more than any other group, realize that life itself is dependent upon vigorous physical activity, and follow this precept in their practice of recommending early mobilization of the involved parts in most operative cases. Programs of activity are prescribed for the paraplegic for uninvolved body segments. At the same time the doctor is alert concerning the need for activity of the normal person.

Today, more and more, people are turning to commercial organizations for assistance in physical activity, so as to compensate for the many labor saving devices which require less energy and to offset the lack of big muscle activity in their vocations. Transportation by automobile is substituted for walking. Shorter working hours leave more free time which is usually taken up with sedentary pursuits. True, serious attempts are being made to offer stimulating recreational activities of a physical nature, but many participate without due regard as to their own physical limitations or to consideration of their immediate condition. Such programs must be based upon the individual's specific needs and competencies, under the direction of qualified persons who serve as maintenance engineers. Activities for this group might well be instituted during the summer or vacation months when both school facilities and personnel are more readily available. Such provision might possibly serve to stimulate the interest and continuance of these pursuits. In this way there might evolve the desire for other more individualized recreational activities, presuming that all would first have the advantage of bringing their physical condition to a state of readiness.

It may be seen from the presentation of changing perspectives that for the developing and maintaining of effective citizenry, there needs to be a continuing emphasis upon provision for all age groups, in order that the string of life may be lengthened, and so that the significance of the spirit may be appreciated in relation to the psychosomatic values to the individual. These persons who have so much to offer with their wealth of experience and understanding must be made to realize that no greater thrill can come to them than through the experience of finding greater happiness in being needed. The fact that many are cognizant of these implied obligations has been evident from the expressions of leaders throughout this nation to the extent that serious considerations are being prepared for effecting such fruitful measures. Only in this way may it be said that we are punching holes in the dark and lightening the way for a more effective citizenry.

RECOGNITION OF IMPERATIVE NEEDS FOR ADEQUATE FITNESS PROGRAMS

During the stress of national emergencies as well as in the Universal Military Training Program, the urgent demand for able manpower becomes an indispensable requirement, although the same hypothesis in regard to similar needs is likewise a requisite for civilian pursuits. True, the inadequacies in respect to the physical fitness and preparation of individuals for the tasks required, are brought into prominence more readily during war periods than in peacetime, yet it is an irrefutable fact that a large majority of the people are below par physically in many respects.

In facing the issue it is difficult to accept any alternative, for these data as disclosed in the subsequent pages can neither be disregarded nor overlooked in the face of the evidence revealed. It is apparent that measures must be taken for the amelioration of the causes through adequate preventive programs in medicine, physical education and the home.

That leaders are cognizant of the significance of the dual problem and the portent at times of emergency inherent in these findings, together with more recent research investigations, has been exemplified in the statements of several qualified authorities quoted in the publication, *Fundamental Exercises for Physical Fitness*,[6] in 1943. These statements evidenced the priceless ingredients of frontier thinking, integrity of belief and sincerity of purpose intended to tickle imaginations to the extent that people are motivated to investigate for themselves more desirable ways of life. These leaders have sought to encourage the providing of better opportunities for all, and now urge the diligent pursuance of a course which may influence future actions and human welfare.

Generalizing from a single analogy, namely, the armed services or war period point of view, is perhaps overstressing an era in which the haste of preparation is most demanding. The need in terms of immediacy at such a time is for a product without flaws and in peak physical condition, with the ability to perform arduous tasks over long periods of time. It is clearly apparent that concern should be felt for dilatory practices which allow young men and women to become a figure in the statistics of inadequacies, an indictment against many systems now malfunctioning. Criticism has been particularly directed toward overzealous leaders who ignore the basic law of vulnerability in trauma producing activities when participated in beyond the maturational age.

Programs, like people, must have stability and balance, with a prospectus conducive to continuous re-evaluation as to concomitant factors and outcomes. Blueprints for building such programs must be drawn from the considered judgment of qualified persons, who have based their opinions upon research findings and observations as to what is believed to be most desirable practice. Guide lines may then be formulated to provide for the wide range of needs through experiences most conducive to the best advantage of all.

The leadership of the American Association of Health, Physical Education, and Recreation is a source of satisfaction because of its increased emphasis on determining scientifically the essential requisites, relative merits of various activities, judicious procedures for administering its offerings, and integrative planning of endeavors with the fields of medicine, education, public and private agencies. This association is not satisfied to accept a laissez-faire policy.

Orthopedic surgeons, pediatrists, school and family physicians, likewise perceive their mission and tasks, recognizing that improvement in the health status of the child is the best prevention for many ills and deficiencies of adult life. Structural deviations and bad biomechanics from faults in growth and development are a definite factor in the production of such later ailments as sciatica, cervicodorsal neuritis, bursitis and arthritis. Such postural deviations as flatfeet, backknees, knock knees, pelvic tilts from short legs, scoliosis and many other such conditions, produce a wear and tear demand and cumulative effect that ultimately endangers health and impairs efficiency at all ages.

VARIANCE IN POSTURAL CONDITIONS

In his classification on a postural basis of college entrants in 1923, Lloyd T. Brown found a definite correlation between the student's health status and his postural condition. Brown's classification rated the various relative ranks as A excellent, B good, C poor, and D as very poor mechanical use of the body. This survey indicated a high proportion of from 80 to 85 per cent in the C and D groups, with the greatest number of illnesses, operations and early nutritional and physiological faults being present in these groups as based on this scale.[7]

Research over a considerable number of years in various situations in California, and covering a wide span of age levels, has revealed authentic statistics concerning the diverse types and incidence of conditions which call for special attention accruing among high school and college age men. Such cases were classified as to posture, feet and ankles, weight divergencies, medical conditions according to the physician's diagnoses, and those persons with poor muscle tone and development. Only those cases of second or third degree severity, 15 pounds below or 20 pounds over normal (according to the Pryor Width-Weight Index Tables),[8] medical conditions referred by the physician, and those cases considered extreme as to lack of physical development, or physically illiterate as to motor skills, were included in the data.

At Alameda High School, Alameda, California, from 1932 to 1937, with an annual enrollment of approximately 2200 students, 1200 of this number being boys, 1473 entering freshman boys were examined and an average of 57.16 per cent or 842 students with 1290 different divergencies and 448 duplicate conditions were found to need special physical education. Of this number the following classifications were recorded: 337 posture, 641 feet and ankles, 237 weight deviations and 75 medical cases which were referred to such classes. In this residential city of about 30,000 at the time of this survey, no previous corrective instruction had been offered to these students. This community might be considered as a representative cross section of the average residential area.

In three semesters between 1940 and 1942, at San Diego State College, San Diego, California, where there were about 2200 students enrolled annually, approximately one-half being men, 761 freshman men were examined. There were 70.4 per cent or 517 men needing attention with 1369 divergencies and 348 duplicate conditions among this group. Among these cases there were found to be 614 posture, 559 feet and ankles, 300 weight deviations, and a small proportion of medical referrals which were considered underpar from a physical standpoint. This example would appear to show that prevailing conditions present at the college level had not been outgrown during the school years, although some educators contend this will happen. Apparently either the developmental activity programs had been remiss or the significance of the problem unrecognized regarding necessity for early diagnosis and need for preventive measures which should have been taken.

According to Leroy Weir, one of the pertinent facts revealed in World War II was, that, of the first 2 million men examined under the Selective Service, 900 thousand were refused. Rejections increased from 30 per cent at age 21 to 70 per cent at age 35, this figure indicating that regression in physical ability of most young adults is more pronounced than their age justifies. The vast majority of those who were free from physical defects, in the bracket between the ages of 18 to 20, were not in condition to undergo immediate military training. It is recognized that such rejections were for all types of reasons, and, therefore, the data are not analogous to the other illustrations herein presented, but rather indicate the extent and proportion of conditions which prevail in the nation.[9]

Indicative of the similarity of findings previously shown for the schools of California, are the facts derived from postural examinations from June, 1942, to February, 1943, of the United States Naval Aviation Cadets at St. Mary's Pre-Flight School, St. Mary's College, Moraga, California. This screening was conducted in order to ascertain the need for developmental instruction, and from the survey it was considered essential that classes for this purpose be included as a part of the physical training program. As the manpower needs increased there was evidence of a lowering of standards by the Cadet Selection Boards, and conditions multiplied proportionally. Weight deviations and medical cases were not included at this time but later became a part of the responsibility delegated by the Medical Department for inclusion in such classes. Since these cadets represented all parts of the nation, it was evident that the resulting information was not unique to any one part of the country. Foot, knee and ankle conditions seemed to predominate among the causes for concern, and this implies the possible after effect of the depression years with improper footwear or poor nutrition, and considerably less exercise in walking.

A study of the recorded data discloses that of the 4,832 men examined in the sampling, 61.73 per cent, or 2,983 cadets had 8,403 divergencies with 5,233 duplicate conditions. The breakdown of the 2,983 needing work included the following weaknesses: 6,298 posture, 1,828 feet and ankles, and 277 with poor muscle tone for efficient functioning. The analysis was made by three different officers who had considerable previous experience in judging posture, and was carried on by means of personal observation of each cadet, using a posture screen. Through a follow-up study of photographs showing the anterior, posterior and lateral views by all three officers independently of each other, the individual ratings were then compiled for a composite judgment as to the presence of a specific condition.

Studies by the Department of Physical Education at Yale University, in 1954, show utilization of Photometric photography in posture evaluation of freshmen students.[10] This research confirms the findings as to the importance of postural analysis as a measure for early discovery of potential growth divergencies, whereby the physician may recommend prescriptions as to preventive and adapted procedures to be followed. In collaboration with the medical profession, investigations are being conducted to ascertain any significance or relationship to the health status.

General screening tests in the schools, in the hands of examiners of reasonable skill, will usually show at least 75 per cent of the group with faults of total or segmental deviations in pupils' body alignment according to those who make such examinations. An orthopedic specialist might add another 5 or 10 per cent to this figure, for it is common knowledge that a majority of children have some postural faults or growth divergency. After such a test or class inventory is made, it is obvious that if an improvement is to be attempted, this large group cannot be handled as separate individuals because of time involvement but may be cared for individually within a group under proper class organization. Even if a developmental or adapted program is set up, it cannot cope adequately with the general problem alone.[11]

There are those who contend that posture is a relative matter which is essentially of esthetic value and has little relation to the health status, and maintain there are comparatively small numbers of young people who have anything structurally or functionally wrong with them. Parents, orthopedists, physicians, teachers, physical educators, therapists, and others who deal with the health and physical problems of those of school age, question such shallow thinking for they see the actual cases and their implications in later life.

The answer would seem to be that, after the posture and fitness inventory, the program potentials must be studied and evaluated in terms of the therapeutic possibilities for development that are needed. All exercises and activities should be assessed on the basis of whether they are beneficial or detrimental. For example, all those that activate the antigravity muscles fall in the favorable group and all others should be minimized, neutralized or discarded. If they are of special value for other than their therapeutic influence, they may be included, but their deleterious effects on postural faults should be offset by a preponderance of movements to correct such deviations. As to games and stunts, these should be modified as to maturational age, time range, force and type, so as not to over-emphasize fatigue factors or over-development of muscle groups that are promoting deviations.

THE ROLE OF THE SCHOOL'S AND
ADMINISTRATOR'S RESPONSIBILITY

The school approach to the therapeutic problems and needs is that of an educational liaison agency, which provides a service for the teaming of all contributing resources that will bring to bear the combined contributions essential for the development, prevention, correction of potential difficulties, convalescence, and maintenence of health status.

It is not intended to imply that education will provide a panacea for all ills, nor to assume that the full responsibility for the amelioration of all divergencies is that of the school. There is definite agreement on the part of teachers that they are limited in certain preparation of a medical nature which is not their job, that professional ethics should and must be observed, and that many other circumstances rightfully prohibit their assuming the role of the physician.

As administrators and teachers, there is a place in the ascertaining of the (a) extent and type of apparent needs, (b) recommendations of school and family physicians, nurses, counsellors, classroom teachers and parents, (c) essential implementation necessary in conference with the school health council as to referrals and best possible procedures, (d) potentials available within the situation and determination as to whether the service lies within the school's jurisdiction, (e) estimated costs for the operation of an adequate program and the possible source of additional funds that may be necessary.

A compass is needed which will point the direction, and while the needle may fluctuate in various ways in accordance with the circumstances and point of view in various communities, there should evolve, under capable leadership, important changes resulting in the physical improvement of the people through such an approach.

Much has been said about the evident need for providing services which will assist the general educational program. Physicians are merely anxious that teachers do not overstep their known competence, and also that they may understand when they should consult the doctor or school nurse. When such restrictions are observed, the concensus favors the organization of special classes.

Most physical education departments do not have either specially trained instructors or separate rooms for such purposes, which are necessary for best results. Additionally, their regular classes are in most cases already too large to allow for the individual attention needed under such a program. If administrators and teachers are interested, there are opportunities to do something about the majority of cases found in any school. Ordinarily many instructors are conscious of their chance and anxious to help these individuals even in large classes.

Those most acutely aware of pupils' needs should continuously urge the teacher education institutions to offer their trainees, who include both the general classroom teacher and the physical education major student, sound ground work along the lines of nutrition, physiology and a background of adapted or developmental physical education. There should be inculded observation and contact with the physician, health service and health education offerings, so that future teachers may be better prepared to plan their activities and to obtain the maximum good for the greatest number. If this is done, more effective and constructive results will be obtained through the classroom teachers, who are largely responsible for carrying out the specific directions and suggestions of both the school physician and the physical education supervisors.

There should be less tendency, especially at the elementary and junior high school level, to lean toward the sports and athletics approach and emphasis on school prestige as a complete physical education program offering. Furthermore, major consideration should not be aimed solely at fostering the welfare of the normal and strong through competitive activities that are likely to occupy so much of the personnel's time that weaker and more needy pupils get little attention. Too often in special classes, the only program, if provided, is of a formal exercise nature, and needs to be implemented through adapted activities which include table tennis, paddle tennis, golf, regular tennis, archery, bowling, swimming, rhythmical activities and the like for those who are able to profit through general conditioning activities. In specific divergencies or restricted cases, general sports activity will accomplish little of value or may even cause real harm, thus necessitating definite neuromusclar reeducation and limited activity.

It is a healthy sign to see more physical education students being prepared for work at the elementary level, yet in most school situations throughout the nation, the physical education is conducted by the classroom teacher. It, therefore, behooves the college and university teacher-education institutions to give their students a dynamic approach to the skeletal and organic needs of the children, many of whom may need special developmental work. Without this understanding, these future teachers may not consider the needs of all their students and are likely to succumb too easily to various pressures, giving to recreation and athletics an undue proportion of the program content, their efforts and time, to the neglect of many needy.

Prospective teachers should be helped to understand that their work, beginning at the elementary school child age, is of much greater importance than only the development of academic skills. Teachers must be taught to recognize potential difficulties, fatigue, muscular insufficiencies and other functional deviations as items for reference to those responsible for following through with such cases.

If physical education is to be of major value in the lives of students, well balanced programs of guidance and development are important. Usually, members of the health and physical education staffs are the spark plugs for fostering the cooperation of all in school and community planning of this nature. Ordinarily, it is a three way effort of the team character involving (*a*) school administrators and all teachers, (*b*) parents, through the Parents and Teachers Association and Dads Clubs, and (*c*) the children themselves.

Teachers in practically every subject area can contribute to the major objectives which deal with mental and physical health, nutrition, body chemistry, physics in relation to structure and function, health education, growth and development and skill in performance. At varying times during the school year, such subjects as english, art, domestic science, social living, and dramatics offer forms of action which assist in the comprehension, and further develop the motor skills of expression together with their importance. This type of planning will call the child's attention to the marvels of his development and should aid in the motivation leading toward an attack on his own personal problems.

This is the challenge confronting the school boards, administrators, teachers, parents, medical profession and others of the community. With the realization of the vital importance for providing complete programs in behalf of children, there should result more comprehensive offerings as a result of the expressed desire of all concerned.

ATTAINING OUR PHYSICAL POTENTIAL

Throughout the lives of people, both individually and nationally, there are opportune moments or periods for buying stock as an investment in the future America. There are so many who are operating in the red, attempting to balance their receipts and budget their health expenditures in keeping with what they have of vitality. All through the ages of a person there is a potential which keeps going on and which is his maximum at that time, so that in his span of life there are certain re-occurring possibilities for peak effectiveness.

By continued effort and straining, individuals seek to acquire powers existing but not yet actualized, powers within themselves capable of coming into full being at some future time. An individual's physical ability potential varies constantly according to his age, physical and mental health status and environment. A nation's physical potential varies according to the degree to which each individual attains maximum physical efficiency at various age levels. It is hard to impress a need unless outside one's self, yet it has been found that under the stimulus of emergencies the adrenals of a nation are stimulated and its people rise to supreme possibilities.

Under the concept of mechanics in the term body mechanics, there was produced a static and not a dynamic approach to posture. The result was that efforts to make bodies conform to a fixed mold, neglected the individuality in respect to variances, and formal calisthenics became the vogue and order of the day.

With the changing times, the pendulum has swung to the other extreme, expecting play and sports alone to furnish the instrument for rectifying all difficulties. While such media have their place in the improvement of the normal individual's physical fitness, they must be properly conducted and not be accepted as the only device for the improvement of specific weaknessess nor be considered a complete regimen within the realm of all in respect to personal needs.

A procedure should be maintained in which the values needed for best synchronized neuromuscular, joint balance and skilled performance should be the goal, in order to obtain a more healthful and adequate basis for body and mind functioning. Such a process would be likely to effect a realistic background for greater success in vocational, recreational and athletic pursuits, soundly based upon engineering principles, policies and procedures, and make available a dynamic and efficient instrument for mental, emotional, physical and social expression. In this way all would be better able to live for a purpose and enjoy life more fully.

Stanley Hall's saying, "There is no emotion without motion," is still a realistic observation. When the body is considered as an instrument of expression and muscles are thought of as extensions of the brain and more than mere motors to move the body about, it is realized that personality and posture are intimately associated. A teacher, whose posture is not good, cannot be as effective a salesman of the ideas and ideals of health and physical education as one with good posture. The story told through the illustration in Figure 1 is obvious. The child or person with a fatigue slump looks lazy, weak or sick; at least he does not convey the impression of poise, well being and vitality that emanates from the photograph

3

of the young lady showing the change which has taken place over a period of time in Figure 2.

All teachers, especially those in the health, physical and recreation education fields, should realize that they carry a share of responsibility for the actual physical fitness of all students, in addition to the usual objectives of their special area of emphasis. They should assist in selling the student, whether he be a child or adult, the idea of being an effective and skillful person with possi-

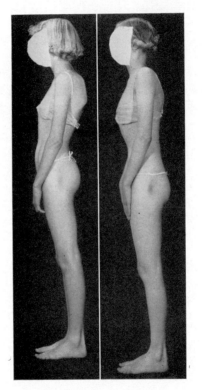

Fig. 1.—Fatigue slump

Fig. 2.—Evidence of change in health status

bilities of excelling being increased by the possession of a well balanced body. The individual's sensori-motor mechanism will be more alert and responsive, than if a large percentage of his energy must be expended in overcoming the neuromuscular handicaps and lessened endurance caused by poor posture.

It should be emphasized that in the past, many, if not most, of the basic theories and practices in physical education, as applied to the amelioration of specific divergencies and suggested by various authorities, were entirely sound and quite worthy of being reconsidered by present and future teachers and students. There is a certain tendency these days to jump the gun, as it were, and to be too easily led into fads and fancies because their proponents speak with glibness and an air of authority. Consequently, it is advised that there be a careful perusal of older teachings in a historical evaluation.

During the past 45 or more years, there has been maintained a rather close personal association between the Orthopedic Hospital of Los Angeles and the physical educators, health services, education system and universities in this city. As long ago as 1910 or thereabouts, a course of lectures was given to doctors, nurses and physical educators in the city school health service, and sufficient interest was aroused to awaken a request for a development of the therapeutic approach to the diagnosis and care of postural and growth divergencies. At this time, Sven Lokrantz, M.D. was recommended to Susan Dorsey, City Superintendent of Schools of Los Angeles, California, who was sympathetic to the idea of establishing corrective centers in various city schools, and the aforementioned doctor was appointed for this purpose.

Thus, it may be seen that the present status of remedial and health activities in this area has been a direct outgrowth of the efforts of past years when beliefs and theories were put into practice. Year after year this locality, while no isolated example, has gone on to further develop the health and physical education programs, and a greater appreciation of the importance of body mechanics has evolved, becoming an accepted part of the curriculum at all levels in the educational system.

It would seem to be true that in the frontiers of the mind, repose the keys to happiness, and that through the dedicated leadership of all who see realistically and in an unbiased manner the *constructive values for service*, lies the *opportunity* for paying the rent for the space one occupies. There must be constant re-evaluation of objectives, seeking the answer as to how life may be made more meaningful for children, youth, adults and senior citizens. For national security there should accrue, as a result of such long range thinking and effort, a greater dividend of potential human resources, thereby fostering the true ideals of democracy.

REFERENCES

1. JOINT COMMITTEE OF AMERICAN MEDICAL ASSOCIATION AND THE ASSOCIATION FOR HEALTH, PHYSICAL EDUCATION AND RECREATION: Exercise and Fitness, J. Health, Phys. Educ., Recreat., *29*, 40–43, 1958.
2. WHITE HOUSE CONFERENCE REPORT: New York, Century Company. 1930, 1931, cited by Los Angeles City School District, *Education of the Physically Handicapped*, school Publication, No. 215. Los Angeles, California, 1931, p. 7.

3. Young, Carl Haven: Meeting Needs of the Individual, J. Health and Phys. Educ., *11*, 71, 1940.
4. Aviation Training Division, Office of the Chief of Naval Operations, U. S. Navy: *Mass Exercise, Games, Tests,* compiler-writer, Carl Haven Young, Annapolis, Maryland, United States Naval Institute, 1943, 235 pp.
5. V-5 Association of America: *Conditioning Exercises, Games, Tests,* 3rd ed. by Karl C. H. Oermann, Carl Haven Young, *et al.,* Annapolis, Maryland, United States Naval Institute, 1960, 280 pp.
6. Colestock, Claire and Lowman, Charles LeRoy: *Fundamental Exercises for Physical Fitness.* New York, A. S. Barnes and Co., 1943, pp. 2–7.
7. Brown, Lloyd T.: A Combined Medical and Postural Examination of 746 Young Adults, Am. J. Orthoped. Surg., *15*, 781, 1917.
8. Pryor, Helen B.: *Width-Weight Tables.* Stanford University, California, Stanford University Press, 1940, 15 pp.
9. Weir, Leroy: Postwar Health and Physical Education, J. Health and Phys. Educ., *15*, 263–64, 1944.
10. Blesh, T. Erwin, Meyers, Carlton R. and Kiphuth, Oscar W.: *Photometric Photography in Posture Evaluation of Yale University.* New Haven, Yale University Press, 1954, 17 pp.
11. Lowman, Charles Leroy, Colestock, Claire and Cooper, Hazel: *Corrective Physical Education for Groups.* New York, A. S. Barnes and Co., 1928, Chapter I.

The above references are not repeated in References for Extended Reading

REFERENCES FOR EXTENDED READING

American Association for Health, Physical Education and Recreation. *Developing Democratic Human Relations.* Washington, D. C., American Association for Health, Physical Education and Recreation, 1951, 562 pp.
   Chapter IV: Democratic Leadership —Rosalind Cassidy.
Daniels, Arthur S.: *Adapted Physical Education.* New York, Harper Bros., 1954, 538 pp.
   Chapter II: Society and the Disabled.
Irwin, L. W.: Changing Concepts in Posture Training, J. Health and Phys. Educ., *18*, 522–573, 1946.
Joint Committee of American Medical Assocation and American Association Health, Physical Education and Recreation. Exercise and Fitness, J.A.M.A., *166*, 1744, 1958.
Kozman, Hilda Clute, (ed): *Group Process in Physical Education.* New York, Harper Bros., 1951, 418 pp.
   Chapter I: Physical Education Today,
   Chapter II: Living in a Democratic Society,
   Chapter III: Developing a Democratic Personality,
   Chapter IV: Educating for Democratic Living.
Licht, Sidney, (ed.): *Therapeutic Exercise.* New Haven, Conn., Elizabeth Licht, 1958, 893 pp.
   Chapter XVI: History.—Sidney Licht.
MacCarthy, Shane: "Fitness and the Future," in *Fitness of American Youth, Report of the Second Annual Meeting of the President's Council on Youth Fitness.* Washington, D. C., United States Government Printing Office, 1958, pp. 27–33.
Michael-Smith, H. (ed): *Management of the Handicapped Child.* New York, Grune & Stratton, 1957, 276 pp.
Rasch, Philip J., and Burke, Roger K.: *Kinesiology and Applied Anatomy.* Philadelphia, Lea & Febiger, 1959, 456 pp.
   Chapter I: The History of Kinesiology.
Rathbone, Josephine L.: *Corrective Physical Education.* 5th Ed. Philadelphia, W. B. Saunders Co., 1955, 318 pp.
   Chapter VI: Exercise in Medicine.
Rogers, James Frederick: *What Every Teacher Should Know about the Physical Condition of Her Pupils.* Pamphlet No. 68 (revised) Washington, D. C., U. S. Office of Education, 1945.

RUSK, H. A., and TAYLOR, E. J.: Physical Disability: A National Problem, Am. J. Pub. Health, *38*, 1381–1386, 1948.

SELLWOOD, JOHN J.: The Integration of Physical Education with Physical Medicine and Rehabilitation Relative to the Preparation of Professional Personnel. Unpublished Doctor's dissertation, The University of California, Los Angeles, 1952. 282 pp.

STAFFORD, GEORGE T.: *Preventive and Corrective Physical Education.* New York, A. S. Barnes and Co., 1950, 312 pp.
Chapter I: New Hope for the Handicapped.
Chapter II: Physical Medicine.
————: *Sports for the Handicapped.* New York, Prentice-Hall, Inc., 1947, 334 pp.
Chapter I: Introduction.
Chapter II: The Need for Adapted Sports.

STAFFORD, GEORGE T., and KELLY, ELLEN DAVIS: *Preventive and Corrective Physical Education.* 3rd Ed. New York, The Ronald Press Co., 1958, 395 pp.
Chapter I: Fitness for the Art of Living.
Chapter II: The Physical Rehabilitation Team.

VAN DALEN, DEOBOLD B., and VAN DALEN, MARCELLA M.: *The Health, Physical Education, and Recreation Teacher.* Englewood Cliffs, New Jersey, Prentice-Hall, Inc., 1956, 436 pp.

WESSEL, JANET A.: *Movement Fundamentals.* Englewood Cliffs, New Jersey, Prentice-Hall, Inc., 1957. 270 pp.
Chapter I: Your Fitness.
Chapter II: Your Physical Potential.

WHEATLEY, GEORGE M., and HALLOCK, GRACE J.: *Health Observation of School Children.* New York, McGraw-Hill Book Co., 1956, 488 pp.
Chapter I: Seeing the Child as a Whole.

YOUNG, CARL HAVEN: Broadening the Corrective Program, California J. Second. Educ., *15*, 87–88, 1940.
————: Challenging Portals in the Profession, J. Health and Phys. Educ., *18*, 647–649, 1947.
————: *Directional Goals for Clinical Therapy Experiences.* New York, Association for Physical and Mental Rehabilitation, 1958, 39 pp.
————: What the Services Teach Us About Physical Education, California J. Second. Educ., *20*, 9–15, 1945.

CHAPTER 2

Development and Adjustment in Structural Pattern Problems

FOR an effective citizenry, there must be a concern by all for the development and adjustment of the individual, whether it be for the purpose of the individual himself or for the sake of society. For whatever reason or purpose, if he is to be educated, something must be known as to (*a*) how he resembles others, (*b*) in what regard he differs from others in respect to the so-called normal organism, (*c*) the kinds of variances and degrees of these differences, and (*d*) techniques and methods for determining divergencies and remedial procedures.

It is seldom that teachers in health, physical and recreation education, together with the many others working with children, youth and adults, come in direct contact with the pre-school age child, except from an observational and theoretical course standpoint. Generally, insufficient knowledge of the mechanism of growth in infancy and the details of developmental deviations and variations of the musculoskeletal system in the earliest years and their implications for later life, may, because of the lack of understanding, be detrimental to the leaders' utmost effectiveness.

It is necessary for best results to know the natural processes of growth as determined by the structural functional organization conferred by heredity. Also, environmental influences, prenatal and postnatal of both intrinsic and extrinsic factors, affect the growth process and cause certain changes.

Nutritional aspects of the mother's condition during pregnancy, as well as that of the child after birth, probably have a very definite causative relationship to skeletal faults. An early philosopher once said that, "If strong be the frames of the mothers, the sons will make laws for the people." Recent studies infer that nutrition plays a part in the structural development even on an inherited basis.

Understanding of the physiological process of maturation is especially important so that parents, physicians, educators and other leaders working with youngsters may take advantage of this favorable period. This stage of life is so vital in the growth and development of the individual that deviations in the normal pattern must be discovered early and essential measures be taken for rectifying real and potential conditions. In a portion of such cases, habilitation or adjustment is advised as the best immediate procedure, since many will need to learn to live with what they have throughout life.

PERIODS OF INFANCY AND CHILDHOOD

It is not alone the postural problems of adolescence and the post adolescent age which need solving if an effective and healthy adulthood is to be achieved, for an essential factor to this end is an understanding of how the individual "got that way" to start with, and what might be done to prevent ensuing difficulties.[1]

In infancy, congenital divergencies, such as clubfeet, dislocation or subluxation of the hips, and other anomalies of development, are usually discovered by the physician, although they must be sufficiently obvious for the parent to notice that something seems wrong so as to warrant a seeking of medical advice.[2]

However, minor grades of deviation may pass unobserved until the walking stage, and thus be overlooked. Faulty foot positions are especially prevalent, such as adductus of the forefoot that later produces the common "pigeon-toed" gait, or mild dysplasia or growth changes in the hip joint. The former may be a hold-over from the intrauterine position of the feet and legs before birth, or be due to faulty positions in sleeping during early infancy. The child may sleep on his face with the knees drawn up under him, with the feet turned inward, or with the thighs abducted in the frog position with the feet turned outward. The former position is conducive to developing a toeing-in or adducted condition, the latter or toeing-out position leads to later production of flatfeet and tibial torsion. Orthodontists call attention to the likelihood of the development of malocclusion of the jaws from the pressure on the cheek and jaw when sleeping in a prone position.

All babies should be closely scrutinized to see whether or not the creases on the back of the thighs, the gluteal folds and the creases, from groin to crotch are symmetrical. If they are not, x-ray pictures should be taken to see if the heads of the femora are in the proper position and if the hip sockets are normal, (Figure 3). If there is an abnormality of this sort, this may be an early forerunner of subluxation or dislocation of the hips. Such an untoward result can easily be prevented if discovered early enough. There is also undoubtedly a tendency toward the production of bowlegs from the use of too bulky diapers.

Since bowlegs and knock knees are very common, it is wise to test the child by bringing the knees or ankles together. If the ankle bones touch and the femoral condyles do not, then a certain degree of bowlegs exists. Likewise, if the knees touch and the ankle bones do not, a knock knee deviation is present. If this condition is noted before or shortly after the walking stage, shoe correction should be made by wedging the inner border of the heels of the shoe, in order to tilt the body weight to the outer side of the feet. The same correction should be made for both types of deviations, the purpose being for physiological and not mechanical reasons.

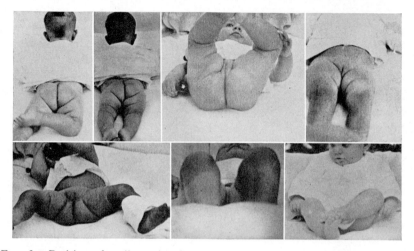

Fig. 3.—Positions for diagnosis of congenital dislocation or dysplasia of hips of infants. Note symmetry or asymmetry of thigh creases and those of groin and buttock. (All photos age 4 months.)

It is known that in many cases leg malalignment will be outgrown, and to relieve a mother's mind, many doctors tell them that growth will take care of the matter. If this were so, why should physicians, in checking a group of healthy adults such as are found in college and university physical education classes, find just as many such deviations as are found in childhood? Why did they not "outgrow" them?

X-ray films of the bones of the foot after birth show the ossifying centers for the os calcis (the heel bone), the astragalus (the ankle bone), and the cuboid on the outer border present at birth. The other tarsal bones, namely, the cuneiforms and the navicular or scaphoid, which later becomes the keystone of the arch, are in a cartilaginous state and will not be seen until 3 to 4 years after birth. Nature apparently intended that the weight should, as early as possible, be carried on the structurally, more advanced, outer border. When weight is so borne, the resistance of the gravity thrust through the leg bones promotes faster growth on the concave areas, and, hence, is the physiological reason for tilting the shoe heels outward for both bowlegs and knock knees.

Normally, the line of gravitational stress should pass from the anterior hip bone through the patella and into the foot through the middle of the ankle joint to a point between the first and second toes. However, most babies tend to be flatfooted, and if any deviations in the legs are present, such as knock knee, bowleg or tibial torsion, this thrust will go toward the midline and push the ankles inward. This makes it difficult for the muscles of the sole to force the foot up and out, and thus produce an arch. Pronation goes with the valgus position and fosters the production of low arches and, later, flatfeet.[3]

It is a normal maturational sequence, during the walking period of infancy, to have the baby crawl for several months on all fours. This helps to exercise the big pelvic and trunk muscles. A baby that crawls will have a straighter spine and better balance when he essays walking.

At a later stage, anteroposterior postural deviations become noticeable, especially in children who have been allowed to sit up too early. The rounding of the back and the prominence of the abdomen tends to promote faulty spinal and chest development.[4]

Babies should be allowed to arrive naturally at the walking stage and not be stimulated and encouraged to stand or remain upright on their legs. Proud parents should restrain their impulse to dandle the child on its feet, or to set the child in a spring seat and allow him to push on his feet with the knees apart. Walkers for this reason may have a deleterious effect if utilized too early with babies. The anxious parents should not worry if a stout baby does not walk until 18 months or 2 years of age. Probably mother nature knows best and will start the urge to walk when she gets ready. In case of doubt, parents should consult the pediatrician or orthopedist so as to make sure regarding the normal development of the child.

Too early encouragement of the standing position before proper muscle strength is developed is a factor in producing or contributing to poor leg alignment and too much stress on the feet. Likewise, it enhances the need for compensatory curves due to demands for segmental weight adjustment in order to achieve body balance. This may cause fixed positions of the upper structure to become stable or permanent and with later growth change to interfere with the stability and alignment of the body, thus producing strain.

If the child's weight is too great for the strength of the ligaments and muscles of the feet, the proper raising of the arches is interfered with in their development. When sitting on the floor in

play, it is important to prevent assumption of the frog-like position, that is, with the knees flexed and the heels beside the trochanters, as this mannerism tends to accentuate tibial torsion,
everted and abducted feet. In either knock knees or bowlegs there
is a compensating valgus position of the feet. On the other hand,
sitting in a tailor-fashion is a corrective position and should be
encouraged.

The use of flimsy, soft-soled baby shoes which give no support
is controversial. Since the child is having a hard enough time
learning to balance properly, it is felt advisable to provide a firm,
welt-soled shoe which, although heavier, will mean less strain on
the leg and balance muscles because of the harder, more stable
surface. Furthermore, if severe pronation exists, the heavier sole
allows for heel correction, whereas the soft-soled shoe does not
make this adjustment possible.

During the walking stage in early childhood, especially from the
first to third years of age, the way the shoes wear should be watched
closely. If the back seam of the shoe tips inward and the sole
wears more on the inside, it is a signal that the weight is falling
on the soft bones and ligaments of the inner aspect of the arch.
This may mean that a potential flatfoot is in the making.

According to the law of bone growth, the internal architecture
and the external shape are changed in accordance with the way
the weight is borne. Then the rationale of tilting the shoe heels
so as to put the weight on the outer border may be seen. This is
also the basic reason for all exercises in physical education to be
given in the fundamental position of weight being placed on the
outer borders of the feet.

Of late years, the increased attention being paid to the teaching
of proper ways of walking has gradually begun to bear fruit.
Children should understand the natural use of the feet in walking
with the toes pointed straight ahead or in a nearly straight position.
Even a moderate amount of toeing-in is preferable to the toe-out
position with the pronated ankles and poor arches.

It is not advisable for those with strong tendencies to pronation
and relaxed arches to go barefooted except for short periods on
soft or flexible surfaces, such as the beach or upon the lawn.
Likewise, the constant wearing of soft-soled tennis shoes should be
frowned upon since they evert the foot and give little support.

When scooters, speed wagons or skates are used, youngsters
should be taught to change from one leg to the other as a propellent,
since the constant action on a single limb causes a shortening of
one leg, a tilting of the pelvis, overdevelopment of one side in the
musculature, and as a result a lateral curvature of the spine
develops. Teachers sometimes overlook the fact that students

have parents, and it is through the medium of the Parent-Teachers Association, that word should be conveyed as to the importance of the effect of such practices.

Most models for ready made clothing have faulty shoulder girdles and poor posture, and thus there is no assurance that such clothing will necessarily fit all children. Clothing weight usually tends to hang out on the tip of the shoulders instead of being supported on the root or base of the neck. There is a similar tendency for garments for both sexes and all ages to be narrow over the chest and wide in the back. When such clothing is heavy, which is necessary in cold climates, there is excessive weight to be carried, thus causing even greater forward sag in the shoulder girdle than would ordinarily be the case in warmer climates.

Shoes are much better shaped and constructed now than formerly, but are still too short or too narrow and with pointed toes.[5] These crowd the toes, create bunions, develop hammer toes, and injure the metatarsal arches. Too often the heel counters are much too wide, allowing for a rotation of the os calcis which is a factor in pronation and flatfeet. In girls' shoes, the sandal or platform type with no counter is deficient and does not support the foot laterally at the heel or arch. If foot structure is normal, this does not make as much difference, but when faulty foot and leg alignment exists, as in the majority of young children, plus the shift of body weight on the forefeet because of faulty trunk posture, the danger of potentials for later disability increases. With this understanding, parents especially, will not accede to special pleadings of the child, or to manufacturers' sales talk as to vogue, and economics will be stretched to meet necessary needs which may prevent future difficulties.

Many small deviations of alignment and postural faults that have been overlooked previously become increasingly evident during the elementary school level in the 6 to 10 year age bracket. These changes are most noticeable in trunk deviations, such as round shoulders, round and hollow back, tilted pelvis with varying grades of lateral curvatures, and fatigue slump. There are a variety of predisposing causes which are due to (a) rapid growth in the presence of faulty nutrition, excessively heavy work or overloading beyond the years, (b) tilted pelvis from a hereditary short leg or pelvic asymmetry which occurs in about 50 per cent of the people and produces secondary lateral curvatures, (c) defects of hearing and/or vision and their relationships, (d) influence of faulty positions and function during games and other play activities and (e) incorrect seating, sitting on one foot, carrying books and such loads upon one hip, and ill-fitting clothing.

These are especially vulnerable years in which the foundation for the future effectiveness is established. There is need for three approaches, namely, observation, experimentation and application with the observer being a seer, the experimenter a doer, and the applier an expediter and teacher.

It is so much easier to float or drift in the tranquil and tepid waters of popular opinion, accepted practices, yes, even mediocrity, if in the majority of instances such constructive efforts are not being exerted, than to strike out and surge through the shoals and rapids for the sake of a belief or ideal which may be in opposition to present "let well enough alone" procedures.

Children are the cherished heritage of every nation and in them one sees what might have been, investing through their efforts in the hope that the dream of well being for all may become a reality. Alexander Meiklejohn once said, "But if man sees the way and does not go; if he has found a principle and does not follow it, what shall we say of that? If that occurs, then life is broken in two."

TRANSITIONAL STAGES OF ADOLESCENCE AND YOUTH

One of the most important and far-reaching concepts advanced in relation to stages of growth is that concerned with maturation. Psychologists describe this process as levels of development of the individual which are reached, during childhood and adolescence, at various periods as a result of the interaction of growth processes reacting with the environment. Body movement, physiological changes, behavior and the learning process would appear to be subservient to a pattern of genetic sequence, which is probably conditioned by the actions or effects of the environment. These intrinsic organic factors bring about daily changes in growth trends and actions, and make difficult the process of education and the establishment of best patterns to follow in respect to any established norms of procedure.

Differences of opinion exist as to the extent environmental influences affect the development, but it would appear to be obvious that favorable conditions do facilitate proper growth. Dentists have found that teeth which formerly appeared at certain ages are now cut at a much earlier age, and that 6-year molars often appear as early as 3 years of age as a result of improved nutrition and better dental care. This would seem to verify the hypothesis that while the hereditary potentials may be present, such a condition will not prevail unless the environmental influences are favorable.

During the junior high school years there is a speeding up of growth, physiologically and structurally, which is especially evident in the growth of the trunk of the body.   The gangly awkward stage of rapid increase of leg length gives way to the organic needs of growing up, and the body is on its way toward sexual maturity. Consequently, it is the dangerous age because of the "vulnerability of fast growing cells" during a stage of rapid growth in which living organisms are most susceptible to injury, according to the dictum of Murk Jansen[6] (Fig. 4).

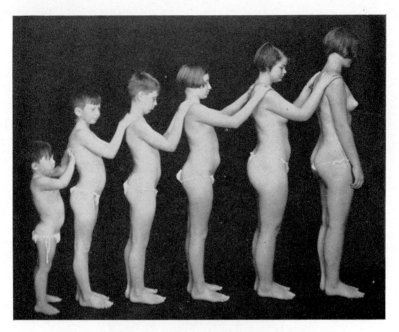

Fig. 4.—Nutritional influence on enfeeblement of growth

Because so many children at this age are in a stage of semi-fatigue and physiological inadequacy, there is a tendency to droop easily into the so-called "fatigue slump" with forward head, drooping shoulders, increased dorsal curve and compensatory sway back.   This is caused by a muscular insufficiency in the antigravity muscles that are responsible for keeping the body erect (Fig. 5).   Consequently poor sitting positions, incorrect lighting, poorly adjusted chairs and desks, and the concentrated study which aggravates the forward head position, all tend to perpetuate such faulty postural habits, and change the structural pattern.

One hears so often that posture is only a static condition, but until it is applied, action in terms of function is lost as a component part of posture.   Young people at this stage are extremely active,

and rightly so.   One finds them engaged in activities which require
some control and reasoning regarding how best to perform.

Young children find it more convenient in bicycle riding to
place the arch of the foot on the pedal rather than the ball of the
foot, because of the broader surface being centered there.   This
develops a tendency to pronate the ankles and to stretch the plantar
muscles of the arch.   All bicycles should have the pedals equipped
with toe clasps to hold the toes in place and to prevent this practice.
Parents need to be especially alert to this habit, and when young-

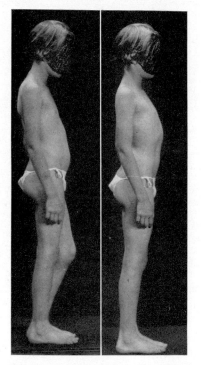

Fig. 5.—Correction of posture slump

sters are shown that professional riders use the ball of the foot
for greater power and speed, this practice may be more easily
changed.[7]

Both boys and girls should realize that when they are playing
golf, they should shift the golf bag from one shoulder to the other
from time to time.   Caddies, especially those who are quite young,
usually form the habit of carrying the heavy bag of clubs on the
left shoulder, particularly when right handed, in order to be able
to pass the requested club to the golfer.   In this way the supporting
shoulder girdle muscles become stretched and often a low shoulder
is the result.   Influence of other activities are seen in Figure 6.

Girls with younger children in the family are prone to lift and carry the toddler on the hip, which may cause strain or permanent damage. Thus, habits are formed in the common functions of daily living which influence the later body structure. The attitude of such young people may be shown through the motto of Father Flanagan's Boys' Home which says, "He ain't heavy, Father, he's my brother."

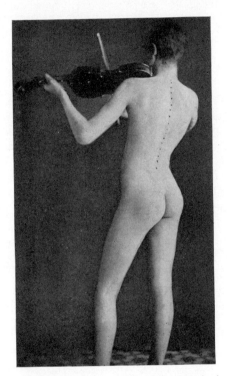

FIG. 6.—Beginning Asymmetry of back due to playing violin.

This is a period in which there is a tendency to promote the so-called heavy "body building" activities, and participation in interschool competitive sports. Too strenuous activity is believed to promote joint injuries and growth damage to the cartilages while they are developing. These are not necessarily acute injuries, such as strains, sprains or fractures, but rather small repeated trauma to these vulnerable areas which may not appear to be important until later years, yet are cumulative in their toll. These traumas are most likely to occur in individuals whose physiological age is not proportional to the chronological age, in other words, their structural strength is not equal to the work load which is placed upon it.

Discrepancies in weight and height, or musculoskeletal ineffici-
ency due to poor body mechanics, increase the wear and tear
factor out of all proportion to that caused by such activities in
the more normally aligned bodies in better physiological balance.[8]
Therefore, the classification method of grouping on a height,
weight, age basis for competitive sports is controversial, since the
taller, heavier boy may be the one whose structural development
is not equal to his chronological age.

Expressions pertaining to interscholastic competition should not
be interpreted to imply that there is opposition to competition
within a school when adequately supervised and controlled by
competent instructors. Rather, that there are limits beyond which
those in the growing years should not be extended. This is in
keeping with the experience of those who observe most frequently
the results of excessive strain and stress.

Girls at this age with secondary characteristics, such as early
and heavy breast development, may increase the shoulder girdle
sag, resulting in anteroposterior spinal deviations. This may be
due to either the drag on the shoulders from increased weight of the
breasts or the added downward pull from poorly fitted or improperly constructed brassieres. Tight brassieres with straps that
ride far out on the tips of the shoulders pull them downward and
forward. This displaces the arm weight forward of the gravity
line, widens the interscapular distance and necessitates increase
of the dorsal spinal curve and compensatory forward head.[9] Thus,
adaptive shortening of the pectoral muscles and stretching of the
scapular adductors (the rhomboids and lower trapezius) produce
muscular and ligamentous imbalance in the posterior shoulder
girdle. The ordinary gymnastic and athletic activities
tend to habituate this malalignment, and a vicious circle is perpetuated which may in later years provoke symptoms of cervical
strain and neuritis. The strapless breast support places much
less strain on the shoulder girdle.

The wearing of proper shoes at this age, assumes major importance because of the increases in height and weight out of proportion
to muscular and ligamentous efficiency. Hence, the many already
existing foot and leg deviations are made worse. Increased consciousness of dress and styles encourages fashion fads, such as
narrow and higher heels, pointed and open toed shoes, many too
narrow in the toes and wide across the ball of the foot with a minimal heel grip, which are sought by girls of this age level. The
moccasin-tread bedroom slipper ballet or loafer type footwear with
very low heels and with no heel counters, are much desired by
both boys and girls, and may be equally disastrous in promoting
foot strain. Such type of shoes lacking in heel support, causes

rotation of the os calcis, and thus fosters pronation and inner knee strain.[10]

Of special relevance in this period is the need for changing from the sensible lasts of childhood to the more adult type of shoes. Consequently, in many instances the fitting problem proves difficult, while again economy requirements on the part of many parents and the gregarious desires of the children to follow the social demand produce a conflict.

Increase in the incidence of bad feet is likely to be furthered in sports and athletics by similarly faulty athletic footwear, such as basketball and tennis shoes which have little support for either heel or arch, spiked track shoes with no shank or heel support, forcing the running and weight wholly upon the ball of the foot, baseball and football shoes commonly made on a general last with no concern for widths and which do not fit the individual's foot.

It has been said, that, "If you want to forget everything else, wear tight shoes." However, increase in size is not enough. The normal foot is straight on the inside, hence the shoe should be the same, the waist or throat should be eased with a snug fit under the arch which gives support, and while the shank needs to be firm, it should still be supportive. Perhaps most important is the necessity for a heel counter which is suitable to the individual's foot and not so wide that it permits sliding or rotation of the heel itself. All of these items are present in fine shoes, but it may require the purchase of combination lasts with varying sizes from "A" to triple "A" in widths. Rubber heels are also recommended to soften the shock of today's hard surfaces.

With such a base of operation, children would undoubtedly feel like the man, who, when asked how he was today, replied, "If I felt any better, I'd be dangerous." Since fitness is a civic responsibility, and raising the general level in the prime years is our responsibility, every community needs to concern itself with making sure that the compelling necessities of the moment are provided in some manner. In this way, all will be helping others to realize their own potentialities, and none will be paralyzed through the indifference of the people.

ADULT AND SENIOR LEVELS OF MATURITY

People everywhere have become so enamored with the searching for material gains, together with the desire for recognition and the resultant adulation, and likewise, the demands of modern life in terms of expenditure of energy have grown so great, that many become casualties of civilization. They no longer have time to live, while their most priceless ingredient, namely health, is being spent without regard for personal cost.

4

There is need to know not only what society is doing to people, but also what it can do for and with people. Only those who are not satisfied with the routine attitude are conscious of the critical necessity for greater insight as to the interrelationship between cause and effect.

The intelligence and inventive genius of mankind must be utilized for the benefit of all, and this involves greater understanding and research as to what is best. Rudyard Kipling once said,

> "I keep six honest serving men:
> (They taught me all I knew)
> Their names are What and Where and When
> And How and Why and Who."

Experimentation should be conducted to determine (a) the amount and sequence of growth which takes place in early adulthood, (b) the physiological and structural stages of change during adult and senior years, (c) the elasticity and tone of muscle and ligamentous tissue in respect to the maintenance of fitness, (d) the significance of biochemical deficiencies and nutritional demands, (e) the effect of weight discrepancies, work programs, malfunction and serious illness in the crucial periods of maturity, (f) the importance of activity to growth and maintenance of health status, and (g) how much and what specific kinds of physical activity are beneficial and for whom, in regard to the adjustment and survival factors for these age levels.

Greater inquisitiveness is required in order to derive authoritative data which may make life more productive and enjoyable. Present knowledge and practices have been based largely upon the observation of conditions which come to the attention of the medical profession as a result of functional and other handicapping difficulties.

In the meantime, there is demand for expediency in applying what knowledge is available, although knowing what to do is not alone enough. It is imperative that the individual appreciate the importance of the problem, for it is questionable whether the majority of persons realize or understand such matters sufficiently to take the trouble to find out what to do, or to entice others to do something for themselves.

In some cases, the problem is that of adjusting the individual demands to the personal structure and capacity. It would seem wise in all instances to take inventory of each person's physical resources as to fitness and skills, and to examine critically and meticulously the media which may prove to be best adapted and most advantageous in realizing his objectives.

Orthopedic surgeons see the results of many injuries during the adult and senior years, accumulating from such activities as strenuous contact sports, athletics involving stress situations, inappropriate occupational endeavors, and aftermaths of military service, which have been characterized by duty beyond the individual's power. These are often due to improper consideration of the stage of skeletal maturity and type of structure in relation to certain body characteristics, faults in alignment, improper performance of movements, or indulgence in play, work or avocations not conducive to the individual's framework and musculature.

For example, it is worth reiterating that a low percentage of acute traumatic injuries does not mean that injury is not being done. Adolescence is not a short stage of development. The processes of maturation take time and such changes may continue into early adulthood, hence the adaptability of the youth cannot be judged by body form nor weight alone. The fact that a boy or girl is 6 feet tall and 160 pounds in weight during his or her freshman year in high school or even in college, is no evidence that the epiphyseal cartilages are closed, or that the glandular, neurological or cardiovascular systems have reached the period of organic balance. These young people may be physiologically retarded, structurally, organically or both. Thus, activities predicated on weight, height, and apparent muscle strength, may render them more susceptible to injury than they would be a year or more later in life.

Those who are engaged in coaching, physical education, recreation, and as participants, including industrial and other occupational endeavors in earning a livelihood, are prone to think in terms of muscle action only, overlooking the fact that the only bony connection between the upper and lower segments of the body is a small disc of bone about the size of a silver dollar. This is held in place by two small articular processes and the ligaments that bind the last lumbar vertebra to the sacrum.

In the face of this insecurity of the base, the muscular effort needed for stabilization is greater in individuals with an asymmetrical development, than in cases of normal structural development and symmetrical alignment. Increase in weight, stature, and muscular development is no criterion that the individual is structurally sound and can take the stresses produced by strenuous endeavors, either in contests or work situations.

Increased muscle strength may make an asymetrical person feel that he can do as well as his fellows and so he can as far as pure muscle force is concerned, but the premium is much too high for the rate of interest received. The laws of physics and mechanics require stability of the base in direct ratio to the load put upon it by the motor action. Hence, the possibilities and probablities of strain or injury are increased in direct proportion. If you increase muscular strength when the segments of the body are out of line, you may also increase the malalignment.

Cognizance should be taken of those sports or work situations during the adult years which are one-sided in nature, involving lateral, posterior or anterior movements to the exclusion of the antagonistic muscle groups in the action (Fig. 7). Such motions

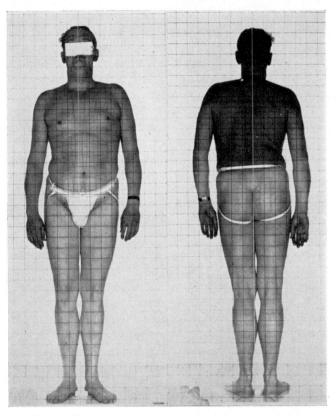

FIG. 7.—Body malalignment due to vocational activity

tend to develop one side of the body more than the other, or utilize one aspect of the musculature as in flexion or extension, while the agonist group is under a stretching influence.

It appears sound to bridge the gap for such activities by fostering the development of antagonistic muscles, other than those engaged in the movement itself, to compensate and offset the unnatural pull, and equalize the opponent muscle balance. Furthermore, such equalizing of stability is a vital force in the increasing of performance results, while avoiding the pull of gravity on the joint structure and ligamentous mechanisms of the body structure.

In this connection it is logical to keep the individual's later years in mind and not accentuate those activities which produce symptoms later on and promote early aging of the joints leading to concomitant or attending distress.

Nearly everyone in the adult years has a shadow, a vulnerable spot or chink in his physical armor which lends itself to certain restrictions of program. Habits are formed in the common pursuits of life which restrain the actions and movements, when, if no physiological conditions are present which may be harmed through specific exercise, might in many instances be contraindicated if such activity is conducted under wise counsel.

Joseph B. Wolffe makes a plea for the promotion of interdisciplinary collaboration, "to explore ways and means of synthesizing the roles of physical educators, physicians, physiologists and scientists in allied fields."[11] He further expressed the opinion that in the schools lie a rich field for investigation for all the span of life. "Here is a situation which is made to order for study and planned action on the part of physical educators, who are, every day, in the very laboratory where the human material is at hand."[12] Jointly working together with the orthopedist and others concerned, there is a chance to consider not only the physically underprivileged, but also the convalescent and temporary deviations from physical normality, and thus apply this information to those not in school.

The follow-up of former students who were known to have had some sort of difficulty, and the follow-through into adult and middle age to discover what had been done for amelioration and adjustment for a full and rich life, might reveal some pertinent guide lines as to what procedures should be recommended. Such a search for improved means for adaptation to stress, fatigue, improved performance, and attainment of potentialities might thus lead many out of the haze of the unknown possibilities.

Robert S. Goodhart claims that "the prevention and management of degenerative diseases associated with aging and the care and rehabilitation of the aged have become matters of major individual and public health concern in the United States. Incapacitation at an early age, because of premature senility or degenerative disease, now represents an economic loss and burden that this country can ill afford." He says further, . . . "Prevention of deterioration and incapacity should be the ultimate goal, not rehabilitation. Aging is a continuous process throughout the life of the individual. . . . Life is a constant struggle between anabolism (tissue construction) and catabolism (tissue destruction). When anabolism exceeds catabolism, the individual is growing. When catabolism exceeds anabolism, it can be stated that the individual has begun to age."[13]

Physiological diminution would apparently be largely responsible for the many changes which take place in the older persons, although there may be some question as to whether this is the cause or effect of structural and functional insufficiency. When calcium is stolen from the bones and deposited in the cartilage, does this account for the posture of older persons, or may this process be delayed by adequate big muscle movement which prevents such regression. This implies that good posture may make more facile the flow of circulation and hence contribute to better physiological function.

C. Ward Crampton refers to the process of de-aging, "The average man of fifty or sixty is commonly from five to ten years 'older' than he need be. As a man ages, his body becomes a documentary record of his past years. 'The old man is a walking hospital.' He shows accumulated damages, defects, tissue poisoning, stagnation, and starvation with half-cured illnesses and infections. These are the results, not of time, but of the hazards that occur from accident, illness, strain, ignorance, or neglect in the passage of time. Our enemy is not age; it is damage, largely avoidable, largely correctible."[14]

Crampton further claims that "At any age, forty, sixty, or eighty, there are accumulated burdens, defects, and deteriorations which in large part can be discovered and identified by thorough examinations. The evils disclosed by examination may often be partly or wholly removed or neutralized. At the same time unutilized sources of vitality and power may be disclosed and developed to great advantage." . . . "Contrary to the unquenchable race-old hopes, there is no simple, easy way back to youth nor one remedy for aging."[15]

In relating these geriatric concepts regarding the elderly patient as well as the senior person in respect to the structural pattern problems, the principle should be enunciated that adjustments can be effective only to the extent that others are willing to facilitate the use of the skilled knowledge which is imparted to them. As one oldster remarked, "Growing old isn't so bad after all, when you consider the only other alternative."

The attitude of many toward aging in the past has been expressed in "My Aching Back."[16]

My Aching Back

As people grow older, they get aches everywhere,
While doctors contend, its just age causing wear.
So they give each sharp pain, a fancy new moniker,
Called nephritis, arthritis, colitis needs toniker.

Now the folks become smart, quit groaning, act gay,
Know that no one is interested, in whatever they say.
Every pill on the market, is tried for relief,
Only druggist doth prosper, yet continues their grief.

When the gall bladder acts up, physician decides,
Operation is needed, probes and explores from inside.
Nothing wrong, yet removes, to prevent apprehension,
Though the stitch still remains, psychosomatic from tension.

So it's best to keep quiet, and save up your dough,
For it's nothing but aging, for the doc told you so.
Enjoy life as it comes, forget all the grief,
Perhaps when a hundred, you'll get some relief.

Seriously, the development and adjustment in structural pattern problems, may be viewed with much concern. The significant influence of every contact is multiplied many fold, and the choice of activities and vocations, when there is a chance for selection, oftentimes predetermines the pattern as to wear and tear later on.

Maturity profiles are often but the reflection of periods of immaturity, which have influenced the muscular and structural development. However, adjustment to such problems is contingent upon the meaning and values accepted by the individual. Whatever is achieved for a better life, rests largely upon the leader's insight, who, recognizing the meaning and extent of such problems, informs others and offers the opportunity for those who are interested in solving them.

REFERENCES

1. LOWMAN, CHARLES LEROY: Posture in Early Childhood, California and Western Med., *41*, 382–385, 1934.
2. LOWMAN, CHARLES LEROY, COLESTOCK, CLAIRE and COOPER, HAZEL: *Corrective Physical Education for Groups.* New York, A. S. Barnes and Co., 1928, Chap. II.
3. *Ibid.*, Chapter VIII.
4. FITZHUGH, M. L.: Some Effects of Early Sitting on Body Mechanics of Infancy and Childhood, Physiotherapy Rev., *23*, 8–13, 1943.
5. LOWMAN, COLESTOCK and COOPER, *loc. cit.*
6. JANSEN, MURK: *Feebleness of Growth.* London, Hodder and Stoughton, 1921, pp. 19–35.
7. LOWMAN, CHARLES LEROY: Feet and Body Mechanics, J. Health and Phys. Educ., *11*, 137, 1940.
8. ————: The Vulnerable Age, J. Health and Phys. Educ., *18*, 635, 1947.
9. ————: Heavy Breasts as a Factor in Production of Faulty Posture, J.A.M.A., *78*, 173–175, 1922.
10. LOWMAN, COLESTOCK and COOPER: *loc. cit.*
11. WOLFFE, JOSEPH B.: "Future Basic Research Relating Physical Education to Sports Medicine," *College Physical Education Association*, 59th Annual Proceedings. Washington, D. C.: College Physical Education Association, 1956, p. 117.
12. *Ibid.*, pp. 119–120

13. GOODHART, ROBERT S.: "Nutrition and the Aging," *New Channels for the Golden Years*. New York State Legislative Document (1956) No. 33, Albany, N. Y., New York State Legislative Committee on Problems of the Aging, 1956, pp. 81–82.
14. CRAMPTON, C. WARD: Medical Services in Aging and De-Aging, J. Assoc. Phys. and Ment. Rehabilitation, *9*, 41, 1955.
15. *Ibid.*
16. YOUNG, CARL HAVEN: "My Aching Back," *Kiwanis Club Bulletin of Westwood Village*. Los Angeles: Kiwanis Club of Westwood Village, Nov. 18, 1955, p. 1.

The above references are not repeated in References for Extended Reading

REFERENCES FOR EXTENDED READING

ANSON, BARRY J.: *Atlas of Human Anatomy*. Philadelphia, W. B. Saunders Co., 1950, 518 pp.

BROWN, WADE H.: "Constitutional Variations and Susceptibility to Disease," *The Harvey Lectures*. Baltimore, The Williams and Wilkins Co., 1930, pp. 106–150.

CALIFORNIA RECREATION COMMISSION: *Recreation for Older People in California*. Sacramento, California, 1951, 68 pp.

COMFORT, ALEXANDER: *The Biology of Senescence*. London, Rantledge & Paul, 1956, 257 pp.

COWELL, CHARLES C.: *Scientific Foundations of Physical Education*. New York, Harper & Brothers, 1953, 260 pp.
> Pages 204–220: The Relation of Physical Education to Health.

DEARBORN, WALTER, and ROTHNEY, JOHN W. M.: *Predicting the Child's Development*. Cambridge, Mass., Science Art Publishers, 1941, 360 pp.

DE LONG, EVERETT W.: Contrasenescence, J. Appl. Nutrit., *9*, 415–421, 1956.

DICKSON, FRANK D., and DIVELEY, REX L.: *Functional Disorders of the Foot*. Philadelphia, J. B. Lippincott Co., 1953, 345 pp.
> Chapter IV: Primary Causes of Foot Imbalance.
> Chapter VI: The Foot of Childhood.
> Chapter VII: Foot Imbalance in Childhood.
> Chapter VIII: Foot Imbalance in Adolescence.
> Chapter IX: Foot Imbalance in the Adult.
> Chapter X: Foot Apparel.

FITZHUGH, M. L.: Some Effects of Early Sitting on Body Mechanics of Infancy and Childhood, Physiotherapy Rev., *23*, 8–13, 1943.

FRANCIS, ANDREW J.: Bases for Selection of Activities for Senior Citizens, Unpublished Research project, The University of California, Los Angeles, 1957, 73 pp.

GOFF, C. W.: Posture in Children, Clin. Orthop., *1*, 66–79, 1953.

GORDON, I.: The Healthy Child: Its Many Disguises, Brit. M. J., *1*, 611–622, 1951.

HOBSON, WILLIAM, (ed.): *Modern Trends in Geriatrics*. London, Butterworth, 1956, 422 pp.

JEFFREYS, R. J.: *Life Will Begin at 100*. Columbus, Ohio, Capitol College Press, 1955, 239 pp.

JOHNSON, WINGATE M.: *The Years After Fifty*. New York, McGraw-Hill Book Co., Inc., 1947, 153 pp.

JONES, H. E.: Those Physical Changes of Adolescence, Nat. Parent Teachers, *52*, 8–10, 1957.

KELLY, ELLEN D.: A Comparative Study of Structure and Function of Normal Pronated and Painful Feet Among Children, Res. Quart., *18*, 291–312, 1947.

LEE, J. MURRARY, and LEE, DORRIS MAY: *The Child and His Development*. New York, Appleton-Century-Crofts, Inc., 1958, 624 pp.
> Chapter III: Physical Maturity and Motor Control.

LERRIGO, CHARLES HENRY: *The Better Half of Your Life*. New York, J. Day Co., 1951, 270 pp.
> Chapter VII: Exercise after Forty.

LICHT, SIDNEY, (ed.): *Therapeutic Exercise*. New Haven, Conn. Elizabeth Licht, 1958, 893 pp.
> Chapter XXIII: Exercise in Foot Disabilities.—Joseph H. Kite.

McGRAW, MYRTLE B., and BREEZE, K. W.: Quantitative Studies in the Development of Erect Locomotion, Child Development, *12*, 267–303, 1941.

MOREHOUSE, LAURENCE E.:   A Conditioning Program for Sedentary Men, J. Assoc. Phys. and Ment. Rehabilitation, 7, 39–43, 1953.

MORTON, DUDLEY J.:   *Human Locomotion and Body Form*.   Baltimore, The Williams and Wilkins Co., 1952, 285 pp.
    Chapter VII: The Feet as a Base.
    Chapter IX: Mechanism of Foot Balance.
    Chapter XI: The Foot in Walking.
——————:   *Oh Doctor, My Feet*. New York, D. Appleton-Century Co., 1939, 116 pp.

NAPIER, J. R.:   The Foot and the Shoe, Physiotherapy, 43, 65–74, 1957.

NATIONAL SOCIETY FOR THE STUDY OF EDUCATION.   *Adolescence, 43rd Yearbook, Part I*. Chicago, University of Chicago Press, 1944, 358 pp.

NEW YORK STATE JOINT LEGISLATIVE COMMITTEE ON PROBLEMS OF THE AGING: *Age is No Barrier*. New York, New York State Joint Legislative Committee on Problems of the Aging, 1952, 171 pp.
    Pages 136–139: Rehabilitation of the Aged—Promise or Reality.
                                                    —Michael M. Dacao.
    Pages 133–135: Rehab. in Com. Prog. for the Aged.—E. J. Taylor.

NEW YORK STATE JOINT LEGISLATIVE COMMITTEE ON PROBLEMS OF THE AGING: *Growing with the Years*.   New York: New York State Joint Legislative Committee on Problems of the Aging, 1954, 159 pp.
    Pages 133–134: Exercises for Senior Citizens.—Ruth Doing.

PRYOR, HELEN B.:   *As the Child Grows*. New York, Silver Burdett Company, 1943, 400 pp.
    Chapter VIII: The First Year of Life.

RASCH, PHILIP J., and BURKE, ROGER K.:   *Kinesiology and Applied Anatomy*. Philadelphia, Lea & Febiger, 1959, 456 pp.
    Chapter XXI: Kinesiology in Daily Living.

SHOCK, NATHAN WETHERIL: *Trends in Gerontology*. Stanford, California, Stanford University Press, 1957, 214 pp.

SIMMONS, KATHERINE: *The Brush Foundation Study of Child Growth and Development II, Physical Growth and Development*, Monographs of the Society for Research In Child Development, Vol. 9, No. 1.   Washington, D.C., National Research Council, 1944.

SMITH, ETHEL: *The Dynamics of Ageing*. New York, W. W. Norton, 1956, 191 pp.

STIEGLITZ, EDWARD J. (ed.):   *Geriatric Medicine*. 3rd ed., Philadelphia, J. B. Lippincott Co., 1954, 718 pp.
    Pages 67–90: Anatomic Changes of Normal Aging.—Jean Oliver.

TANNER, J. M., *et al.*:   Aberdeen Growth Study I.   The Prediction of Adult Body Measurements from Measurement Taken Each Year from Birth to 5 Years, Arch. Dis. Childhood, 31, 372–381, 1956.

TIBBITTS, CLARK, and DONAHUE, WILMA, (eds.):   *Aging in the Modern World*. Ann Arbor, University of Michigan, 1957, 175 pp.
    Pages 47–66: The Human Machine at Middle Life.—Donahue.

TIBBITTS, CLARK, (comp.):   *Aging in the Modern World, Supplement I*. Ann Arbor, University of Michigan, 1957, 246 pp.
    Pages 56–64: The Personal Challenge of Aging.—E. J. Stieglitz.

WETZEL, N. C.:   Assessing Physical Condition of Children; Components of Physical Status and Physical Progress and Their Evaluation, J. Pediat., 22, 329–361, 1943.
——————:   Physical Fitness in Terms of Physique, Development, and Basic Metabolism, J.A.M.A., 116, 1187–1195, 1941.
——————:   The Baby Grid, J. Pediat., 29, 439–454, 1946.

WHITE, P. D.:   The Role of Exercise in the Aging, J.A.M.A., 165, 70, 1957.

WILLIAMS, ROGER JOHN: *Biochemical Individuality*. New York, John Wiley and Sons, Inc., 1956, 214 pp.
    Chapter I: Biochemical Variation.
    Chapter III: Anatomical Variations—Significance.
    Chapter IX: Miscellaneous Evidences of Individuality.

YALE UNIVERSITY CLINIC OF CHILD DEVELOPMENT: *The First Five Years of Life*. New York, Harper & Bros., 1940, 393 pp.
    Chapter III: The First Year of Life.
    Chapter IV: From One to Five.
    Chapter VI: Motor Development.

CHAPTER 3

Integration of Organic and Musculoskeletal Function

WHEN lifetime efficiency and health status of the body are considered geriatrically as a continuing period from birth to death, there is a better appreciation of the conditions and forces that produce physical wear and tear, and the need for preventive and maintenance efforts.

Just as an engineer in projecting a bridge or building must visualize and strengthen areas required to withstand special stresses, so must those in physical education and other ancillary services recognize that they are dealing with a mechanism that requires the same attention. Architects must also take into consideration the future life of buildings and consequently make allowance for the prevention of excessive attrition, using perception in anticipating possible needs for the future. In the same manner, those working in human engineering must appreciate the individual's present needs while preparing him to meet effectively regular requirements of the future with allowance for the excessive demand which may be necessary.

Regard for the various types of individual must be considered. For instance (a) the lithe person with muscular hypertension, shown by increased reflexes, evidences more postural deviations and emotional instability, and (b) stout people are more prone to be phlegmatic, and sluggish with hypo-tonic reactions, slow metabolic rate as manifested by a tendency to obesity and postural deviations, a condition incidental to the weight, with faulty body chemistry seeming to prevail. Whereas those of medium type apparently have the least illnesses, the fewest evident divergencies, and might be considered to be the nearest to normal.

GROWTH AND DEVELOPMENT CONTINGENT ON MANY FACTORS

In an endeavor to arrive at a better understanding of the individual or organism, it is worthwhile reviewing a few of the many factors which, combined, largely determine the growth and development possibilities. The differences between individuals

(58)

come about through the growth potentials and the favorable experiences made available to the organism. It is well to recognize the coordinating influence of every aspect, including the organism and environmental agencies. Such a concept makes more effective the integrative procedures conducive to development, maintenance and adjustment.

GROWTH OF THE ORGANISM

The stabilizing nature of the body makes more favorable the action at various stages of development of individuals, such levels being reached at different periods as a result of the interactions of growth processes with the environment. Individual rate of growth is usually fairly constant, although changes appear to come in spurts. Although the inherited potentials may be present, greatest possible growth and development do not prevail without favorable environmental climate. Apparently there are critical periods in the development of organisms when they are more susceptible to the influence of extrinsic factors, and it is imperative that such opportunities find favorable conditions for assisting in the speeding up of the growth process.

All parts of man are tied together in a network, that is, the human organism is thought of as a highly complex ensemble of mental and physical traits that are intertwined and interdependent. As one part functions, all other parts are affected, they exert a reciprocal influence upon one another and are mutually affected by intrinsic and extrinsic factors.

Psychosomatic implications must be evaluated, since the physical and mental aspects are parts of the same organism, and a sound program of physical education or rehabilitation must be sufficiently comprehensive. Due consideration should be given to all factors affecting the growth and development of the human organism as a whole and as a functional unity.

Through insight into what the well balanced individual should possess in the way of physical and mental qualities, one is able to recognize and avoid the development of undesirable states which lead to personal degeneration, disintegration and disorganization. For the normal, the aim is for adequate functional, structural and postural adjustment in keeping with the social strata in which the individual lives. For those less fortunate or gifted there is need for modified activities related to interest, skill capacity, association with others, avoidance of environmental stress and re-adjustment of programs. Whether stimulation of the organism is from within or by means of the environment, the factor of activity is essential to growth and is considered by some synonymous with learning.

NATURE OF GROWTH

Insight as to the nature of growth is a fundamental requisite in order that the greatest good may be accomplished with a minimum of effort and maximum of results. Educators as well as those of other areas are especially interested in discovering what the potentialities of people are today, to what extent they are attaining these possibilities, and how education can best assist in the process. From this standpoint one of the important gaps in our knowledge calling for a solution is that of establishing maturation levels as they pertain to the growth process. In this respect such data should also reveal to those concerned with physical development, important steps which might be taken, while others working toward habilitation and rehabilitation measures will have greater insight and information as to why and how they should best proceed.

A real opportunist realizes that definiteness of a task sets up a challenge with tensions constituting a drive toward completion of of a task. Progression of goals is likewise pertinent, and each man must be approached on a level of least frustration for all are not stubbornly and richly born and many pay a large price for impatience. Realization of such factors help in the enriching of many human needs.

Differentiation between growth and development is necessary to understand the changes which take place in the organism.[1] *Growth is a quantitative affair*, an increase in size, a matter of accumulating content. The organism grows physically with the increase in height, weight, or bulk of muscle, but the mind does not increase in the number of cells or lobes much after birth. It is not possible for growth to take place without movement or activity of some sort, for while the potential may be present, there must be a receptive environment to create capacity.

Development is a qualitative affair, which takes place with changes in physiological and mental abilities or acquisitions. Individuals acquire ability and develop their performance in such a way as to show such important steps as (a) differentiation which is the recognition of a detail or pattern, (b) integration, or the organization of discretely perceived things or actions into meaningful patterns, which gives larger plans of action and understanding and when such takes place is known as insight, and (c) precision that is a change within a pattern of behavior which leads to definiteness, economy of effort and strength. All of these developmental processes likewise take place in the learning of muscular movements resulting in the increased skills and performance of action, while actual changes in size may result as a concomitant of such activity.

Developmental changes which occur in the organism, in any adequate study, must include a statement concerning the decline of physical vigor, for with the slowing up process of growth in the young there is a corresponding increase in strength and skill until middle age. With the passing of this period there is gradual loss of strength, changes in skill, and often regression of the dominant element in the individual's thinking and feeling. This process is affected by the metabolic and physical activity, delicate physiological balances and bio-chemical changes, environmental factors and other unknown elements. The decline of physical and mental ability varies with individuals and what they may do to postpone such decline through intelligent practices based on known facts, although there are naturally continual and inevitable changes which take place with aging.

Growth physically is apparent, and the progressive ability of the child to master more difficult tasks, is evidence of some underlying developmental process as yet not fully comprehended. It is known (a) that growth is the product of the interaction of the organism, a continuous and gradual rather than saltatory process, (b) that it proceeds most rapidly in the early years and appears to follow an orderly genetic sequence, (c) that relative growth rates tend to remain constant from infancy to maturity, (d) that growth is probably a process in which differentiation and integration play a parallel, though not always, a co-ordinate role, and (e) that the effect of specific training varies with the stages of maturation reached by the organism and will proceed regularly in the face of wide variations in environmental conditions.

FACTORS AFFECTING GROWTH

With the clarification of the principles of growth, it should be noted how the normal growth processes may be interfered with or promoted. Realization of hereditary tendencies make it possible to be on guard in some instances. On the other hand environmental factors, including illness or accidents, affecting the individual physiologically and psychologically, may be controlled to an extent for children by parents and by the clear thinking adult.

Heredity is the determiner of potentials for growth with which all are endowed and is of vital importance. The life career is maintained or guided by the physiological process of maturation, the regulatory mechanism of the organism, which preserves the balance of the pattern and the direction of growth. The behavior of the individual offers an indication as to the level of development. This is a part of the hereditary aspect which is a safeguard against variations in environment and gives a gradual development in all aspects up to the age of senescence.

Biological factors determine the differences in individuals even within a family as established by the Mendelian Law. The principle may be stated, in the presence of a dominant factor, the recessive one is present but does not show. This accounts for instances where two parents of inferior intelligence or stock produce a brilliant or smart child, providing the dominant genes cover up the recessive characteristics. However, offspring are affected if they mate with recessive types. In summation, the genes determine the direction of growth processes, while inheritance provides the start and direction of growth.

Studies of maturation[2] as revealed by factual evidence seem to be conclusive that (a) constitutional growth factors are very important in mental development, (b) differences in the rate of maturing appear very early in life, and (c) there is a good deal of consistency in rates of maturing in individuals, with respect to some mental functions at least, when viewed at different stages of growth. A constitutional factor is not necessarily an hereditary one, even if traced back to earliest infancy. It is not really known as to how much the level of maturity manifested by the child at birth owes to possible unknown factors in his pre-natal environment, and how much to the germinal complex. Consistency in rate of growth over long periods of time is of itself no more conclusive. It is conceivable that the constancy of the intelligence quotient, for example, may simply reflect a rate of development conditioned or set by non-hereditary factors in the early life of the individual.

There are two types of heredity to consider, namely, the biological which includes the physical, social, emotional and mental growth, all of which are transmitted through the medium of the germ plasm of the parent stock, and the social heredity into which an individual is born, such as the family, community and total environment. The latter is extremely important because of the interaction with the organism and can be separated only in analytical thinking, for in actual natural situations such separation would lead to instant death of the organism. Environmental factors support, inflect and modify, but do not generate progressions of development.

The potential for growth capacity is dependent upon environment, the function of which is to raise the latent power of capacity. Children from homes in which there is more culture, learning, and provision for greater opportunities for development are superior to those children from more limited economic and social strata.

The impact of the mental phase is meaningful in that it affects the judgment in situations where there is a choice which might do much to prevent unfavorable conditions from arising and in correcting others. Standards of living do not necessarily always help, since people become more prone in urban living to huddle in their hutches or apartments with sedentary pursuits, and to postpone exercise or physical activity for tomorrow.

Favorable environmental situations can do much in changing certain hereditary factors. Children with crooked teeth can have them straightened. Anomalies or birth injuries may be corrected through orthopedic surgery in imperfections such as webbed fingers or toes, club feet, upside down stomachs and a multitude of other like conditions. Glandular deficiencies react favorably to treatment, as do certain eye difficulties, and by means of immunology and other remedial treatment such cases as diabetes, resistance to disease, asthmatic tendency and many other conditions can be relieved or overcome.

Unfavorable environmental climate can likewise affect the organism negatively in many ways, (a) restriction of educational opportunity, (b) illness contracted such as poliomyelitus or other like diseases or infections, and (c) emotional conditions due to the type of situations with which people are faced. For example, physical strain, economic stress, excessive competition, routine or stifling work may contribute to mental aberrations or even insanity.

There are several types of environmental factors which promote or deter, depending on how they are utilized and classified, such as cultural which is subdivided into political, religious and social; physical including geographical, climatic and government; and institutional encompassing the home, school, community, and others which affect people at some stage of life.

INDICES AND STAGES OF GROWTH AND DECLINE

Personality may be considered as a psychosomatic manifestation, and the concept of self, as the individual experiences it, is virtually indistinguishable from the image of the body. Original perceptions in infancy and childhood are limited almost exclusively to the body. Earliest experiences are comprised of sensations, and it is likely that throughout life, despite radical changes, an individual's concept of self retains some of these initial impressions. Posture, gait and facial muscles serve to reveal something of the individual's characteristic attitudes. The tendency to over-value physical appearance serves to reinforce the importance of the body image.

SKELETAL AND MUSCULAR CHANGES

The most evident aspect of physical development is growth in body bulk, which is marked by two major waves; first in the prenatal and infant period, and second at the time of puberty. There is rapid increase during the intrauterine period in body bulk, to be followed by a doubling of weight in 5 months after birth, and a tripling in 12 months. There is then a slowing until puberty when it increases at a rapid rate for many months. Between the 12th and 17th years, the average boy's weight increase is equal to that of the preceding 10 years.

Average weight does not show as marked a change in the early years but proceeds rapidly from adolescence. The trunk is very long at birth and continues to grow rapidly at first but little during childhood and adolescence, finally lengthening materially after 17 years of age. The head does most of its growing before birth and the rest of the body soon after, for by 6 years of age the head is 93 per cent as large as it will be, and is 98 per cent of its final size by 12 years. Bones of the face seem to take turns in growing, with noticeable changes taking place through adolescence. In this period the bodily proportions are not right, for the legs are too long and the arms and legs are gangling, but there is an added depth of chest and a broadening of the shoulders as maturity is approached.

Muscular changes are constantly taking place, with a shifting in structure from the fat flabby bulky muscle to a later stringy and flexible one. As the years proceed, there is added range of motion and considerable additional strength which gradually decreases. Inability of the muscles to support the structure may cause much trouble which often remains throughout life.

Termination and decline of growth appears to be around later adolescence, as the bones increase in size only about 1 per cent, the muscles along with the vital organs about 4.5 per cent, the total weight approximately 7 per cent, while the strength increases nearly 25 per cent. The slowing down of old age is marked by a gradual change, when the weight and height decrease slightly. From middle age, strength and skill slowly regress. There is wide differences of opinion regarding the actual ages of such changes, for sex and racial characteristics as well as retention of maintenance fitness, bio-chemical and physiological factors cause variations.

PHYSIOLOGICAL CHANGES

These modifications are characterized during the passing years in the systems of the body. However, for the sake of brevity they are not described in detail since the major emphasis is being directed toward the muscular and skeletal systems. It is readily accepted that each of the following has definite impact and relationship to all other parts of the body, and is inseparably conjoined with structure, growth and function.

These systems are (a) circulatory in all its ramifications, (b) digestive with its responsiblity for supplying nutrients for growth, development and function, (c) respiratory as developed in proportion to the demands of the organism, (d) neural complexities related to the ability to think intelligently and do abstract mental work so essential in life, (e) glandular functions so extensive in application and without which there would be no life, and (f) differences among various bodily organs which are cited to illustrate the complexity of growth and to impress as to the importance, and inevitable displacement that sometimes prevails among the organs and thus affects the body function.

PSYCHOLOGICAL CHANGES

Findings concerning the changes which take place in the individual's mental growth and decline assume added significance when one realizes the great number of individuals who are confined or require treatment at some period of life. Added meaning takes place with an understanding of the import in seeking to make sure that needed changes occur. However, only a brief condensation is possible, since detailed description is out of context with the major theme and only mere mention of pertinent points is possible at this time.

Mental ability grows rapidly during childhood and adolescence, reaching a peak somewhere between the late teens or early twenties. Some psychologists contend that this stage is reached at a much later date. Many believe that there is a gradual decline of mentality soon after, and that by 55 years of age mentality has receded to about the 14-year level, although there is little real evidence to support this belief. Ability to learn, as shown by some experiments involving actual learning situations, shows a similar growth and then a slow decline.

Data on ages of persons involved in publishing books, producing inventions and conducting scientific work, show maximum productivity to be reached in the thirties.[3] Some findings show best work to be produced early in life, while other studies place the age of master work in the late forties. And yet leaders in political, business and professional life are usually well over 50, which would suggest that either ability does not begin to decline as soon as the research indicates, or that the accumulation of knowledge and experience, along with a maturing of judgment more than

5

compensates for the first decline. However, records and tests do indicate a definite decline after 60 years of age, although there are numerous exceptions to this rule.

Although the innate capacity is the major factor in accounting for individual differences in ability, the importance of social and economic circumstances and education cannot be overlooked as affecting the degree of developed intelligence and the rate of gradual loss.

Suggestions based on present knowledge of the growth and decline of ability point up the need for (a) earlier reaching of life work by the most able, and adjustment after middle life to declining years or powers, (b) deliberate effort through education and other social means to increase the general intelligence and to stay the general lessening of mental powers in the later years, and (c) exerting serious concern to adapting life at each age to the potentialities of that period, that each may, in its own way, be most fruitful.

Differences in opinion as to indices and stages of growth and decline keep us on an even keel just as a tide keeps the ocean from going too far in one direction. Individuality then, is the tide, and the sun and moon alone cannot be depended upon to control it for us. All must learn to do that for themselves and make the necessary adjustments according to the indigenous powers with which they are endowed.

INTERRELATIONSHIP IN STRUCTURE— FUNCTION DESIGN

Basic understanding in terms of procedure should be recognized from the foundation laws and principles as beacons, which are inseparably associated with growth, structure and adjustment of function. For instance, bone changes its internal architecture and external shape according to the ways in which the weight is borne or the stress is applied, as stated in Wolff's Law of bone growth.[4]

The importance of having environmental conditions conducive to proper bone development during the years when bones have their period of greatest growth cannot be overestimated. Incorrect seating, improper shoes and clothing for example, all cause stress to be placed incorrectly on the bony structure, resulting in a divergence from the normal course of skeletal growth. All activities during the growing years, such as play, work, sleeping conditions, facilities and equipment in childhood and adolescence, should be supervised and directed so that the weight is properly borne and the stress is applied where best supported to assure proper structural development.

All bones do not receive their entire growth nor become completely matured or ossified until the early adult years.[5] Until the late teens they do not correspond definitely to the activity of the glands of internal secretion, which largely control the maturation of the body. Growth cartilages or epiphyseal lines close at various periods, while the epiphyses near the joints and diaphyses or shafts of the bones fuse early or late in relation to the stage of organic and structural maturation.

The carpal indices are like sign posts which point out the distance traveled toward maturity. The small bones of the wrist ossify at different ages, hence, x-ray photographs of the wrist indicate whether skeletal development is normal or delayed, that is, whether physiological age is in proper relation to chronological age. At about 7 to 9 years of age these bones have usually assumed their mature shape, but they must still grow in size, and continue this process until about the fifteenth to seventeeth year.

Long bones grow in size and length at different rates in accordance with the periods of growth increments. Their growth plates may not be completely fused until the age of 21 years or even later. The pelvic bones and spine do not complete full ossification until approximately 16 or 17 years of age, and occasionally as late as the twenty-fifth year. Such factual information is given added importance in emphasizing the value of continuing developmental and rehabilitation measures throughout school life, and gives wise counsel as to why severe bodily contact in sports may be harmful.

Structure and function are vitally interrelated according to biological law. Just as a tree that is exposed to the wind develops a hard, twisted bark on that side and bends away from the force of the wind, so does the body framework develop in keeping with the stress applied which changes the segmental alignment. The shape of various bones is often the result of the stress of all the muscles attached to them, plus the force of weight bearing. A muscle becomes larger and more powerful from use and weaker from disuse, and hence, the need for unilateral development of antagonistic muscle groups. In direct proportion, the anchorage of large powerful muscles has to be rougher, heavier, and more extensive than that of small ones.

The importance of the application of this principle to the control of environmental influences during the period of greatest growth cannot be overestimated. For instance, if a child's feet are not properly shod before 7 years of age during the formative period, they are likely to be more seriously injured than they would be later in life during the same length of time. A faulty diet causing malnutrition will result in a more serious handicap at one time than another, depending on the lack of constituents needed for organic health or bone growth during certain stages. For example, condensed milk, unless fortified with mineral materials, may bring on rickets when fed to a baby, whereas, such feeding in a 10-year-old child would not produce the same disastrous results.

Orthopedic surgeons and physical educators should never forget the Law of Vulnerability of fast growing cells as it applies to the immature boy or girl. Its author, Murk Jansen,[6] stressed the fact that during stages of rapid growth, cells and tissues are more likely to be injured by forces applied to them than after growth has been completed. While intensified programs of physical education are viewed with great satisfaction, everyone must recognize the possibility for great good or harm being inherent in such activity. All over the nation machines are being worked to capacity, and to keep them operating properly, engineers and mechanics must keep them correctly aligned, their joints and bearings well lubricated, with their foundations leveled to an exact degree and heavy enough to meet the leverage stresses applied to them.

Technically, the human machine is more efficient than any inanimate one, yet does not differ in a structural sense, since the body as an operating instrument is subject to the same laws. It should be common knowledge that as Brigadier General Louis H. Renfrow, Deputy Director of Selective Service said before the Military Affairs Committee of the American Legion's National Security Commission in Los Angeles on September 1, 1956, "more than 2,200,000 young men have been rejected by the armed forces since the Korean War. The percentage of those rejected is 30 to 35 per cent."[7] It may well be implied that a large number of these rejections were due to structural faults, since the statistics reported previously found approximately 70 per cent to have some postural divergency.

Disturbed body mechanics are evident to the expert examiner in a high percentage of all persons examined. This fact should be taken into account in the modification of physical education, athletic and recreational programs especially for the late elementary and junior high school age levels. Many strenuous activities tend to increase the wear and tear on the bearings and joint cartilages. This means that the aging process is fostered, appearing in later years as a factor in producing symptoms of joint stress or arthritic changes in addition to segmental instability.

Many already know these facts and make little effort to avoid the discrepencies, being like the unknown author who wrote,

To get his wealth, he spent his health
And then with might and main,
He turned around and spent his wealth
To get his health again.

Milton has said, "Nature had done her best, do thou thine." It is not the days in your life that count, its the life in your days, and these are all too short years to be wasted. It is much easier to prevent than to repent and strive to retrace the steps which have been lost through neglect.

INTEGRATION OF ORGANIC ACTION AND SKELETAL FUNCTIONS

In connection with physical education in particular and all skilled movements in general, the functional use of various body segments may require finely coordinated effort, whereas those segments whose functions are for grosser movements, such as weight bearing or leg action, do not demand the same type of control. It may be seen that there should be an appropriate sequence in all activities.

There is a definite integration of organic activity in respect to blood supply, respiration, digestion, glandular, and neurological control, which must all be related and taken into consideration. For instance, any work of skill calling for increased attention, with requirements for highly coordinated effort, is more fatiguing and causes greater demand on the brain and nervous mechanism than big muscle mass work. For this reason fine work should be of short duration or fatigue and harm may result. On the other hand, muscle mass work needs an increased blood supply and, if prolonged, or too severe, may result in harm to the cardiovascular mechanism and heart lesions may result from such augmented stress.

The natural balance that exists between organic capacity and motor or neural output should also be borne in mind, and the different types of bodies must be considered from this standpoint in terms of stress. People of the thin, lithe, high speed type have certain differences both skeletally and organically and, being temperamentally and neurologically unlike the medium or stout types, should be managed according to their individual needs even within groups.

VARIANCES IN HEIGHT AND WEIGHT INDICATIONS

Removal of the causes of poor posture, structural weaknesses and functional efficiency, is a fundamental principle underlying all therapeutic procedures. In correcting such faults, all contributory causes, such as malnutrition, obesity, incorrect habits of sleeping, sitting, walking, eating and the like, must be altered.

Some authorities consider 7 per cent underweight as the danger zone for young children for it indicates lessened resistance and increases susceptibility to disease. In respect to nutritional factors in the lithe type child, judgment must be exercised. This is especially true where such children have parents who are also thin and lithe, and the child should not be considered necessarily unfit unless definite stigmas of malnutrition and growth faults are also in evidence. The problem of the obese child is of pertinence since the added weight in accordance with the joint structure may have even greater significance to the later body structure than to that of the thinner child. Someone has defined obesity as being a little short for the weight, while malnourished is underweight for the height.

A widely accepted means for determining nutritional status in terms of body structure is that which is known as the Helen B. Pryor, *Width-Weight Tables*.[8] This classification is based upon thousands of cases which have been treated statistically and utilizes the thoracic and bi-iliac diameters, plus age and height. Therefore, the basis is determined as to normal weight and deviations upon the individual's framework.

INTERDEPENDENCE IN MUSCLE ACTION

A muscle is composed of thousands of muscle fibers bound together by connective tissue and surrounded by a sheath of the same tissue, and are usually attached to the periosteum but may be fastened to the bone itself. The origin is mostly by fleshy attachment, while the insertion is invariably by means of a tendon, although both attachments may be tendinous.

Muscle action is what a muscle will actually do, what it can accomplish in its position and by its leverage when called upon by the nervous system. Generally, when a muscle contracts, the insertion moves nearer to the origin, and when a muscle relaxes the reverse is true. When a muscle contracts, it shortens and bulges sidewise, that is, each separate fiber swells out laterally, the sarcolemma (delicate elastic sheath which invests every striated muscle fiber) stretches and the whole muscle feels hard. Each time an exercise is repeated the muscle sheaths become more distensible. The power of a muscle depends upon the sum of the cross-sectional areas of all the muscle fibers. A comparatively slender muscle, in-so-far as its gross appearance is concerned, may thus have a cross-sectional area and power far in excess of what one might suppose, depending largely upon its internal structure and arrangement of the muscle fibers.

MUSCLE TONE AND PHYSIOLOGICAL ELEMENTS

Some muscle units are in a constant active state described as muscle tonus, which is a normal state of healthy muscle tissue.

It is the condition that exists in the muscle when it is receiving impulses from the nervous system. In "tonus" the fibers work in shifts, some of the fibers contract for a while and then another group take over the work so that tension can be maintained for a period of time without extreme fatigue. The slack can be taken up quickly when needed, and it may be observed that in the trained athlete, muscles are smooth and stringy, an evidence of tonus.

Best and Taylor describe tonus "As a result, chiefly of the work of the Sherrington School, the word 'tone' or 'tonus' as applied to skeletal muscles has acquired a clearly defined meaning . . . Muscle tone is the steady reflex contraction which resides in the muscles concerned in maintaining the posture characteristic of a given animal species. To use Sherrington's words 'reflex tonus is postural contraction . . . and its seat is therefore mainly in the *antigravity muscles*'."[9]

Physiological constituents in muscle tone consist of the receptor-effector system and is called a reflex arc, which makes up the neuromuscular functional unit of the organism. All parts of the reflex arc are capable of being affected by stimuli and are for the purpose of transforming energy into impulse. The sensory-motor pathway is as follows, the receptor or sense organ receives impulses through specialized nerve endings, traveling by way of the afferent or conducting path from the periphery to the center via the sensory nerve to the synapse or space in the cord where the axone meets the nerve center. Association neurones are found in the spinal or central nervous system returning the response to the impulse, thence to the synapse or junction on the way out to the motor nerve, by means of the efferent or conducting path from the center to the periphery via the motor nerve. At the myoneural junction or nerve end plates in the muscle units, the action is picked up by the effector muscle or motor unit which acts through the neural stimulation. In this manner muscle action takes place, and it may be seen that good posture as well as muscle function depends upon many associated groups of skeletal muscles.

TERMINOLOGY OF MOVEMENT

Flexion is the movement at a joint, in which the angle of articulation of its component bones is decreased. It is produced by muscles (flexors), so attached as to bring their point of attachment or origin on one member closer to the point of insertion on another; an example being the action of the biceps in flexing the forearm on the arm at the elbow.

Extension is the action of an opposed group of muscles (extensors), which move the joint toward its straight or neutral position, or in some instances carrying the part farther into a hyperextended position. An illustration is the gluteal muscles, extending the thigh on the pelvis or to the limit of backward movement which would be hyperextension.

Abduction is the changing of position of a part away from the mid line of the body (brought about by abductors or in opposition to the adductors), in restoring the part to a neutral position from that of adduction. It is shown in the deltoid muscle as it abducts the arm at the shoulder joint.

Adduction is the carrying of a part toward the midline of the body or away from the abducted position. For instance, the pectoralis major is the adductor of the arm at the shoulder and acts in opposition to the deltoid muscle.

Rotation is the movement of one part on another by moving on its long axis, referring expecially to the ball and socket joints, as in the shoulder and hip. Rotation in these joints is spoken of as inward and outward from the neutral position in the sagittal plane or from front to back.

Supination and Pronation. In the motions of a rotatory type, these movements are more limited in extent and refer to the palmar (palm) or plantar (back) aspects of the hands and feet. A representative would be the pronators which move the hand or foot surface upward or palmar, or surface downward or plantar, and the supinators in the opposite direction.

Circumduction is the direction of movement occurring at such joints as the hip, shoulder, and wrist, and which allows the part to be carried continuously from one plane to another as in adduction elevation, abduction depression or adduction flexion or abduction extension.

The execution of a movement is known as muscle action and consists of the following:

Concentric action takes place when a muscle is contracted and shortened, as in the action of the biceps in elbow flexion.

Eccentric action proceeds when the muscle contracts and is lengthened, as in the biceps, when the arm extends with a weight in the hand (placing a weight on a table), acting as the antagonist in controlling speed of action.

Static action results when a muscle contracts and remains the same length, as in the action of back muscles in maintaining an erect position of the trunk. This is a stabilizing action against gravity and is brought about through the maintenance of the continued state of tonus in the antigravity muscles, and is caused by reflex action. This is the so-called stretch reflex, which is brought about by pressure or tension as proprioceptive impulses that stimulate the muscles to act.

Agonist-antagonist action takes place when opponent muscles tend to balance each other and thereby maintain appropriate position of the body parts in their more or less fixed posture. However, when a part is to be moved to a new position by the agonist muscles, that is, from the state of tonic contraction into the state of phasic contraction, the antagonist must automatically receive a let-go impulse which is adjusted in accordance with the factors of speed, range and force required by the needs of the action. Morehouse and Miller clarify this issue as follows: "During the actual execution of movements, postural tone in the antagonist muscles must give way; this temporary abolition of tone is known as reciprocal inhibition."[10]

MECHANICS OF BONY LEVERS

The bones of the skeleton are articulated at the joints, which are the points at which motion takes place. The muscles or motors of the musculoskeletal system are attached near the joints in such a way that their attachments, or the points of application of their force obtains the best leverage. There are three classes of levers in the body. These are (*a*) first class levers in which the fulcral point lies between the weight arm and the power arm, as in the action of the triceps on the forearm, (*b*) second class levers have the fulcrum at one end and the weight lies between the end and the power, as in the action of the calf muscles on the heel in rising on the toes with the toes being the fulcrum, and the weight being applied at the ankle joint between the two and (*c*) third class levers have the fulcrum at one end and the power is between the end and the weight, as with the biceps in flexion of the elbow.[11]

Range is the extent of the arc of motion through the largest number of degrees permitted by the mechanical adjustments at the joint.

Duration is the length of time in which movements are continued or repeated, and should be appreciated in relation to the production of fatigue, coordinative factors of skill and muscle action involved, as in fine or gross movements. Rhythm or speed of movement should be based on the need or purpose for which an exercise is given.

Force is the relation of effort to output and should be considered as to the quality of effort, also, as to form and control. Form is spoken of in relation to the total pattern of movement in connection with any motor performance. This involves the neuromuscular response as to alertness or time reaction, the ease and grace of movement, the definitiveness, precision and accuracy of the movement necessary to the production of controlled action.

Form in this sense, is essentially the vehicle of expression of the emotions, and muscles may be thought of as extensions of the brain for conveying significant meaning in relation to the environment.

As may be readily seen, muscle action is interdependent upon many elements for movement, including the structure of the muscle and fibers itself, the neural system, organic action, and balancing function of opponent muscles. Coordinated together, the body is enabled to move about and to accomplish the many intricate tasks with which it is confronted. Only when all parts are operating efficiently is it possible to accomplish feats of skill or endurance.

JOINT STRUCTURE AND MOVEMENT

There are two major sections to the skeleton. First, the axial portion which includes the head, vertebræ, hyoid bone, sternum and ribs. Second, the appendicular section as the extremities consisting of the arms and legs.[12]

As far as the joints are concerned, those of the upper extremities are light in construction compared with those of the legs. Because of the prehensile use of the arm and hand, they have a great range of movement in the shoulder joint. In fact, the main characteristic of the shoulder girdle and its appendages the arms, is mobility. This is essential to the highly complex action of the hands. From an evolutionary standpoint, it has been thought that much of the development of the human brain was brought about by the development of the use of the hands.

Because of the greater variety and character of highly coordinated movements, the muscles of the arms and hands require a more intricate neuromuscular arrangement than that of the coarser, larger muscles of the body and legs. Effective performance of the hands and arms depends on the position and balance of the shoulder girdle and its joint structure, which is the chief base of action from which the arm muscles act. Hence, the essential need for good postural alignment in relation to the trunk. Another important fact is that structures of a very complex and highly integrated neuromuscular apparatus are extremely vulnerable to injury because of the high degree of coordinative action involved in their functioning.

In the lower extremities the need for stability and weight bearing characterizes the articulation of the legs with the pelvis. The hip joint is a deep socket called the acetabulum which allows a remarkable degree of motion in all planes, but not to the same extent as the more shallow shoulder joint. To ensure stability further, the joint is bound by heavy ligaments and operated by large, coarse-fibered heavy muscles.

Support and locomotion then are the chief functions of the lower extremities. The attachments of the appendicular portion of the skeleton to the axial portion is by means of two girdles, namely, the shoulder girdle and the pelvic girdle. The former is the lighter and is quite movable, whereas the latter is a ring closed at the symphysis pubes by a cartilaginous bumper, bound together by ligaments. Posteriorly, the lateral pelvis bones (the os innominata) articulate with the sacrum by irregularly ear-shaped joints (the sacroiliacs), which allow but little motion and transmit the body weight to the legs.

SKELETAL ARTICULATIONS

In order to have a clear idea of the dynamics of body action, it is important to consider briefly the joints which are analogous to the bearings of an inanimate machine. The chief components of joints are bones, cartilages, synovial lining, ligaments, tendons, and muscles with, additionally, the essential nerves and blood vessels.

There are four main types of articulations (1) the ball and socket type, (2) the hinge type, (3) the saddle or compound type, and (4) the sliding type. Examples of these in order are (a) hip or shoulder joints, (b) knee and elbow with their hinge action, (c) compound or saddle joints, such as the metacarpo-carpal of the thumb and the astralo-calcaneal joints of the feet, and (d) the ankle which is an example of the sliding joint as is also the sub-patellar articulation in the trochlear groove of the femur.

The surfaces of the bones, where they come together, are sheathed by a covering developed as a cartilage. This forms a pearly, shiny-smooth surface which, when lubricated, allows the bones to move on each other with minimal friction. This specialized layer of the mesodermal or middle embryonal layer, from which all structural tissues are formed, acts also as a buffer and has enough resilience to absorb shocks incident to activities such as jumping and falling. Beyond a given limit this layer is subject to injuries, either minute cracks or fractures or areas of compression from sudden or continuous overaction of the muscles or the gravitational load.

The ends of the long bones are enlarged or bulbous at the joint ends. This allows for attachments of the tendons through which the muscles act to produce stability or motion. All around the joints is a ligamentous capsule whose fibers are thickened along the lines of greatest stress, and contain a certain percentage of elastic fibers which take up the shock from tension at the extremes of the range of movement.

Movement beyond the normal physiological range will over-stretch these ligaments and produce a strain. A greater degree with tearing of the fibers would be known as a sprain, which allows one bone to slide off the other but returns to its normal position when force is discontinued. If it does not return to normal position, the injury is called a subluxation. Still greater slipping, which obliterates the normal continuity of the joint, is a complete dislocation. In cases with deviations of posture, the malalignment of the joints involved, renders them more susceptible to injury than if their muscles and ligaments provide a balanced control on all sides of the joint.

Within this ligamentous capsule, and lying on a protective fibro-fatty cushion, is the synovium or synovial lining which is made up of a thin layer of cells on a connective tissue base. This tissue secretes the synovial fluid which lubricates the joint. This fluid is straw-colored and slightly viscous, which, colloquially, is sometimes called the "joint water." The synovium lies in folds or reduplications of the fatty layer mentioned above, which allows it to stretch to the physiological extreme of motion when the joint is opened, and to fold up like a bellows when the joint is closed.

Because of an undue amount of compression from a strain or fall, or from repeated small trauma occurring from movements such as deep knee bends, the folds of the lining of the joints may be pinched again and again. This process may go on until a synovitis is caused. This is most common in the knee, and in time a fibrous tissue reaction is caused which is evidenced by a grating or crackling crepitation on movement. Thus, the so-called football knee is disclosed, although this condition is not unique to any one sport. It is also developed very commonly in women from wearing high heels because of the unbalanced strain placed upon the knee in such a postion.

These examples illustrate the accumulation of micro-trauma to joint structures, which may or may not be appreciated during the school years, since the trouble may not appear until long after the completion of school. Here is illustrated again the acceleration of the aging process which may be advanced materially during the growing years and in persons whose postural deviations are not remedied.

GROWTH AND DEVELOPMENT OF JOINTS

Just above the ends of the long bones, which form the joints is a transverse area called the epiphysis or growth cartilage, and on the opposite side of this line of cartilage is the diaphysis or shaft. Ossification of these growth centers is continuous until the stage of sexual maturity arrives.

There are two factors of stimulation to bone growth, namely, gravitational stress and muscle tension. The stresses thus applied to the bones and joints account for their conformation or shape, and this is in accordance with physical laws previously cited. Skeletal growth, though in a sense continuous, is more rapid at certain stages of development. Such growth is influenced by many factors, such as hereditary tendencies, nutritional states, activities, bio-chemical influences and organic functioning. Consequently, the shape of the component elements in the joints may be altered unless the growing centers are properly nourished, and the mechanical stresses applied to them are properly balanced under control in relation to their work load.

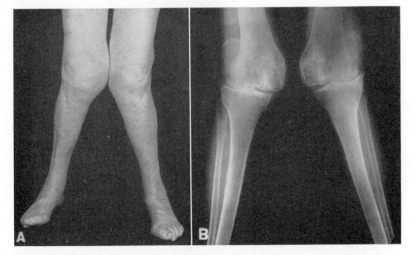

Fig. 8.—*A*, Knock knees extreme at 70 years of age. *B*, X-ray picture shows changes at knee, lateral lipping and marked narrowing of cartilage

Sensitivity of these growth centers is greatest during those periods of rapid growth, and therefore, they are most vulnerable during the formative stages. This is the reason why parents and teachers should be most cautious in regard to the character of the activities given youngsters in the growing years,[13] and why special consideration is recommended in regard to prevention and correction of faults in body mechanics in connection with developmental and adapted physical education. As an illustration of the effects of stress in relation to the configuration of joints, consider the common knock-knees.

The line of the knee joint is approximately at right angles to the line of weight bearing, and, under normal conditions, such as the slight increase of internal angulation in the female because the pelvis is wider, there is a proportionate modification of the angulation of the joint line. However, if knock knees exist, the line of gravitational stress will pass through the joint on the outer side. In early years, if the deviation is only of a mild grade, the femoral and tibial epiphyses will be stimulated to grow more rapidly on

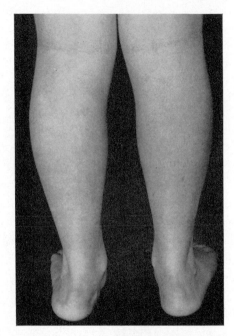

FIG. 9.—Valgus ankles—1st degree.   Knock knees, flat arches.

that side and thus tend to correct the angulation. However, if the internal lateral ligaments become increasingly stretched, allowing the deviation to increase, there will be too much compression of the growth plates on the outside and a corresponding release on the inner condyles, so that the shape will change accordingly. Such an extreme condition is found in Figure 8.

Sometimes when the arches lower and the ankles pronate, the shift of support to the soft springy foot ligaments will reduce the bony resistance below the knee as well as add a lateral and rotatory thrust inward on its ligaments. Figure 9 indicates a valgus or pronated ankle condition. If the angle of the neck of the femur with the shaft tends to increase toward a right angle, the weight thrust from above likewise throws a lateral stress on ligaments.

These tend to stretch more and allow the inner aspect of the knee joint to gap more and increase the compression on the outer condyles until their growth is retarded. This makes it impossible for the deviation to be overcome naturally.

Picture what happens when a child increases his body weight during a period when muscle strength cannot keep pace with rapid growth, or consider the effect of intensive muscle activity with the application of greater force on these joints. Such occurs in severe contact sports or excessive weight bearing activities, also when increased and strenuous programs are advised in accordance with height and weight classifications. These illustrations may give some idea of the wear and tear increase from ill-advised activities in the presence of postural faults and particularly during this "so-called" vulnerable age level.[14]

JOINT STABILITY

Bony configuration of the joints and its mechanical limitation to motion beyond a normal range have been discussed, as has also the relation of the supporting ligaments to stabilization of them. In some joints there is a further protection against injury from undue stresses through the involvement of ligaments. The two joints so protected are the knee and hip joints. In the former, the cruciate ligaments check the forward and backward sliding movement and help to maintain the locked position back of dead center when standing. In the hip joint, there is an internal check ligament called the teres ligament which fastens to the middle of the head of the femur and is attached as a tether to the floor of the socket.

Other internal structures in the knee joint deserving of mention are the semilunar cartilages which lie in the inner and outer margins of the joint line. They are triangular in cross sections and curve around the margin of the condyles in a halfmoon shape. Laterally, they are attached to the capsular ligaments, but the thin internal margins float free. These serve to deepen the shallow cup of the tibial condyle and make for stability both in standing and during motion.

Fracture and displacement of these ligaments are very common incidents in athletics, especially in football, skiing and soccer, or where sudden cutting in direction or blows from the side of the leg occur. The downward, inward thrust with a rotatory force against the resistance of the ground or floor, when the substance of the shoe will not allow for any giving action, is the movement which causes such injuries generally. Consequently, any elongation or laxity of the ligaments on the inner aspect, due to faulty leg alignment or rotary stress from pronating ankles and relaxed arches, are a predisposing factor to knee injuries.

Generally speaking, personnel working in physical education and body building programs are not devoting adequate time and consideration to the basic structure of the body framework. The major emphasis is upon the motor apparatus and the technical aspects of skill development and size of muscles. In consequence, there may be insufficient appreciation of the basic bio-physical laws that govern and affect the bearing of the human machine and functional adequacy.

It is not enough to know the origin and insertion of skeletal muscles nor to have a fair comprehension of kinesiology, unless there is sufficient realization of the way joints are developed, how they work in relation to the rest of the body, and what stresses can be applied to these joint bearings with safety, in accordance with the age, growth status, and fitness index.

In summation, it is clear that individuals thrive best when there is total interaction of the body in ratio to the frugal expenditure of energy demands. Organic, skeletal, and muscular integration is similar to that of an efficient committee working together for dear life. Not as Don Quinn, the writer for the television show Halls of Ivy, in the program presented by Ronald Coleman in April 1952 gave when he said, "A committee is a group of the unfit, appointed by the unwilling, in order to do the unnecessary."[15] Somewhere in each one there is a right combination, if it can be found, and our effectiveness will then depend not on how old we are today, but how we are when we are old.

REFERENCES

1. MILLARD, CECIL V.: *Child Growth and Development in the Elementary School Years.* rev. edition; Boston, D. C. Heath and Co., 1958, 512 pp.
2. MARTIN, WILLIAM E. and STENDLER, CELIA BURNS: *Child Development: The Process of Growing Up in Society.* New York, Harcourt, Brace & Co., 1953, 519 pp.
3. PRESSEY, SYDNEY L. and KUHLEN, RAYMOND G.: *Psychological Development Through the Life Span.* New York, Harper Bros., 1957, 654 pp.
4. LOWMAN, CHARLES LeROY, COLESTOCK, CLAIRE and COOPER, HAZEL: *Corrective Physical Education for Groups.* New York, A. S. Barnes and Co., 1928, p. 81.
5. *Ibid.,* Chapter IX.
6. JANSEN, MURK: *Feebleness of Growth.* London, Hodder and Stoughton, 1921, pp. 19–35.
7. RENFROW, LOUIS H.: News item in *Los Angeles Times,* September 1, 1956.
8. PRYOR, HELEN B.: *Width-Weight Tables.* Stanford University, California, Stanford University Press, 1940, 15 pp.
9. BEST, CHARLES HERBERT and TAYLOR, NORMAN BURKE: *Physiological Basis of Medical Practice.* 6th ed., Baltimore, The Williams & Wilkins Co., 1955, p. 962.
10. MOREHOUSE, LAURENCE E. and MILLER, AUGUSTUS T., JR.: *Physiology of Exercise.* 3rd ed., St. Louis, The C. V. Mosby Co., 1959, p. 74.
11. LOWMAN, COLESTOCK and COOPER: *op. cit.,* Chapter IX.
12. *Ibid.,* Chapter X.
13. LOWMAN, CHARLES LEROY: A Consideration of Teenage Athletics, J. Health and Phys. Educ., *12,* 398–399, 1941.

14. KANSAS PUBLIC SCHOOLS: Survey of Inter-School Tackle Football in Junior High School, Kansas City, Board of Education, February, 1958, pp. 7–8.
15. QUINN, DON: Television Production *Halls of Ivy*, starring Ronald Coleman, April, 1952.

The above references are not repeated in References for Extended Reading.

REFERENCES FOR EXTENDED READING

BALDWIN, ALFRED L.: *Behavior and Development in Childhood.* New York, The Dryden Press, 1955, 619 pp.
    Chapter XV: Maturation.
BAYLEY, N.: Individual Patterns of Development, Child Development, *27*, 45–74, 1956.
BAYLEY, N. and ESPENSCHADE, A.: Motor Development and Decline, Rev. Educ. Res., *20*, 367–374, 1950.
BEST, C. H., and TAYLOR, N. B.: *The Living Body.* New York, Henry Holt & Co., Inc., 1952, 792 pp.
    Chapter XI: The Physiology of Nerve and Muscles.
BRECKENRIDGE, MARIAN E., and VINCENT, E. LEE: *Child Development.* 3rd ed. Philadelphia, W. B. Saunders Co., 1955, 497 pp.
    Chapter I: Some General Principles of Development.
    Chapter II: Influences on Growth: Physical.
    Chapter IV: Influences on Growth: Nutrition & Routines.
    Chapter VII: Growth and Use of the Body: Physical Growth.
    Chapter VIII: Growth and Use of the Body: Motor Control.
BRINLEY, ELDON D.: Interscholastic Football in the Elementary School, The Texas J. Sci., *4*, 464–470, 1952.
CARLSON, A. J. and JOHNSON, VICTOR: *Machinery of the Body.* 4th ed., Chicago, University of Chicago Press, 1953, 663 pp.
    Chapter IX: The Action of Muscle and Nerve.
    Chapter X: Mechanisms of Correlation—The Spinal Cord and Brain.
COMMINS, W. D., and FAGIN, BARRY: *Principles of Educational Psychology.* 2nd ed., New York, The Ronald Press Co., 1954, 795 pp.
    Chapter III: Human Variability and Growth.
    Chapter IV: Growth and Maturation.
COWELL, CHARLES C.: *Scientific Foundations of Physical Education.* New York, Harper & Brothers, 1953, 260 pp.
    Pages 39–72: The Nature of the Individual.
    Pages 74–93: Genetic Growth and Development.
CROW, LESTER, and CROW, ALICE: *Adolescent Development and Adjustment.* New York, McGraw-Hill Book Co., Inc., 1956, 570 pp.
    Chapter II: Biological and Cultural Heritage.
    Chapter IV: Physical and Psychological Growth.
————: *Human Development and Learning.* New York, American Book Co., 1956, 578 pp.
    Chapter II: The Fundamentals of Human Development.
    Chapter III: Physical, Mental and Emotional Development.
CUNNINGHAM, DANIEL JOHN: *Textbook of Anatomy*, edited by J. C. Brash. 9th ed., London, Oxford University Press, 1951, 1604 pp.
    Pages 333–401: Section on Arthrology (Joints).
    Pages 403–484: Section on Myology (Muscles).
CURETON, T. K.: Weight and Tissue Symmetry Analyses, Suppl. Res. Quart., *2*, 331–347, May, 1941.
DAVIS, ELWOOD C., and LAWTHER, JOHN D.: *Successful Teaching in Physical Education.* New York, Prentice-Hall Inc., 1948, 617 pp.
    Chapter XII: Individual Similarities and Differences:
                Implications for Physical Education.
DEARBORN, WALTER, and ROTHNEY, JOHN W. M.: *Predicting the Child's Development.* Cambridge, Mass. Science Art Publishers, 1941, 360 pp.

DUVALL, ELLEN NEALL: *Kinesiology.* Englewood Cliffs, N. J., Prentice-Hall, Inc., 1959, 292 pp.
　　　Chapter II: The Human Framework.
　　　Chapter III: Muscles and the Neuro-muscular Mechanism.
　　　Chapter IV: Mechanical Relationship of Muscle and Bone.
EDWARDS, LINDEN FOREST: *Concise Anatomy.* 2nd ed., New York, McGraw-Hill, 1956, 502 pp.
　　　Chapter II: General Osteology.
　　　Chapter III: General Arthrology.
EWERHARDT, F. H. and RIDDLE, GERTRUDE F.: *Therapeutic Exercise.* Philadelphia, Lea & Febiger, 1947, 152 pp.
　　　Chapter II: Analysis of Joint Motion.
FORD, ADELBERT: *Foundations of Bioelectronics for Human Engineering.* Navy Electronics Laboratory Report 761. San Diego: U.S. Navy Electronics Laboratory, 4 April, 1957, 119 pp.
FOREST, ILSE: *Child Development.* New York, McGraw-Hill Book Company, Inc., 1954, 291 pp.
　　　Chapter III: Infancy.
　　　Chapter IV: Early Childhood.
　　　Chapter V: Growth Levels.
　　　Chapter VI: The Physical Growth of Children.
GARRISON, KARL C., and GRAY, STANLEY J.: *Educational Psychology,* New York, Appleton-Century-Crofts, Inc., 1955, 505 pp.
　　　Chapter II: The Nature of Growth and Development.
　　　Chapter III: Physical Growth.
GREULICH, W. W., and PYLE, S. I.: *Radiographic Atlas of Skeletal Development of Hand and Wrist.* Stanford, California, Stanford University Press, 1950, 190 pp.
HUBBARD, A. W.: Muscular Force in Reciprocal Movements, J. Gen. Psych., *20,* 315–325, 1939.
HURLOCK, ELIZABETH B.: *Adolescent Development.* Rev. ed., New York, McGraw-Hill Book Co. Inc., 1956, 703 pp.
　　　Chapter III: Body Changes.
JERSILD, ARTHUR T.: *The Psychology of Adolescence.* New York, The Macmillan Co., 1957, 438 pp.
　　　Chapter III: The Changing Body.
　　　Chapter IV: Physical Activity and Ability.
KOZMAN, HILDA C., CASSIDY, ROSALIND and JACKSON, CHESTER O.: *Methods in Physical Education.* Philadelphia, W. B. Saunders Co., 1952, 557 pp.
　　　Chapter II: Your Pupils: Growth and Development.
KROGMAN, W. M.: The Concept of Maturity from a Morphological Viewpoint, Child Development, *21,* 25–32, 1950.
LEE, J. MURRAY, and LEE, DORRIS MAY: *The Child and His Development.* New York, Appleton-Century-Crofts, Inc., 1958, 624 pp.
　　　Chapter III: Physical Maturity and Motor Control.
LICHT, SIDNEY, (ed.): *Therapeutic Exercise.* New Haven, Conn.: Elizabeth Licht, 1958, 893 pp.
　　　Chapter I:　The Motor Unit.—Christian Coers.
　　　Chapter III: Mechanical Anatomy of Motion and Posture.
　　　　　　　　　　　　　　　　　　　　　　　—Michael A. MacConaill.
LOWMAN, CHARLES LEROY: The Relation of Postural States to Competitive Sports, The Physical Educator, *9,* 67–68, 1952.
McCLOY, C. H.: Anthropometry in the Service of the Individual, J. Health and Phys. Educ., *5,* 7–11, 1934.
MATTHIAS, EUGEN: *The Deeper Meaning of Physical Education.* New York, A. S. Barnes and Co., 1929, 88 pp.
　　　Chapter II: The Essence of Physical Education.
MEREDITH, H. V. and KNOTT, V. B.: Changes in Body Proportions during Infancy and Pre-school Years; Shelic Index, Child Development, *9,* 49–62, 1938.
MURPHY, GARDNER: *Personality.* New York, Harper & Bros., 1947, 999 pp.
　　　Chapter III, Heredity and Individual Growth.

NATIONAL RESEARCH COUNCIL OF THE RESEARCH SECTION: *Measurement and Evaluation Materials*. Washington, D. C.: Amer. Ass'n Health, Physical Education and Recreation, 1950, 138 pp.
 Chapter II: Anthropometry and Body Mechanics.

NATIONAL SOCIETY FOR THE STUDY OF EDUCATION: *Adolescence, 43rd Yearbook, Part I*. Chicago: University of Chicago Press, 1944, 358 pp.
 Chapter I through VII.

NORTHWAY, W. H.: Injuries to Joints, Arch. Phys. Therapy, *23*, 467–473, 1942.

OLSON, WILLARD C.: *Child Development*. Boston, D. C. Heath and Co., 1949, 417 pp.
 Chapter I: Growth and Development.
 Chapter II: Growth Periods and Educational Programs.
 Chapter III: The Expression and Nurture of Physical Growth,
 Chapter IV: Motor Development and Play.
 Chapter VII: The Child as a Whole.

QUIMBY, R. H.: What a Man Should Weigh, Res. Quart., *5*, 91–109, 1934.

RAND, WINIFRED, SWEENEY, MARY E., and VINCENT, E. LEE: *Growth and Development of the Young Child*. 6th ed., edited by Marian E. Breckenridge and Margaret Nesbitt Murphy, Philadelphia, W. B. Saunders Co., 1958, 548 pp.
 Chapter I: Current Concepts and Theories of Growth and Development.

RASCH, PHILIP J. and BURKE, ROGER K.: *Kinesiology and Applied Anatomy*. Philadelphia, Lea & Febiger, 1959, 456 pp.
 Chapter II: The Framework and Joints of the Body.
 Chapter III: The Structure and Action of Striated Muscle.
 Chapter VII: Simple Machines.

RATHBONE, JOSEPHINE L.: *Corrective Physical Education*. 5th ed., Philadelphia, W. B. Saunders Co., 1955, 318 pp.
 Chapter II: Anatomy and Mechanics of Joint Action.

SELLWOOD, JOHN J.: Relationships of Growth and Developmental Patterns of Posture, J. School Health, *25*, 190–196, 1955.

SHERRINGTON, CHARLES SCOTT: *The Integrative Action of the Nervous System*. New Haven, Yale University Press, 1947, 433 pp.

SIMMONS, KATHERINE: *The Brush Foundation Study of Child Growth and Development II, Physical Growth and Development*. Monographs of the Society for Research in Child Development, Vol. 9, No. 1. Washington, D. C., National Research Council, 1944.

STAFFORD, GEORGE T., and KELLY, ELLEN DAVIS: *Preventive and Corrective Physical Education*. 3rd ed., New York, The Ronald Press Company, 1958, 395 pp.
 Chapter III: Biological Foundations.

STEINDLER, ARTHUR: *Kinesiology of the Human Body*. Springfield, Illinois, Charles C Thomas, 1955, 708 pp.
 Lecture IV: The Physical Properties of Cartilage,
      Muscles, Fascia and Tendons.
 Lecture V: On the Mechanics of Joint and Muscle Action.
 Lecture XI: Pathomechanics of the Lumbrosacral Junction.

STRONG, O. S. and ELWYN, A.: *Human Neuro-anatomy*. 3rd ed., Baltimore, The Williams and Wilkins Co., 1953, 442 pp.

THORPE, Louis P.: *Child Psychology and Development*. 2nd ed., New York, Ronald Press Co., 1955, 709 pp.
 Chapter IV: Physical Growth and Health.

WAKIM, KHALIL G.: The Physiological Aspects of Therapeutic Physical Exercise, J.A.M.A., *142*, 100–108, 1950.

WELLS, KATHERINE F.: *Kinesiology*. 2nd ed., Philadelphia, W. B. Saunders Co., 1955, 516 pp.
 Chapter III: Fundamental Principles of Motion Levers.
 Chapter IV: Fundamental Principles of Force and Work.
 Chapter V: The Joints: Their Structure and Function.

WHITE HOUSE CONFERENCE ON CHILD HEALTH and PROTECTION: *Growth and Development*. New York, Century Company, 1932.
 Part III: Growth and Development of the Child.
 Part IV: Appraisement of the Child.

WRIGHT, W. G.: *Muscle Function*. New York, Paul B. Hoeber, Inc., 1928, 188 pp.
 Chapter I: General Principles of Muscle Action.

CHAPTER 4

Pertinence of Relationship in Body Segments

THERE is serious contention on the part of many authorities as to what is normal in regard to the segmental alignment of the human body. It is, however, an accepted fact, that there is much variance in respective individuals and that while a static measuring stick cannot be justified exclusively in gauging the structural merits of all on the same basis, there is need, nevertheless, for some instrument of comparison.

Normality in one may be contrary to that of another, generally speaking, and the effective operation under working conditions is an additional judgment to be determined. Hence, it is of meaning to consider each individual within his own orbit. An inspection type of check-up similar to an automobile inspection would at least seem in order to ascertain (a) how the tires are standing up, (b) if the air cleaner is functioning properly, (c) whether there may be too great a load or too little for the size of the undercarriage, or (d) perhaps there is need for a tune-up or even a complete overhaul. It is impossible, as in a second hand car, to get much of a trade-in toward a new one.

An inventory taking of stock should be a requisite for time passes pleasantly, eventfully and quickly—all too quickly when you are well—but harshly and slowly when nature complains. These bodies are yours or perhaps those of others whom you love, and unless something is done about such matters while these lives are in progress, so much of opportunity is lost but not forgotten. Within accessibility of all are competent specialists, orthopedic services, and in many school situations adapted or developmental programs in physical education.

BASIC BODY MECHANICS

An understanding of the statics, kinetics and dynamics of the musculoskeletal system requires a reasonable knowledge, or at least some comprehension, of engineering. Arthur Steindler has given outstanding evidence of this fact in his book, *Kinesiology of of the Human Body*.[1]

(84)

Any definition of good posture must take into consideration the proper relationship of the various body segments which should be in alignment, under or over each other. That is, so related to the gravity lines laterally and anteroposteriorly that a minimum of energy needs to be expended to maintain the body as near as possible in a state of equilibrium which is unique to each individual's specific characteristics. The body, in anything but recumbency, cannot be in a fixed static state as a box or table. Therefore, it must be maintained in balance by the continuous action of the large masses of antigravity muscles whose function is to hold against the downward pull of gravitational forces.[2]

The most effective position of all body segments is that in which they are maintained in a relation to each other with the least expenditure of energy. The body position is related to its environment by the registration of visual, auditory, tactile and kinesthetic sensations over the afferent sensory nerve tracts to the brain or spinal cord. Position is retained or altered by stimuli through the neuro-motor mechanism to whatever muscles need to be activated. This is the dynamic aspect of good posture. In order to obtain the most effective development of coordinated skills through this action, there must be a clear understanding of the best base position for the skeleton and its various segments from which muscle action takes place in respect to individual variances.

Sometimes the things which are done in the name of education and in recreational pursuits, are like trumping your partner's ace. It is often observed that some people are travelling counter-clock-wise in using unwise practices, and after a while there must either be repairs or else the clock runs down. None are so vain as to believe that immunity to segmental troubles are any ones sole prerogative, for illness or injury may strike suddenly and unequivocally, and such may be a personal warning to you.

How marvelous to have the grace of a bird in flight or to be able to play with the abandon of a porpoise in the sea. On the other hand, how depressing it must be to hobble and grope about, seeking and asking only for balance.

The building up of muscle mass does not always imply good posture, an observation which is quite apparent to those who regularly judge students either in posture contests or when viewing people under duress conditions of handicaps. Some high school lads who have specialized in strenuous sports activities show magnificent development of the arm and shoulder girdle, but this increased arm weight in the presence of a basic slump in the trunk only tends to increase the dorsal curve and forward head position.

The end result in later life may be recurrent neck pains and backache or neuritis over the shoulders and arms. From the standpoint of simple mechanics, such development is analogous to putting a 100 horse-power motor in an automobile whose chassis is in bad alignment. This causes more rapid and excessive wear in moving parts and bearings. In humans the increased wear and tear is on the ligamentous and cartilagenous substances of the joints.

It should likewise be remembered that organic factors as related to posture have static and dynamic aspects. The position of the organs at rest as well as changes in their position during functional activity is related to skeletal alignment. An example of this contention is shown through the fact that the heart and lungs cannot act with optimum efficiency in the presence of a forward head and shoulders or a pronounced round back.

Good body mechanics refers to the function of all the parts of the human body, including bones, joints, muscles, viscera, and nerves. This naturally involves the general physiology of the total body and each phase has reciprocal impact upon each of the others. Consequently, if development of skill as well as muscular and organic endurance are related to good postural alignment, everyone, especially physical instructors and coaches, should be interested in the improvement of basic underlying faults in body mechanics of both a skeletal and organic nature.

If each one of us would but ask himself, what can I do, then the battle would be joined. There are those who know but do not tell, and there are those who tell but do not know. An old Arabic saying goes, "He who knows and knows that he knows, is wise. Follow him." This is the challenge all must face, to find the way, and seeing it to take action. As an unknown writer expressed it, "He who would do some great thing in this short life must apply himself to the work with such a concentration of his forces, as, to the idle spectators, who live only to amuse themselves, looks like insanity."

Do not be discouraged with the task of preparation ahead, for such a journey is like a long flight of stairs. You can take only one step at a time, and each one made shortens the climb until the top is in sight. The search for knowledge is often gained only after arduous effort and toil, and when experience is also added, the sum total is in many cases the answer. This is what parents, teachers, physicians and *you* can do in fulfilling your duty to yourself and to your fellow man.

NORMALCY IN GRAVITATION ALIGNMENT

Good posture is natural, graceful, unstilted, unassumed and constant without reflection. Best body mechanics is considered as a mechanized correlation of the various systems, and normal may be said to be obtained when synchronization is most favorable to total function. Figure 10 is an example of normal dynamic movement. Posture is one characteristic which assists nature in compensations but it is often overlooked as an active disabling agency, since the adjustive qualities of the body may recompense or counter balance variations causing such hidden clues to go unnoticed.

Discovery of predisposing symptoms or actual presence of weaknesses reverting to posture as a causative element is largely dependent upon prescribed formulas ascertained by competent authorities who have tested their beliefs in the crucible of time. Knowledge of anatomy is accepted as comparatively stable, with *Gray's Anatomy* as an authentic reference source. Ideas as to determinants of functional states of the body are more flexible since they are more difficult to observe and establish. For this reason there are numerous leaders who have expressed their opinions and formulated various methods in judging symmetry and from whose thinking reliable guides have been selected and presented.

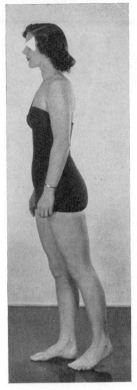

FIG. 10.—Normal Dynamic Movement

GRAVITY LINES

The *center of gravity* of the body is described by Lovett as follows, "In the erect position, the center of gravity of the body lies in front of the ankle joints, which are held from dorsal flexion in this position by the gastrocnemius muscles. The center of gravity lies also in front of the knees, which are held in position by the hamstrings and quadriceps extensor muscles. The center of gravity lies also anterior to the sacroiliac joints and most of the vertebral joints."[3]

The anteroposterior or *gravity line* in relation to the lateral anatomical landmarks is described by Davis as falling through the "Front of outer ankle bone (fibular malleolus), back of the patella, middle of great trochanter, middle of shoulder tip, and to the tragus of the ear."[4]

The relationship of the lateral halves of the body to the *center line* is referred to by Bancroft in her discussion of the "vertical line test."[5]   A simple rule for determining the lateral gravity line or center line is to erect a plumb line from a point midway between the heels, through the cleft of the buttocks, through the mid points of all the vertebræ, and through the mid occipital protuberance. In checking the leg line, the string should pass from a point just between the big toe and the second toe, through the middle of the ankle joint, through the middle of the knee cap, and then to a point approximately just inside the anterior superior spine of the ilium.

When body segments do not conform to the above measures in an ordinary position of rest, a proportionate degree of faulty mechanics are considered to exist.   Since the individual is in a mild state of disequilibrium in relation to gravity, he must compensate for the weight deviation by shifting a corresponding mass in an opposite direction in order to keep his balance.   This may be due to underlying structural deviations such as a short leg, or a muscular weakness that allows a segment or part to shift because of an inability to neutralize the pull of gravity.

POSTURAL POSITIONS

Since emphasis is usually placed upon prescribed fundamental postural positions[6] in physical education and orthopedics, there needs to be a rounded statement concerning the requisites believed most essential in each position.

Standing in an erect position commonly known as "attention" is the result of reciprocal innervation by antagonistic muscles exerting their action in all planes for the adjustment of body balance.   The basic factors are standing tall and without strain, with the head up, chin in, neck flat, chest high, shoulders in gravity line, which are held well back with the raising of the chest, pelvis tilted down in back and rotated up in front, abdomen is automatically tucked in and flat, knees slightly flexed to avoid strain, and the feet pointed forward and about 4 inches apart with the weight on the outer borders.   Flexion of the knees and rotation of the legs and feet outward while tensing and relaxing of the abdomen will assist in prevention of the pooling of the blood, which so often causes service personnel to faint when held in a static position for long periods without relaxation.

The average goal to be sought in the "habitual" position is similar to the previous one, which can be best attained with a minimal amount of effort and the least degree of stress.   In the "rest" position which is similar to "at ease," the feet are spread about 1 foot with equal weight distribution borne on the perimeter at three points—the heel, outer border (fifth metatarsal), and across the head of the metatarsals to the inner side where the first and second metatarsal heads of the foot are the major points of contact.

Emphasis should be placed upon avoidance of incurring a hollow back, since it is felt that psychologically the attention should be upon the back and not the front. With the rotation of the pubic bone upward the abdominal muscles are shortened, while extending the dorsal spine raises the rib cage, and thus flattens the back. Standing tall, with the head back and eyes straight ahead, is, undoubtedly, conducive to erect posture and consequently less tiring.

Sitting should be a restful position if the segments of the spine are aligned one upon the other, and properly supported. Too often the tendency is to round the back and protrude the head forward, with a consequent buckling at the middle of the body causing the back muscles to overstretch, resulting in the sliding forward and down in the seat to relieve the back and neck strain.

For most effective position the head should be erect, chin held in, with the lower portion of the back and pelvis resting against the back support, shoulders relaxed and comfortably braced against the back of the chair, with the feet flat on the floor and pointed straight ahead in the rest or reading position. Best results and the least tiring in the active or working position are the same with the exception of leaning forward at the hip joints and not bending at the waist. Frequent periods of rest are advisable to allow for a lessening of shoulder tension, and to raise the chest which cannot avoid a certain amount of cramping and shoulder drooping after long sessions of work in a sitting position.[7]

Proper adjustment of school chairs and desks is essential to the assumption of correct sitting positions. Present practices of constructing chair and car seats with sponge rubber offer very little real support for the pelvic region and the spine. As a result there is an increasing amount of low back and sacro-iliac troubles.

Walking unless properly done is most tiring and may be more of a shuffle indicating abject depression. Emphasis should be stressed upon fully extending the spine, with the head erect and chin in, expanding the thoracic cavity for best aeriated functioning, and arms hanging freely from the shoulders without any rigidity of the shoulder girdle. The feet should swing forward and strike the ground, heel first and lightly with the weight passing over the outer borders and thence to the ball of the foot. At this point the step reflex activates the calf, hamstring, and gluteal muscles which add the propulsive thrust for the next step.

Running is a form of activation which is practically the same as that in the walking position, except that the body leans forward somewhat and the leg and foot alternations are more rapid with lessened deceleration on the resting phase. The leaning in the forward progress of the body weight and the tension on the gluteals, hamstrings and gastrocnemius muscles give the strongest position for such progression. The arms swing at the sides, with the elbows bending more than in walking, their alternation and speed of the swinging action compensating for the leg action and making the balance easier.

Lying in Sleep and Correction are positions which vary as to content and differ in purpose, being used for passive and active reasons. Some are better adapted for relaxation and others for corrective or remedial use, and all are not prescribed for indiscriminate application. The determining factor as to which is the best position to lie in when asleep should not be stated as the "side which is down," for it is certain that persons with lateral curvatures which are exaggerated by assuming the same position with a similar sag in the back may receive considerable harm.

For rest and relaxation there should be various modifications which the body takes without prompting, as shown by actual tests in the United States Naval Pre-Flight School, St. Mary's College, California during the relaxation period of instruction and the checking of cadets in sleep.

Such varieties are as follows.— (*a*) Back lying or *supine* on the back with the arms relaxed and resting by the sides with the legs fully extended, which is the first position taken in teaching relaxation. Variations of this position were with the knees bent in hook lying and the feet spread about 2 feet apart. This position is very useful for resting a tired back and in relieving backaches in those with hollow or lordosis conditions. The flexed hips slacken the pull on the iliopsoas which is tightened and shortened. Hence, when the legs are extended, the pull of these hip flexors on the lumbar spine drags it forward without stretching the shortened lumbar extensors.

(*b*) From the same approximate *supine* position the arms are stretched overhead, with the knees flexed as above, and with a folded towel, pad or board slightly wider than the scapular spines placed under the dorsal curve and is known as the "gravity method." This position is useful for correction of kyphosis and can also lift the rib cage in a funnel or flat chest. Some may not be able to tolerate the arms in the wing position, because of the shortness of the pectorals and anterior shoulder joint, muscles and ligaments, common in round shoulders. Consequently, the time should be short or the arm position modified to an arm at side position.

(*c*) In the *side lying* position on the right side, right knee bent and right arm under the head, the left arm is lying relaxed back of the trunk. This position is useful in stretching the muscles of the waist on the under side in long left curves. The same in reverse on the other side is indicated for opposite condition.

(*d*) A *prone lying* position with the head turned to either side and with a pillow under the abdomen with legs fully extended is useful for hollow back conditions. Persons with pronated ankles and flatfeet should not lie with the toes pointed outward but turned inward to favor the weak tibials and to stretch the tight peroneals.

Occupations require many unorthodox positions which can be compensated for through understanding as to the best manner to carry on the work, and through participation in suitable corrective or recreation activities to offset these vocational demands. Children are especially vulnerable to such habits as carrying books in untenable positions, writing on arm chairs which pull the body radically to one side, and long periods of concentration which foster sedentary habits that are not conducive to good body mechanics.

Cognizance of faulty working conditions has caused steps to be taken in many industries so as to minimize the effects of enforced positions. Schools and parents should be alerted to the attentive effort necessary to prevent poor practices, and also to inform students about possible results which occur from such disturbances.

PHYSIOLOGICAL CHARACTERISTICS

Differences in the characteristics of various body types are of vital significance and should be carefully considered in the physical education field, especially in connection with the therapeutic care in prevention, development and corrective work. Instructional class teachers and particularly coaches must take cognizance of such facts in other phases of various activities as well as in athletic endeavors, where failure to observe such individual differences in regard to program offerings may be detrimental in their effect.

Interest in the anthropological aspects of body build started with Bean, Bryant and Goldthwait and has been greatly stimulated by the later work of Sheldon,[8] whose classification is the most technical and scientific expression of bodily build.

All teachers are advised to study the research of those who have called attention to the importance of the biological approach. In this way they become better qualified and able to understand and cope with the reactions of the differing types, thus adjusting their methods and planning. Realization that there are skeletal, physiological, neurological and mental differences peculiar to each type makes more apparent the reason why group work in classes must be made applicable to individual needs.

There are many who consider that what is past is prologue, and yet if an assessment of the present is made, it is realized that there are many tangents of life which offer a chance for change. From a practical standpoint, a general screening test at the beginning of the school year, in which gross variants of body alignment are noted for follow-through and body types are checked for assignment to specific activities, gives a most useful inventory as to needs of students.

Once an evaluation is made it becomes possible to formulate a plan of action in direct relationship to these needs. When large groups are run through the educational mill on a sink or swim basis, and without the recognition of these individual physical and mental variations, it is no wonder that the quality of the results is so variable. The good of the group is important, but the welfare of the individual is paramount, for in this instance it is a case of the whole being improved through the sum of its parts.

Admittedly, the habitat of persons has great significance and meaning in their physiological development since environmental factors furnish the culture or growth media whereby the hereditary genes may best function. Therefore, body type may not be the only important answer as to structural relationship, for neuro-muscular action, physical fitness, reaction time and the total development of the body all have a definite role to play.

Although it is easy to become opinionated and believe that some one item is causative, it is advisable to appreciate the many variations and the proneness to injury found among the various types. Each has its own distinctive characteristics[9] and when aware of such, due allowance and specific provision may be made which aid in better operation and avoidance of difficulties.

LITHE OR ECTOMORPH TYPE

The consensus indicates that the lithe, lean slender individual is likely to have hyperacting reflexes, quick reactions, and an organic set-up that is correspondingly integrated to these needs. Consequently, he is neurologically, mentally, and physiologically hyperactive and usually has an increased metabolic rate.

Posturally, the slender type is prone to faults of alignment and, because of the suppleness of his musculo-ligamentous structures and easy fatiguability, tends to slump more readily and finds it hard to attain and maintain good posture. Emphasis is essential in order that he may realize that many ills are caused or associated with faulty body alignment in later life. Therefore, he must strive consciously to develop the best postural pattern and habits possible in order to attain present and future effectiveness.

This group can be helped to meet life situations better, if they are given a slowing down program of physical education. The program must have a high interest content but be decreased in range and intensity of effort because of the limited endurance, or a tendency to poorly controlled emotionalism, and erratic physical and mental behavior of the participant, yet be a challenge to the skill and psycho-motor responsiveness. Development of poise and deliberation should be the objective of a program planned to minimize harmful practices and increase beneficial results.

MEDIUM OR MESOMORPH TYPE

It is generally agreed that medium type persons are better adapted structurally, organically, and neurologically to meet the stress of life situations. They have good integration of their operational functions and tend to have many of the better attributes of both the lithe and stout types, although retaining their own particular characteristics which give little reason for special attention.

Usually, such individuals' basic metabolism is stable and constant, musculoskeletal organization is in better balance, and nerve patterns operate more smoothly. They are ordinarily, somewhat slower than the lithe and faster than the stout type, and have better endurance and effectiveness under stress than either.

That there are exceptions among different persons in such respects is evident among athletes performing today. Rather than negating isolated opinions as to trends of peak performance in respect to particular types, it is supportive in that the relationship of hereditary and environmental forces cannot be overlooked in any instance. Better techniques and knowledge are changing the sometimes mediocre performer to an outstanding athlete, but knowing what one has to work with has much to do with the ultimate result and direction to pursue.

Although the fact that such persons as the above are fortunate in being born with less predisposition to traumatic injury or alignment problems, it does not lessen the need for concern and early recognition of potential changes. All are subject to illness or accidents, and it is easy to overlook inefficient function in these individuals, due perhaps to poor development, whatever the cause. They, too, need assistance and attention with their physical problems.

STOUT OR ENDOMORPH TYPE

Judging from appearance it is usually believed that the stout or fleshy group are easy going, phlegmatic, slow reacting, thick skinned and of great power. Such may be true regarding general type but is usually due to the lower metabolic rate, anatomical differences in position of the stomach and length of the intestinal tract, as well as body chemistry which necessitates an adjustment to their requirements. Nervous and mental reactions appear to be retarded, while movements are more deliberate with slower time reaction, often resulting in an apparent sluggish or lethargic attitude because of a lower oxidizing rate or hypo-active thyroid.

Realization as to the physiological state of such individuals makes possible an appreciation of the fact that they must push themselves in order to keep up with the demands, thus predisposing them to common ills and stress more severe than in other types. Their increased adipose tissue and overweight places a heavy burden on the entire system and they appear to be lazy or easy going, which may be due to fatigue since the cardio-respiratory demands from the enormous increase of capillaries requires greater heart strain. They do have great endurance but at a lower tempo, although because of their bulk and size they are expected to accomplish more than other persons.

A program for the management of obesity must be safe, effective, and consistent with known facts, lending itself to personal dignity, not disparagement and ridicule. Obese persons must be shown dietary measures with special attention to water and sodium intake, must understand their vulnerability to postural faults such as knock knees, flatfeet, sagging abdomen, drooped shoulders and round back, and must be taught the importance of a program for their entire lives. This as yet unsolved medical problem calls for a checking of glandular condition, as well as counsel from the physician and parent as to best chemotherapy procedure to follow.

Special consideration should be given to students of the elementary and junior high school age group regarding activities, because such members are likely to have a physiological age, not commensurate with their chronological age. Their growth centers and joints are more subject to trauma, either from the cummulative daily gravitational stress plus muscular activity, or sudden traumas from strenuous or heavy activities involved in weight lifting, football, wrestling, and pyramid building.

Worthy of investigation in relation to athletes is the problem of whether during an intensive sports program, individuals demand a greater intake of food which is often stored as fat or bulk instead of muscle structure. Does this demand become a requisite and then habitual thus creating a problem in later life? Is this a contributory situation to later weight problems in adult life?

The foregoing comments dealing with growth and development in relation to body types are of special significance to teachers, nurses, physicians, physical-health and recreation educators, coaches, parents, and therapists in all fields. Understanding of the various stages and structural aspects are most pertinent, as well as the many influences from within and without the body that modify and condition the growth of the human organism, for such factors are meaningful to the well-being of the nations' greatest resources.

ORGANIC AND STRUCTURAL INTEGRATION

While teachers and therapists are not expected to be able to make diagnoses of pathological conditions, ability to recognize the more serious or contributing causes of such cases is most assistive for referral purposes. Therefore, even a brief statement of the common etiological factors should be of benefit for reference, particularly for those working with young people.

Actual pathological conditions commonly found that cause physical disablement of either a temporary or permanent influence on growth or function are rickets, arthritis, tuberculosis, syphilis, osteomyelitis, poliomyelitis, cerebral palsy, muscular dystrophy, multiple and arterial sclerosis.

Non-pathological conditions which may be potent causes of both structural and organic inadequacy include cardiovascular, cardio-respiratory, visual faults, auditory discrepancies, tonsils, adenoids, and glandular dysfunction. Physiologically the faults of nutrition and assimilation directly affect the integrity and stability of bones, muscles and ligaments, and during rapid growth periods directly influence body mechanics. These elements act through both organic and neuromuscular channels combined.

At certain ages mental and emotional factors, such as shyness, bashfulness, self-consciousness, feelings of insecurity and inferiority may play an important part in respect to posture. The excessively tall stoop to make their appearance less noticeable, particularly where there is muscular insufficiency, while girls embarrassed from large breast development, seek to conceal the characteristic through sagging forward which, plus the heavy weight, drags on the shoulders, all contributing to round shoulders and back.

Habits formulated as early as even the crawling state and further accentuated through one-sided play activities add to the already startling fact that over half of all persons have a hereditary tendency to a laterally tilted pelvis. Positions which tend to increase asymmetry of muscular development and eventual changes in bony structure from a physics standpoint of function must be avoided.

Persons responsible for children should observe and note such tendencies, so that steps may be taken to prevent deviations. Especially pertinent are school influences when children sit for long periods at desks on chairs which are not suitable for them, since the muscles are not as yet strong enough to furnish adequate support.   In addition, the left handed individual must usually write on the right side, lighting may be of a glaring nature and falling on the writing surface from the wrong side.

Too much extra curricular activity, too heavy a school load, carrying heavy books on one side, inadequate sleep, together with poor nutritional habits, are not conducive to well being.   There is an additive effect of such practices which results in neurological and emotional stress, and in turn influences growth faults which may prevail throughout life.

Actual defects and divergencies, at least of a serious nature, will not generally be cared for by the average instructor, therapist or technician.   However, all those in contact with youth, especially, should understand about such conditions and the proper direction to follow.   W. W. Keen once said, "With all our varied instruments, useful as they are, nothing can replace the watchful eye, the alert ear, the tactful finger, and the logical mind which correlates the facts obtained through all these avenues of information and so reaches an exact diagnosis."

POSTURAL STRAIN

History has recorded the exploits of nature in the growing incidence of chronic disability in our nation.   Rather than being an indictment, this is a tribute to the ingenuity of American medicine which has kept people alive long enough to do something about their conditions.   Greater emphasis must be directed to the preventive aspects of the problem, which in time may even reverse the trend from a treatment approach to that which seeks development as an important adjunct to diagnosis and prognosis.

Orthopedic physicians have applied the diagnostic expression of "postural strain" to those conditions involving joints and their supporting structures, and in the sense of the so-called static stress rather than the sudden acute strains.   This is an entity which conveys a definite picture, and may occur in any part of the body and usually has a gradual onset as a background.[10]

Most commonly such conditions of a progressive nature are to be found around the shoulder girdle and cervico-dorsal area, lower

back and pelvis, and in the feet, knees and legs. Its major causa-
tion is the use of body parts to maintain a continuous position
beyond ordinary endurance, especially when there is some malposture of the segments involved. Stress on ligaments, tendons
and muscles is carried to the point where mild inflammatory response takes place around the involved joints with symptoms of a
burning or aching sensation. Gradually there is some limitation
of motion, and a feeling of soreness and stiffness develops in the
muscles. The steady increase of muscle tension reduces the interchange of blood constituents, with cramps and immobility resulting.

Continuance of this hypertensive state because of an accompanying neuritis, may produce fibrotic changes in the muscle sheaths
so that free movement of one muscle over another is restricted.
This is especially true in the shoulder region, resulting in the
so-called frozen shoulder. The same condition is likewise found
to take place in other areas of the body but is not as self evident,
due to the continuous use of the arms in daily movement.

Another instance of this static strain is seen in poorly aligned
feet and legs due to prolonged activity or standing in a limited
area. As the arches relax and the ankles pronate, the ligaments
of the foot stretch, allowing the bones to sag. Thus, an increasing
load is thrown on the muscles which support the body weight in
the increasingly faulty positions.

This undue stress may provoke symptoms quite remote from
the apparent source, and sooner or later indications of discomfort,
soreness or pain takes place in the feet, knees, legs, and even the
back. Since the leg is a shaft, then if the arches fall, the ankles are
pronated, causing the entire leg and thigh to rotate inward. When
this occurs there is a resultant tension on all structures fastening
the leg to the trunk, and in the case of children was formerly
called growing pains when they complained of aching near the
joints.

Such clues are like warning flares for they are often an indication
of some irritation of the growth centers. This situation is known
as osteochondritis or inflammation of the bone and cartilage, and
is found especially in overweight persons with low metabolic rate,
whereas with children ordinarily the physiological age is below the
chronological age. Here the stress is too great for the stage of
development of the epiphyses or growth plates. An illustration
is found in Schlatter-Osgood disease of the upper tibial epiphysis,
generally present in young people.

When these undue stresses, both static and dynamic, continue
over a long period, the condition becomes chronic. Pressure
points gradually thicken, just as the skin becomes calloused from
unusual and repeated pressure, and so do the ligaments become

7

similarly thickened from increased tension or prolonged stress. Thus persistent and undue stress around the margins of the joints, in time, produces irritation of the covering of the bone or periosteum which may result in thickening, lipping or spur formations. This is the forerunner of further arthritic changes which indicate the aging process caused by excessive wear and tear.

It should be appreciated that biological changes are also contributory causes of similar results, for biochemical research has found that body deficiencies may demand supplemental substances to meet the requirements of the system. Evidently there are certain requisites of nature which must be supplied. "May you live as long as you want, and never want as long as you live" is an adage which truly applies to longevity in all its ramifications.

NEUROLOGICAL ASPECTS

Just as patterns are woven into the warp of the cloth, so are intricate forces within made a part of the total being. As postural strain increases to the point of inflammatory reaction, the sensory nerves about the joints begin to register the discomfort and provoke a protective spasm or increased tension in the muscles that control the joint. This guarding tends to further limit motion and may even cause a limp or other involuntary reaction. These symptoms may be only transitory at first and disappear with rest, only to return again when activity is resumed.

When resistance is lowered and a focus of infection or toxemia exists anywhere in the body, the joint area may become involved and further swelling and pain be present in a more aggravated form. Any child who complains of such symptoms should be excused from exercising and the parents notified to consult a physician. Recognition of and concern for such signs may be like the turning of the key in the lock opening the door to the problem before it is serious so that the case is brought to the attention of those who know what should be done.

Chronic postural strain is definitely related to the stability of the joints, and if the muscles that control a joint and help to stabilize as well as move it are not in balance because of the adaptation to faulty alignment, a greater than usual potential danger of injury or increase in strain exists, neurologically. When ligaments and muscles are stretched on one side of a joint, their antagonists are shortened correspondingly and neuromuscular response suffers.

Too rapid attempts at mobility following severe illness oftentimes are conducive to difficulties due to laxity of joint and muscle structures in various types of individuals who have a propensity for strain. The resultant traumas may be deeply involved and their extent in the aggregate vast and unknown, although they may be remotely related to some of the tension problems and implications neurologically.[11]

All possible investments, which make for better balance of the sympathetic and autonomic nervous systems, are of value to the individual since there is less concern and hence greater stability mentally.

FATIGUE PROBLEMS

When considering the subject of joints a word about *fatigue* is not amiss. Too often, the psychosomatic aspects of the sensations and actions that influence the emotions or produce certain objective signs in the person's behavior are thought of alone. However, there is a localized effect of fatigue from the structural standpoint such as occurs in inanimate material when force is applied. Even the musculoligamentous and other skeletal elements such as bones and fascial tissues may develop fatigue.

Teachers of activities should recognize this fact in estimating the degree, frequency, character, and duration of participation, and adjust or prescribe a program within fatigue limits, especially in terms of developmental age with youth as well as chronological age with older people. A person may carry on very easily up to a certain point, but forcing the tiring structures to go on when they have begun to relax and stretch from fatigue, further jeopardizes the organism and the potential weaknesses may become a fact. The result of fatigue is shown in postural slump in Figure 11.

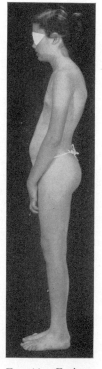

Another element, too often overlooked, is a physiological one. As fatigue increases, the waste products of activity are thrown into the circulation, thence being pumped to the heart by the muscles and diaphragm and in turn sent to the lungs to be eliminated. If there is faulty posture with a fatigue slump and muscles that are tired and full of toxins, then there is a retardation of oxygenation or purifying of the blood so that a much longer time of rest and surcease from work is required. Strain in joints is increased because joints are not sufficiently stabilized by tired structures which allow them to sag further out of position.

Joints in positions of malalignment from the

Fig. 11.—Fatigue slump.

postural sag or from asymmetrical development require increased muscular tension. In the presence of fatigue this may increase and produce a state of muscular hypertension. In this state there cannot be a proper interchange of blood constituents because of the spasm of the capillaries, which may be mild, moderate, or severe and force symptoms all the way from tiredness to actual cramping. This may lead to an awareness which may provoke emotional reactions, which in turn, require a further increase in tension to drive ahead with a resultant greater dynamic and static stress.

It is believed by many that American life today, particularly in large cities, fosters a chronic state of fatigue in children most of the time. When all the school and extra curricular load is considered, the question arises as to how much more physical and mental burden can be absorbed. In this face of change, it behooves classroom and activity program instructors to give considerable thought and attention to the size of the ultimate load which may be safe, while parents must weigh false values and seek a balance sheet safely within reach.

NUTRITIONAL FACTORS

It is becoming increasingly evident that faulty nutrition plays an important role in influencing growth and promoting divergencies from normal, both as to form and function. Any deficiencies in dietary needs are reflected in the developing pattern, with a corresponding loss of energy and lessening of skill performance. Youngsters are prone to spend their allowance for "junk" which has little food value, in fact which is actually harmful. School lunches should be watched to assure that proper quality is provided as well as an adequate choice is made by the child, and that no other activity is allowed during the time set aside for eating, nor immediately following the meal.

Inadequate foods which lack proper proteins, minerals and vitamins make for depletion of bone substances so vitally needed in growth and development. It has been found that fashion has so dictated thinness as an essential of beauty that young girls, especially, are literally starving themselves and stealing the substances from their bodies which are so necessary throughout life.

When scarcity of proper intake is combined with insufficient rest and sleep, a state of tension prevails which is often persistent and leads to secondary conditions not always immediately evident. Such important omissions are everybody's business, and are a reflection of the times which demands quick action and parental concern. Growing up effectively must be taught students, so that they may understand the importance of proper foods in terms of personal needs.

THE AGING PROCESS

The middle and later years are marked by a number of physical and psychological changes which call for an assessment by individuals as to their capacities and limitations. Many in the early adult years are so occupied with meeting their needs for immediate security, that they fail to take count of stock and to exploit their opportunities for planning the future.

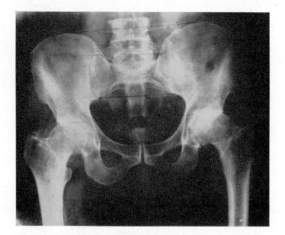

Fig. 12.—X-ray picture showing arthritic hip joints from early osteochondritis of growth cartilage.

Just as in inanimate machines in which the major depreciation comes from wear and tear in the bearings and the members involved with them, the major part of structural stresses in the human machine occurs in the joints. Consequently, the alignment of the joints, the weight of the mass they are required to carry, and the forces applied to them both by the muscle motors and the gravitational stresses, are all elements in the process which accounts for their depreciation.

From the aging standpoint, it is almost a daily occurrence in a physician's office to observe the process whereby otherwise healthy individuals have symptoms referable to the joints, whose age is 5 to 10 years more advanced than the chronological age of the individual. The minute traumas on joint structures due to activities in the presence of faulty posture ultimately accumulate and may account for synovial and other later arthritic changes. Figure 12 shows arthritis in hip joints from earlier osteochondritis of growth cartilages.

"To know what you know and know what you don't know is the characteristic of one who knows" according to Confucius. The field of gerontology crosses the pathways of thought of all sciences and presents innumerable problems as yet unsolved. Only recently has the aging of man as an individual and the basic mechanisms of the process of aging been thought of as a biological consideration. Involutional atrophies and functional alterations of senescence are no less important than growth, development, differentiation and maturation, for they continue simultaneously at varying rates and in variable degrees of speed throughout the life span.

The innumerable experiences and vicissitudes of existence have made changes, which even the skilled clinical pathologists have difficulty in ascertaining as to whether they are due to aging alone or are pathological and therefore theoretically an avoidable process. New measures in the practice of medicine are changing and will change even more in the decades ahead, so that the lights on the horizon grow ever brighter with new hope for those in their senior years.

REFERENCES

1. STEINDLER, ARTHUR: *Kinesiology of the Human Body.* Springfield, Illinois, Charles C Thomas, 1955, 708 pp.
2. LOWMAN, CHARLES LEROY: Faulty Posture in Relation to Performance, J. Health, Phys. Educ., Recreation, *29*, 14–15, 1958.
3. LOVETT, ROBERT W.: *Lateral Curvature of the Spine and Round Shoulders.* 5th ed., Philadelphia, P. Blakiston's Son and Co., 1931, p. 224.
4. DAVIS, G. G.: *Applied Anatomy*, Philadelphia, J. B. Lippincott Co., 1910, p. 492.
5. BANCROFT, JESSIE H.: *The Posture of School Children.* New York, The Macmillan Co., 1919, pp. 6–11 and 283–290.
6. LOWMAN, CHARLES LEROY, COLESTOCK, CLAIRE, and COOPER, HAZEL: *Corrective Physical Education for Groups.* New York, A. S. Barnes and Co., 1928, Chapter III.
7. LOWMAN, CHARLES LEROY: The Sitting Position in Relation to Pelvic Stress, Physiotherapy Rev., *21*, 30–33, 1941.
8. SHELDON, WILLIAM HERBERT: *Atlas of Men.* New York, Harper Bros., 1954, 357 pp.
9. LOWMAN, COLESTOCK and COOPER: *op. cit.*, Chapter IV.
10. ————: *op. cit.*, Chapter X.
11. BRIESEN, HANS V.: A Discussion of Stress and Exhaustion as a Primary as Well as a Contributing Etiologic Factor in Organic Neurological Disease, Military Surg., *101*, 256–290, 1947.

The above references are not repeated in References for Extended Reading.

REFERENCES FOR EXTENDED READING

BARTLEY, S. H. and CHUTE, E.: *Fatigue and Impairment in Man.* New York, McGraw-Hill Book Co., Inc., 1947, 429 pp.
BLAIR, GLENN MYERS, JONES, R. STEWART, and SIMPSON, RAY H.: *Educational Psychology.* New York, The Macmillan Co., 1954, 601 pp.
     Chapter II: The Biological and Social Bases of Behavior.
BOGERT, L. J.: *Nutrition and Physical Fitness.* 6th ed., Philadelphia, W. B. Saunders Co., 1954, 664 pp.
BROCH, H.: *Importance of Overweight.* New York, W. W. Norton & Co., 1957.
CROOK, BILLIE LOUISE: A Scale for Measuring the Antero-Posterior Posture of Pre-School Children, Res. Quart., *7*, 96, 1936.

CURETON, THOMAS K.: *Physical Fitness, Appraisal and Guidance.* St. Louis, The C. V. Mosby Co., 1947, 566 pp.
    Chapter IV: Appraisal of Body Type as an Approach to
           Health and Fitness Guidance.
CURETON, T. K., and WICKENS, J. S.: The Center of Gravity of the Human Body in the Antero-Posterior Plane and Its Relation to Posture, Physical Fitness and Athletic Ability, Suppl. Res. Quart., *6,* 93–105, 1935.
DE LONG, EVERETT W.: Contrasenescence, J. Appl. Nutrit., *9,* 415–421, 1956.
FORD, ADELBERT: *Foundations of Bioelectronics for Human Engineering.* Navy Electronics Laboratory Report 761. San Diego, U. S. Navy Electronics Laboratory, 4 April, 1957, 119 pp.
    Chapter VIII: Effort, Fatigue, Rest and Sleep.
FOX, MARGARET G., and YOUNG, OLIVE G.: Placement of the Gravital Line in Antero-Posterior Standing Posture, Res. Quart., *25,* 277–285, 1954.
GLUECK, SHELDON, and GLUECK, ELEANOR: *Physique and Delinquency.* New York, Harper Bros., 1956, 339 pp.
GOFF, CHARLES WEIR: Orthograms of Posture, J. Bone and Joint Surg., *34-A,* 115–122, 1952.
HELLEBRANDT, F. A., and FRANSES, E. B.: Physiological Study of Vertical Stance of Man, Physiol. Rev., *23,* 220–255, 1943.
HOWARTH, M. BECKETT, *et al.: A Text-book of Orthopedics.* Philadelphia, W. B. Saunders Co., 1952, 1110 pp.
    Section: Neurology in Orthopedics.
JOHNS, EDWARD B., SUTTON, WILFRED C. and WEBSTER, LLOYD E.: *Health for Effective Living.* New York, McGraw-Hill Book Co. Inc., 1958, 507 pp.
    Chapter VIII: Maintaining a Healthy and Attractive Body.
KELLY, ELLEN D.: *Teaching Posture and Body Mechanics.* New York, A. S. Barnes and Co., 1949, 212 pp.
    Chapter V: Good Body Mechanics Described.
KENDALL, HENRY O., KENDALL, FLORENCE P. and BOYNTON, DOROTHY A.: *Posture and Pain.* Baltimore, The Williams and Wilkins Co., 1952, 204 pp.
    Chapter I: The Standard Posture.
KUHNS, J. G.: The Late Effects of Minor Degrees of Poor Posture, Phys. Therap. Rev., *29,* 165–168, 1949.
LANE, JANET: *Your Carriage Madam! A Guide to Good Posture.* 2nd ed., New York, John Wiley and Sons, Inc., 1947, 160 pp.
LICHT, SIDNEY, (ed.): *Therapeutic Exercise.* New Haven, Conn., Elizabeth Licht, 1958, 893 pp.
    Chapter XIV: Sports in Medicine.—H. W. Knipping & H. Valentin.
MASSEY, WAYNE W.: A Critical Study of Objective Methods for Measuring Anterior Posterior Posture with a Simplified Technique, Res. Quart., *14,* 3–22, 1943.
METHENY, ELEANOR: *Body Dynamics.* New York, McGraw-Hill Book Co. Inc., 1952, 225 pp.
    Part III, The Conservation of Energy.
PHELPS, WINTHROP M., KIPHUTH, ROBERT J. and GOFF, CHARLES W.: *Diagnosis and Treatment of Postural Defects.* Springfield, Charles C Thomas, 1956, 190 pp.
    Chapter V: Body Mechanics.
PRYOR, HELEN B.: *As the Child Grows.* New York, Silver Burdett Co., 1943, 400 pp.
    Chapter VI: Fatigue in Child Posture, and Body Mechanics.
RATHBONE, JOSEPHINE L.: *Corrective Physical Education.* 5th ed., Philadelphia, W. B. Saunders Co., 1955, 318 pp.
    Chapter III: A Neuromuscular Basis for Reconditioning.
RESEARCH SECTION OF AMERICAN ASSOCIATION FOR HEALTH, PHYSICAL EDUCATION AND RECREATION: *Research Methods Applied to Health, Physical Education, and Recreation.* Washington, D.C., Amer. Ass'n for Health, Physical Educ. and Rec., 1949, 535 pp.
    Chapter VII: Anthropometry and Body Mechanics, Res. Methods.
    Chapter VIII: Methods of Res. in Experimental Kinesiology.
    Chapter IX: Photographical and Cinematographical Res. Meth.
    Chapter X: Res. Methods in the Mechanics of Sports and
               Physical Education Activities.

SCOTT, M. GLADYS: *Analysis of Human Motion*. New York, F. S. Crofts & Co., 1942, 388 pp.
> Chapter VII: Physical Principles of Total Body Action.

SHELDON, WILLIAM H., STEVENS, S. S. and TUCKER, W. B.: *The Varieties of Human Physique*. New York, Harper & Bros. 1940, 347 pp.
> Pages 30–46: Somatotyping.

SHERMAN, H. C., and LANFORD, C. S.: *Essentials of Nutrition*. 4th ed., Philadelphia, W. B. Saunders Co., 1957, 505 pp.
> Chapter IV: Energy Aspects of Nutrition.
> Chapter V: How to Meet the Energy Need and Have the Body Weight You Want.
> Chapter XVI: Rickets and the Vitamin D.

STAFFORD, GEORGE T.: *Preventive and Corrective Physical Education*. New York, A. S. Barnes and Co., 1950, 312 pp.

STAFFORD, GEORGE T., and KELLY, ELLEN DAVIS: *Preventive and Corrective Physical Education*. 3rd ed., New York, The Ronald Press Co., 1958, 395 pp.
> Chapter VIII: Nutritional Disturbances.

STEINDLER, ARTHUR: *Kinesiology of the Human Body*. Springfield, Illinois, Charles C Thomas, 1955, 708 pp.
> Lecture VI: On the Pathomechanics of Muscle Function.
> Lecture VII: On Body Balance and Body Equilibrium.
> Lecture VIII: On Measurement and Computation of Bodily Motion.
> Lecture XIV: The Mechanics of Posture.

TRUSLOW, W.: Relationship of Foot Strains to Other Body Strains, Med. Times, *58*, 275, 1946.

VAN HAGEN, WINIFRED, DEXTER, GENEVIEVE, and WILLIAMS, JESSE FEIRING: *Physical Education in the Elementary Schools*. Sacramento, Calif. State Dept. of Education, 1951, 1004 pp.
> Chapter VI: Body Mechanics, Postures in Physical Education.

WELLS, KATHERINE F.: *Kinesiology*. 2nd ed., Philadelphia, W. B. Saunders Co., 1955, 516 pp.
> Chapter I: Fundamental Concepts.
> Chapter II: Fundamental Principles of Stability.

WESSEL, JANET A.: *Movement Fundamentals*. Englewood Cliffs, N. J., Prentice-Hall, Inc., 1957, 270 pp.
> Chapter IV: Analyze Your Figure and Vitality.
> Chapter V: Analyze Your Form, Motor Ability, Movement,
>   Working Skills and Playing Skills.

WHITE HOUSE CONFERENCE ON CHILD HEALTH AND PROTECTION: *Body Mechanics: Education and Practice*. New York, Century Company, 1932, 166 pp.

WILLIAMS, ROGER J.: *Biochemical Individuality*. New York, John Wiley and Sons. Inc., 1956, 214 pp.
> Chapter X: Individuality in Nutrition.
> Chapter XI: The Genetotrophic Approach.
> Chapter XIII: Implications for Medical and Dental Research.
> Chapter XIV: Implications for Advance in Psychiatry.

CHAPTER 5

Divergencies in Structure and Function

When one attempts to discover some of the divergencies in growth and development occurring among school children as well as those prevalent in adult life, it is important to realize the frequency with which they are met, the origin and significance of these deviations, and the limiting effects these difficulties may have. Briefly, we need to know that these divergencies exist, their nature, their extent, their effect upon growth and function, and the measures necessary to prevent or remedy them.

"Diagnosis by intuition is a rapid method of reaching a wrong solution," according to the classic statement of Jacob Mendes DaCosta, 1833–1900. While it is accepted that, "Everything that is written in books is worth much less than the experience of a physician who reflects and reasons" as claimed by Rhazes, 850–923, it is important that a blueprint be prepared to guide the builder. The materials presented are intended as a guidance resource in detecting actual defects or anomalies while suggesting recommended procedures to follow for their amelioration.

Whatever the cause may be, knowledge may aid in preventing any further damage or assist those concerned with habilitation to live and work with what they have left. Such conditions arise from several factors such as a defect in the genes, congenital circumstances, or environmental influences. It is our job to care for those we may help, for "Great accomplishments in life are more often due to purposeful activity than to chance," and we do have this opportunity.

As a point of reference before considering abnormalities, it would seem wise to consider what is meant when referring to normality. Normal in this reference is thought of as the regular or usual standard which is most natural to the so-called common type, accepting the fact that there are many variances as to individuals. These are more of an approximate average rather than a fixed standard, and should remain flexible in every sense until further research reveals more accurate standards.

When attempting to determine variations in posture and related conditions, it is realized that more investigation is needed to set points of departure in measurement. The present basis for judging disgressions has been handed down from generations of the past, and it is time that at least a consensus be formulated which would perhaps offer more than a mere rule of the thumb in this respect. Until such time as studies have been completed which are more definite, the best pattern to follow is to be found in the experiences of those who have dealt with such conditions.

Various types of divergencies are classified generally under two heads, the first being known as physiological and the second as psychological. All physical and mental divergencies varying in either direction from the normal are also included.

A structural condition may be said to be that which causes a change in cell structure and is referred to as lethal, in which the individual usually dies, and sub lethal, which produces anomalies with heredity and environment being of equal importance, since either may have causative effect.

Functional conditions are those which are not primarily due to structural defects which appear to be intact, and the divergency is a result of failure to function properly. It is so often the case that postural conditions are judged only from a static relationship, although of greatest pertinence is the ability to move and operate properly. Range and strength of movement as well as coordination is similarly of importance in walking, standing, sitting and daily functions of living.

Suffice to say that the causes of change structurally as well as functionally have limiting effects on efficiency of performance and economy of energy. Psychosomatic implications are constantly observed among those recovering from debilitating illness and from accidents. Remedial measures of necessity must include mental insight and stimulation. Best results can only be obtained when all forces are marshalled in recognition, prevention, development, habilitation, rehabilitation, and evaluation of individuals.

DISSIMILARITIES IN ANTEROPOSTERIOR PLANE

Posture appraisal as to the anteroposterior plane[1,2] is best ascertained from the lateral or side view of the body. From this perspective it is possible to observe the perpendicular alignment in regard to anterior and posterior lists of body balance vertically, segmental disparities in terms of a straight line, and the finite sections of the structure in relation to movement. Various segmentary diversifications are presented together with a clarification of possible cause and effect, with suggestions for prevention and improvement as a means of identifying and clarifying conditions.

FORWARD HEAD

Admittedly, forward head may be induced by an heredi-tary tendency toward an increase in the dorsal curve of the spine or round back, but usually it is an acquired deviation, although it is a compensatory position related to spinal posture. From a therapeutic standpoint, it is important to recognize muscular and ligamentous strain on the neck due to concentration from balancing the weight of the head. To counterbalance the level of the line of vision must, in this in-stance, be in relation to the axis of the ver-tebræ of the neck. Hence, it must be at a greater than normal angle, and the poste-rior neck structures become shorter and the anterior structures become stretched. Figure 13 shows a condition of this nature.

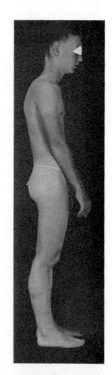

Few persons consider that eye strain means anything more than undue stress on the intrinsic and extrinsic muscles, which alter the position of the eye-ball when changing the focus or direct-ing changes in the visual angle. From the kinetic view, the fixation of attention requires holding of the head still for focus-ing, which means continuous actuation of the neck and shoulder muscles as extrinsic fixators to steady the base of such action. Hence, disparity in neck and shoulder girdle segments entails muscular imbal-ance, and maintenance of attention means increased stress on all these structures causing early fatigue and undue expendi-ture of nervous energy.[3]

Fig. 13.—Forward head and backknees.

Furthermore, if the hands are being used in connection with any act of skill requiring finely adjusted muscular coor-dination, such as writing, holding a book for reading, sewing or using tools, then in order to have a steady base of action for hands and arms, the muscles of the shoulder girdle and head must be stabilized. This throws a further load on the same structures since the degree of fixation is definitely related to the amount of intensity of attention when there is a high degree of interest backed by eagerness, enthusiasm or the creative urge. The elements of speed or drive necessitated by a time factor also constitute further neuro-muscular and emotional elements of stress.

Another element too often overlooked is the matter of balance. Biologically, nature placed the special sense mechanism chiefly in the head, and since the eye is an organ of balance as well as a visual organ, alterations of body position in relation to environment requires an intricate tie-up with the auditory, tactile and kinesthetic mechanism. This is accomplished through various sensory channels which register not only spatial relationships, but also the relationships of respective body segments with each other and with the environment.

Spatial orientation mechanism makes its energy demands on the head, neck and shoulder girdle musculature. Appreciation of these facts is important not only to those attempting to correct postural irregularities, but of concern to coaches and teachers of activity and craft skill in which relaxation and poise are conducive to successful performance and avoidance of fatigue.

ROUND SHOULDERS

Usually when there is a forward head, the weight of the arms also swings the shoulders forward, and because of their almost continuous use in the front of the body, the chest or pectoral

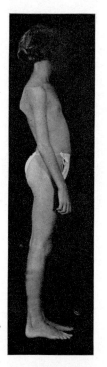

muscles adapt both dynamically and statically to this position. In girls and women, the added weight of the breasts drags still further on the clavicles and helps to accentuate the deviation. In this deviation the tips of the shoulders sag forward of the weight line, swinging on the sternoclavicular articulation.[4]

There is also a rotatory factor in round shoulders, for, as the scapulæ are drawn apart, they rotate on their long axes, making the vertebral borders more prominent. (Fig. 14). The inferior angles tend to point backward as the tips of the shoulders sag down about 1 to 2 inches. The normal scapular interspace, except in very heavily muscled and stout persons, measures about 3 inches. Therefore, if the spacing amounts to from 3 to 5 inches, it may be thought of as second degree or moderate, and 5 inches or over is considered as third degree or severe.

When the shoulders can be actively or passively brought to a normal or flat position, they are said to be relaxed round

FIG. 14.—Round shoulders with rotated scapulas.

shoulders, but when, because of their increased curvature, the clavicles are so short that the scapulæ cannot be drawn back to normal, the condition is classified as rigid.

There is also a deviation quite common to paralysis in which there is muscular imbalance, especially where the rhomboids and lower trapezius are affected. In this case there is not strength enough to adduct the scapulæ to the spine against the gravitational load of the arms. The basis or essential point of attack on the problem is to work on the basic body and spinal alignment in order to alter the essential compensatory assumption of this slumped fatigue position (Fig. 15).

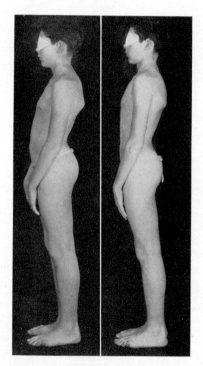

Fig. 15.—Round shoulders, winged scapulas, hollow back.   Two-year follow-up.

However, no series of exercises will accomplish a correction unless all of the above mentioned causes are also given consideration. Rest and nutrition are as essential as postural instructions, while insight and motivation of the individual are also necessary. When there is complaint of pain and limitation of motion in the shoulder area, it is advisable to recommend seeing an orthopedic surgeon because of possible bursal, tendinous, and joint inflammation which are quite common and without proper attention may result in a stiff or frozen shoulder.

An occasional deviation known as Sprengel's deformity is of a congenital type and is due to a failure in embryonal life of the scapula to drop down into normal position. Usually there is a bony or fibrous bridge over the vertebral column which prevents its descent. Exercises are used to no avail and parents should be urged to seek surgical help, which may then be followed by specific activating exercises (Fig. 16).

ROUND BACK

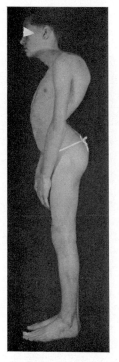

FIG. 16.—Sprengel's Deformity.

A kyphosis condition may be either hereditary or acquired, and is an increase of the dorsal curve of the spine which may be accompanied by a hollow back or lumbar lordosis. In an exaggerated state it may become an almost total rounding with only a short curve of the lumbosacral junction (Fig. 17). This should not be confused with round shoulders which may be found without any vertebral deviation, although practically all round backs are accompanied by compensatory round shoulders and forward head.

The characteristics of the moderately flexible type are due only to postural slump from muscular weakness or poor nutritional status, or as a compensatory position assumed to counterbalance deviations in other segments. The severe form or rigid type will not do so, because the bones have begun to change shape and the deviation is already in a structural deformity stage.

In the rapid speed-up of growth during the pre-adolescent and adolescent stage, these structural changes may develop very rapidly, especially when there is some physiological disturbance of body chemistry in which the ossifying centers are retarded in their development. This produces the so-called osteochondritic round back, with such insidious pressure changes in the vertebræ that it soon appears to be like the round back of old age. The alteration of the shape of the chest and the shortening of the spine allow the internal organs to sag and eventually lead to symptoms of back and neck strain. Where this condition is found, it should be referred for medical attention for no amount of exercise alone will accomplish a correction. In severe cases a cast or brace is applied first, then followed by specific exercises and bracing until the back becomes stable (Fig. 18).

In the flexible stage, attention to nutrition is very important and incorrect habits which accentuate the condition must be avoided. Supplemental exercises in recumbency of a stimulating nature have a tonic effect and swimming on the back using elementary back strokes and the frog kick is beneficial.

The more flexible or myotonic forms should always be referred to an orthopedist, because, in addition to the above recommendation, a brace or corset will be needed to hold any gain which is made by exercises, while medical attention to underlying metabolic conditions will be indicated (Fig. 19, p. 113).

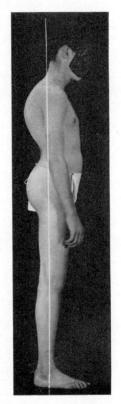

When the curve does not quite straighten out in recumbency, the indication is that the bones are beginning to change shape. Therefore, the condition is in a *transitional* stage which often within a few months changes to a *mildly rigid* form. At a later date it changes to a more *severe rigid* state. All such cases in school should seek the advice of the school physician, who in turn will obtain the opinion of an orthopedic surgeon since the condition is or has been developing into a fixed deformity.

This condition is just as serious or even worse than a lateral curvature, and parents should be so advised and told not to expect exercise alone to correct the condition. Casts, braces and later corsets are necessary to aid in correction. Passive stretching, traction by hands or otherwise, and manipulations are not advised for when

Fig. 17.—Round back.

the back is rendered more flexible without support to maintain the correction gained, it will be made worse.

Early recognition of pathological kyphosis should be considered whenever there is any spasm or soreness in a back which is held rigidly or has a posterior deviation that tends to be more angular or pointed in a given location. Such cases should be checked by the medical service since they might prove to be Pott's disease or a tubercular spine. This condition is less frequently seen today

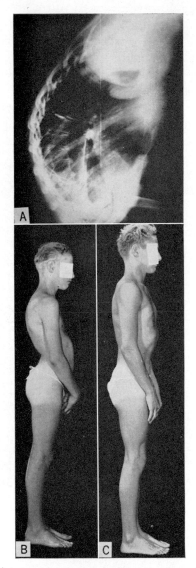

FIG. 18.—A, X-ray picture of kyphosis-transitional stage. Note wedging. B, Kyphosis-transitional stage with beginning wedging of vertebra and cartilage. C, Correction by treatment to moderate long slight round back. Fair return of general alignment.

but should be recognized at once since exercises must not be given because of the serious harm they may cause.

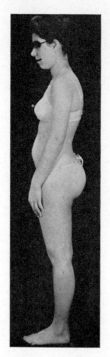

Fig. 19.—Total Round back prolonged into lumbar area.

ROUND HOLLOW BACK OR KYPHO-LORDOSIS

When both the anteroposterior curves have become increased beyond normal with about equal degrees of exaggeration in each curve, the condition is known as kypho-lordosis. In the usual round back, the dorsal curve is longer and the overhang of the shoulder girdle back of the plane of the pelvis segment is not found, as in simple or total round back deviation. Round hollow back should receive the same considerations as previously described, with special attention being given to other segmental compensations. This condition may be found in any of the stages which have been mentioned—postural, transitional, or structural (Fig. 20).

HOLLOW BACK OR LORDOSIS

Swayback is a condition characterized by varying degrees of increased curve in the lumbar area or small of the back. The most important factor in this deviation is the increased forward obliquity of the pelvis and the muscular and ligamentous imbalance

8

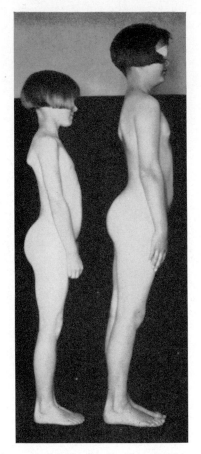

Fig. 20.—Round shoulders, round hollow back.   Note also forward tilt of pelvic segment.
Sisters, 2 years' difference in ages, one lithe, one medium type.

front to back in stature.   For example, the abdominal muscles, which are the most important basic fixators of the trunk anteriorly, become elongated or stretched.   This promotes weakness and faulty position of the internal organs.   Posteriorly the back muscles across the hollow region shorten like a bow string, holding up the back of the sacrum and rotating the pelvis forward (Fig. 21).

Being powerful, the back muscles tend to increase extension of the spinal column and flexion of the hip joints, thus decreasing the effective total range of motion in these two areas.   The posterior spinal ligaments consequently become shortened and increasingly tight, and the anterior ones become stretched resulting in similar ligamentous imbalance in the hip joints.   Such a limitation of the complete range of movement in joints is a common cause of injuries such as strains or sprains, because the components of the joint cannot move through a sufficient range. Therefore, ligaments that have become shortened are more likely to be strained or torn. Sacro-iliac sprains are of this type sometimes, and adjustment of the posture in this relationship together with equalization of leg lengths often corrects such aggravations.

Lordosis is usually accompanied by such compensatory deviations as forward head, cervical lordosis, round shoulders, flat chest, backknees, or flatfeet. Other spinal or diversiform changes

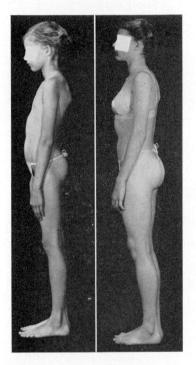

FIG. 21.—Hollow back, prominent scapulas and round shoulders. Shows 5 year follow-up of correction through exercise.

may be moderate or severe in degree (Fig. 22). This circumstance most commonly appears in children during rapid growth, and starts in babyhood when the child makes his earliest attempts to stand up against the pull of gravity. The heavy child with pendulous belly has to lean farther back to carry the weight, while the thin lithe type usually sags because of muscular weakness and natural flexibility.

Caution is directed against the use of such instructions as "chest up" or "shoulders back" which will only cause the child to exaggerate the lumbar curve even more. The military stance with shoulders braced and chest high illustrates this point.

The major principles to observe are (a) care in correcting so as not to make the compensatory deviation worse; (b) start any exercises in the lying position, thence progress to a sitting position; (c) flatten the back by attention to strengthening of the abdominal muscles, with tipping up of the pelvis in front and rotating downward behind; (d) hip flexion in leg raising should be restricted, because the hip flexors or psoas magnus are already too short; and (e) work for control of the pelvic segment as most essential, with muscle tensing of the abdomen and tightening of the buttock muscles.

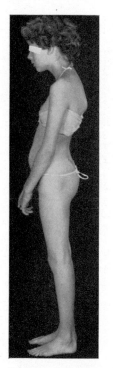

FIG. 22.—Lordosis and other compensatory conditions.

FLAT BACK

A lessening of the ordinary anteroposterior curves of the spine, in which both dorsal and lumbar curves are flattened and the forward inclination of the pelvis is decreased, is known as a flat back. This may be accompanied by forward head and round shoulders and is often present with faulty foot posture. Such a back may be normal for certain individuals, but in indicated cases, attention to general posture, diet, and appropriate rest periods may be necessary.

Care should be taken to minimize the abdominal tensing and gluteal pinch used in correcting other postural faults of the trunk, since they would only increase the amount of flattening. Attempts to produce an unnatural curve in the lower back of such individuals may result in considerable difficulty.

FLAT, FUNNEL AND PIGEON CHEST

The flat chest is often found in the lithe type individual with decreased chest expansion and shortened pectorals together with depressed lower ribs and narrowed epigastric angle (Fig. 23). Those having hollow or funnel chests or pigeon breasts are usually victims of rickets and malnutrition during the early growth period. Similar activity as that utilized for overcoming the flat chest is beneficial in the correction of these cases, although it is much more difficult to obtain results.

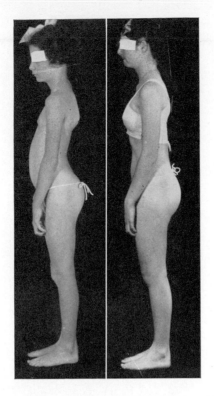

FIG. 23.—Flat chest, relaxed abdomen, round shoulders. Three-year follow-up.

PROMINENT ABDOMEN

Protusion of the lower abdomen is often present in very young children of both lithe and stout types (Fig. 24). In the former, it is part of the muscular laxity and fatigue slump, while in the latter it is due to the increase of weight from excess fatty tissue. It is most common in conjunction with hollow back and an increased pelvis inclination, and with compensatory increased dorsal curve and forward head. It is often seen in cases of faulty nutrition such as rickets, and sometimes indicates a disturbance of the glandular system. Exercise may be used with excellent results for this condition, especially in conjunction with nutritional or glandular treatment (Fig. 25).

PELVIS

The key to the postural problem and likewise to the effective use of the body from both the static and dynamic standpoint is the pelvic segment. Its position and use has an essential bearing on the adjustment and control of the body mass above it as well

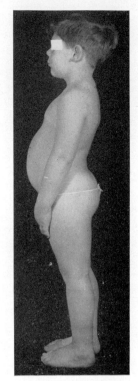

Fig. 24.—Prominent abdomen.

as effect on the parts below. From an evolutionary view, the change from the quadripedal to the bipedal position has made this segment a biologically weak link. The readjustment of internal organs and circulation, as well as the control by muscles and ligaments of the body mass in the erect posture, have apparently not yet reached a permanent status of stability. Consequently, it is felt that a brief discussion may be helpful, particularly to students of physical education, teachers, therapists, and parents.

The pelvic girdle is a closed ring formed by two irregularly shaped side bones which flare upward and outward, known as the innominate bones. Before maturity they are formed in three parts, the wings are the "ilia," the front portion or rim of the pelvis in front are the "pubic bones," and the lower portion on which we sit are the "ischial bones." Between these parts are centers of ossification from which these bones grow.

During childhood and the growth periods up to adolescence, unless the body weight is carried properly, some deviations or actual deformity of the pelvic girdle can be produced. The pelvic ring is closed posteriorly by the sacral bone of pyramidal or wedge shape which is the keystone of the arch and upon which the spinal column rests. The anatomic relationship at this junction, called

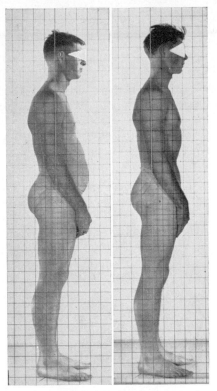

Fig. 25.—Ptosis.

the "lumbosacral joint," and the great variations in shape and size that are found, indicate that the final results of evolutionary change have not become fixed. This area then is especially vulnerable to both direct and indirect injury.

The lower extremities are connected to the pelvis at the hip joint, which is a deep circular socket into which the spherical head of the thigh bone or femur fits. Here again, the head of the femur is attached to the shaft by another *growth center* called the "epiphysis," and as a result any forces, such as gravity load or work stress from activity, may affect its growth. This may also occur in the socket at the bottom of which is another growth center where the three parts of the pelvic bones come together. This junction of the femoral head and neck is especially sensitive to stress and injury, and is a particularly vulnerable point during stages of rapid growth. As a result, incongruities of shape may occur insidiously in both the head and the socket or "acetabulum."

The purpose of this type of joint is to allow a fairly wide range of movement, but at the same time it is essentially responsible for support. It differs from the arm and shoulder girdle relationship in that it is more intimately and firmly related to the trunk.

Its component bones are heavier structurally to carry the super-incumbent weight. The joint is stronger, and the muscles that control it are more massive and of a coarser texture. Hence, they are not so highly specialized from a dynamic kinetic sense as the shoulder joint.

Functionally, the pelvis is considered to have two areas, the false and the true pelvis. The former is composed of the flaring iliac wings which support the abdominal viscera, and the latter, the deep portion which contains and protects the vital pelvic organs, such as the bladder, rectum, uterus, and prostate gland, constitutes the birth canal.

The sides of the pelvis are arched over the sacrosciatic notch, and the two arms or "rami" of the pubic bones act as a tie rod in the front. Each notch is bridged by the ischiosacral arch strongly bound by the sacrosciatic ligaments. This notch lies under the heavy mass of the buttocks or gluteal muscles, and through which run the big blood vessels and sciatic nerve formed by the nerve roots that emerge from the lateral spinal openings of the last two lumbar vertebræ and those of the first three sacral segments. Before passing down the leg as the sciatic nerve, branches are given off within the pelvis that pass around to the pelvic organs and the hip joint, and extend down the inner aspect of the thighs.

Aside from the hip joints, there are two joints located behind, such as the sacroiliac joints whose ligaments bind the keystone and the side members of the pelvic ring. In front where the two pubic bones come together, there is not a true joint but a cartilagin-ous bumper covered by the pubic ligaments. This is nature's way of giving a light framework to support the trunk. It is very light in construction in proportion to the work it has to do.

When this factor is realized, it can be appreciated that any malalignments in this area can be potential troublemakers. Partic-ularly since the heaviest of the body muscle masses are attached to the pelvis, the force of these muscles acting in the presence of postural faults accounts for many wear and tear symptoms in later life. Figure 26 shows a potentially dangerous condition. These difficulties have been fostered by ill-advised big muscle development.

Measurement of Pelvic Inclination, according to Cyriax, reveals that:

> The determination of what constitutes a pathological degree of antero-posterior pelvic tilt is not easy, because even in normal persons that angle is not constant, being subject to a certain amount of physiological variation. . . . It varies in the two sexes, being slightly higher in the female. Furthermore it varies with changes of posture; this is in great measure due to the changes of tension in the ilio-femoral ligament. It is also influenced by alteration in the line down which the centre of gravity of the body passes, *i.e.* whether the body is leaning slightly forward or the reverse.[5]

Authorities indicate that the normal anteroposterior tilt or inclin-
tion of the pelvis in males is from 50 to 56 degrees, while in females
it is from 54 to 60 degrees, as measured on a line from the lumbosacral junction to the symphysis pubes in the standing position.
      Cyriax states, furthermore, that:

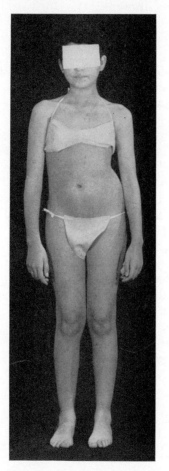

FIG. 26.—Pelvic malalignment.

The following clinical data as regards the bony points of the pelvis
will be found of value:

(a) The relation of the anterior superior spine to the upper margin
of the symphysis pubis. In normal subjects when viewed
laterally, these points should be in the same vertical plane.
Roughly speaking every half inch of deviation of the anterior
superior spine from this plane means a corresponding alteration
in the pelvic tilt of about 9°.

(b) The relation of the anterior and posterior superior spines. In normal males they are in about the same horizontal plane, but in females the latter spinous process is about three quarters of an inch higher. Roughly speaking every half inch of deviation of the posterior-superior spine from the normal means a corresponding alteration in the pelvic tilt of about 5°.[6]

Various conditions increase the forward tilt, such as inward rotation of the leg from pronating and relaxed feet, due to the pull on the pyriformis or rotator muscles which fasten to the upper three sacral vertebræ and hence cause drag downward and forward.

Resultant Effect of Pelvic Variation. Weakness of the abdominal muscles in the presence of tension on femoro-pelvic flexors, and walking and standing in high-heeled shoes cause an effect like walking down hill. The wearer leans back to maintain balance which increases spinal extension and causes a swayback. When there is corresponding tension on the structures attached to its front, the pelvis will be tilted downward in front. The plane of the sacrolumbar junction, according to Steindler, is where "The longitudinal axis of the fifth lumbar vertebra forms with the axis of the upper sacral segment an angle of 120 to 135 degrees. The smaller the angle the greater the weight stress. The greater shearing stress then increases the tendency of the fifth lumbar to slide forward."[7] This is the effect of anatomical pelvic variation.

About 1 in 5 persons have some congenital structural variation of the anatomy at the lumbosacral joint. One common irregularity is a tendency of the last lumbar vertebra to slide forward on the first sacral vertebra. This occurs when there is a developmental defect in the neural arches. The bony discontinuity throws all stress of weight bearing on the ligaments. Consequently, all children with acute or exaggerated lordosis, especially those with a short sharp curve, should be closely scrutinized, because active participation in sports or heavy gymnastics could produce serious injury.

FLEXED AND HYPEREXTENDED KNEES

We would be remiss if we did not mention various knee conditions so often prevalent in this plane. Some individuals walk with their knees in a bent position, never fully stretching the knee joint or using the extensors in walking. This semi-squat position places a tremendous strain on the joints and keeps the flexors in a state of tension resulting in undue fatigue.

More common is the condition known as backknees, which is a state of hyperextension. It is axiomatic that this practice is very often present with heavy persons, since their muscle tone is already weak, thus subjecting the knee joints to excessive load on the cartilages. In some instances, the subject has assumed this pose as a strutting effect and when the significance is explained to him, will work diligently to strengthen the posterior flexors.

In summation, the anteroposterior position is the most important in terms of total balance, conservation of energy output, proper support of the internal organs, efficiency of body movement, and, esthetically, from an appearance point of view.

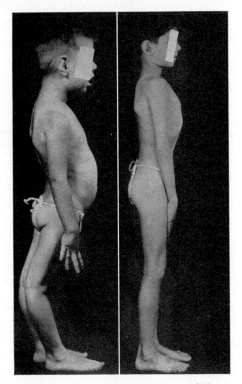

Fig. 27.—Genu recurvatum.   Five-year follow-up.

Basic techniques must be made a part of the armamentarium of those responsible for the prevention of unnecessarily dependent persons, who, through recognition and attention to their possible disablement, may avoid falling into this category (Fig. 27). Therefore, this, the first of two planes of posture evaluation, takes on new meaning.

DISSIMILARITIES IN LATERAL PLANE

Screening of postural discrepancies in the lateral plane is judged from the front and rear view of the body. From this angle the central gravity line of the body separates the two lateral halves, and deviations away from this midline are called lateral faults in alignment. Although for convenience, enumeration is from the top down, this midline or "gravity line" is erected from the floor upward, making a right angle with the horizontal base. Subsequent descriptions clarify nonuniformities with recommendations for recognizing variations and procedures for their prevention.[8,9,10]

HEAD AND NECK

A shift of the position of the head may be due to unilateral deafness or other auditory difficulty, or to some visual fault or eye muscle imbalance in which case one eye may be higher than the other. In both instances the head and neck may turn as well as tilt. Probably the commonest fault is as a result of some lower imperfection in alignment, for when the trunk shifts to balance over a pelvis that is tilted because of a short leg or other reason, the head must likewise have a counter tilt in an effort to bring the eyes into line.

Wry neck or torticollis results in a combination of a tilt and rotation or twist, which is the meaning of torticollis, and may be a result of a congenital condition or unilateral spasm. It might also be caused by a shortening of one of the muscles that turns the head, *i.e.* the sternocleidomastoid, or by a shortening of other lateral muscles. In this state, the head is tipped to one side, and the face is rotated to the opposite side. Correction sometimes requires surgery, although follow-up exercises are necessary to maintain position.

PELVIC DEVIATIONS

Whereas the pelvic segment of the body is the base of the trunk and the connecting section between it and the legs, its importance in relation to general body mechanics must be realized. Since about 50 per cent of all persons have a tilt, lateral or forward or backward, a twist or both, it is essential to know how to recognize these deviations and prevent compensatory conditions (Fig. 28).

Several circumstances may cause these deviations, such as (a) actual intrinsic differences in leg lengths; (b) unilateral arch depression; (c) unilateral knock knee, bowleg, or backknee, in which the difference in angulation at the knee joint tends to lower one side of the pelvis; (d) differences in the angulation of the necks of the femora with the shafts; (e) variations of size, shape or position of the component parts of the pelvic bones or innominate bones; and (f) dissimilarities in size, shape and position of the two sides of the body of the sacrum.

Estimation of such divergencies by measuring from the tip or anterior superior spine of the ilium to the internal malleolus or ankle bone in the lying position does not give a true picture of the pelvic deviation or so-called short leg. Such a method of judging excludes the foot and does not show the effect of weight bearing. It is better to determine this measurement in the standing position, from the anterior spine to the malleolus and also to the floor, next from the mid crest of the ilium to the floor on the side, then in the rear from the posterior superior spine of the ilia to the floor. If

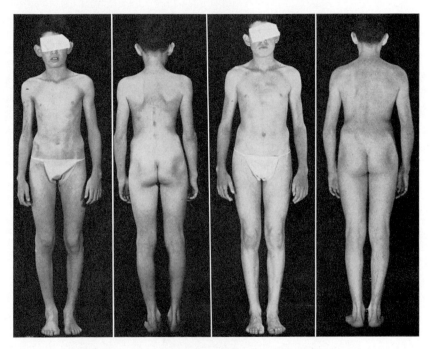

FIG. 28.—Pelvis rotation and tilt. Two-year follow-up.

all these measurements are less on one side than on the other, a plain lateral tilt exists. However, the measurements in front may be equal, but those of the back or side be unequal. For example, the anterior spines may be level and the posterior ones not, or one anterior spine may be higher but the posterior spine of that side lower, while the mid lateral measurements are equal and the waist angles are the same (Fig. 29).

In such a condition there is a twist or torsion technically called "tortiopelvis." If such differences exist during the growth period, there is usually some compensatory lateral curvature of the spinal column. If there is a rotary component in the pelvis, there is likely to be one in the spine. Actual short leg, like any of the

the other variations mentioned, is probably hereditary. Consequently, as early in life as possible, it is important to take steps to ascertain the facts and correct the tilt.

Exercises to correct trunk deviations by strengthening these muscles without correcting foot, leg, or pelvic imbalances will be of little ultimate success and may actually promote deformity. Where expert opinion is not available, the simplest and best thing to do is to use the plumb line, note asymmetries of position and

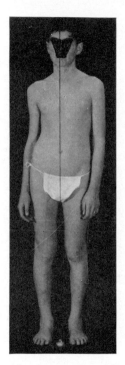

FIG. 29.—Low hip, with compensatory shift in body alignment.

then level the pelvis with a block placed under the heel of the low side. Thickness of the board will likewise show the actual difference in height of the hip. Parents can then be told that a difference in heel heights is indicated, and they in turn can then check with the family physician, pediatrician or orthopedist.

LATERAL TRUNK CHANGES

When any portion of the spinal column bends away from the central gravity line, the condition is one of the lateral spinal curvatures or scoliosis. In recording, these curves are designated in relation to their convex sides. The commonest early curve is a

long convex curve to the left, called a "total left curvature."
When there is a curve to the right in the upper back and to the
left in the lower or waist area, it is designated as a "right dorsal,
left lumbar" curvature. The first type is commonly known as a
"C" curve, while the latter is known as an "S" curve (Figs. 30 and
31).

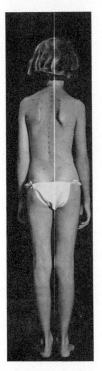

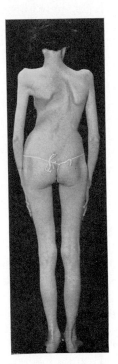

FIG. 30.—"C" curve.   FIG. 31.—"S" curve.

From the developmental standpoint there are two main classifications, "congenital" and "acquired." The first may arise from
malformations of one or more vertebral bodies or of the ribs while
the second comes from postural or developmental growth faults,
or as an accompaniment of some disease process. They may be
further classified according to the degree of deviation as postural
or functional, first degree, transitional or second degree, or structural which is third degree.

Chief causes of pathological curves may follow such injuries as
fractures, sprains, or strains, or may be associated with abscesses
of the pleural cavity as a secondary development, or after operations for resection of the ribs in tuberculosis or empyema of the
lungs. They may also accompany such nutritional disease as

rickets, in which the bones are too soft, or be an aftermath of some form of paralysis such as poliomyelitis or progressive muscular atrophy.

FUNCTIONAL OR POSTURAL SCOLIOSIS

This form of curvature of the spine is chiefly caused by growth faults, such as mentioned under pelvic tilts or short leg, due to heredity, growth discrepancy, from paralysis or after fracture, muscular weakness following exhausting illness or from disturbed nutrition. Other causes include faulty habits of standing, sitting, sleeping, carrying heavy objects on the hip, and may develop as part of the general fatigue so common among rapidly growing children or be due to habitual faults in position assumed at work or play because of accompanying defects of vision or hearing.

Environmental influences such as bad lighting, poor adjustment of desks, or faulty clothing, also play their part. To diagnose the stage in which a curvature may be, the simplest test is that of recumbency. In this position the early or postural curve will disappear with the removal of the gravitational load or dismissal of deviations below. When the curve does not quite straighten by this test but can be corrected by manual assistance or stretching, it is in the transitional stage. This means that the ligaments of the spinal joints are becoming adaptively shortened on the concave side and stretched on the convex, and that uncontrolled deforming factors have begun to change the shape of the bones.

First degree curves may be cured by exercises and appropriate correction of nutritional and fatigue states. Proper motivation as to posture correction by conscious effort is important, plus the elimination of bad segmental positions from short leg or pelvic tilt. On some occasions an arch of one foot may be low, thus causing the short leg, and is amenable to correction.

TRANSITIONAL SCOLIOSIS

A second degree or transitional phase should always be watched for, and may be recognized when it is noticed that exercises are failing to correct the curvature. No time should be lost in getting a medical or orthopedic opinion as to further procedure. By close attention to the history of the case and the multiple causative factors, plus a careful physical examination together with x-ray pictures preferably taken in a standing position with the shoes off, the physician can then determine the course to follow.

The physical educator should not assume full responsibility on his own, even when the school has an adapted section for such cases, but should refer such to the school physician for his recommendation. Special care should be taken with the pre-adolescent students since they are in the last stage of speeded up growth and have no time to lose if correction is to result.

Students have parents, a fact often overlooked by teachers, and the latter should be advised that at this age the curvature will rapidly become more fixed and more difficult to correct unless attention is given to its care. Manipulative treatment to render the curves more flexible is not recommended, unless conducted by competent persons supervised by qualified orthopedists who will be able to hold what correction is gained with appropriate apparatus (Fig. 32).

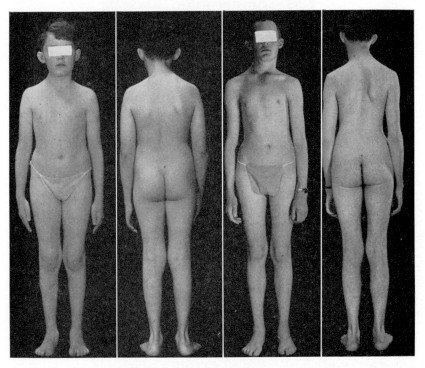

Fig. 32.—Transitional scoliosis. Seven-year follow-up.

STRUCTURAL SCOLIOSIS

Third degree stage of scoliosis can be recognized by the tests previously mentioned. For instance, when the individual is placed in the "Adam's position" and bends forward, the side of the back over the convex area of the curves will be more prominent than the opposite side (Fig. 33). This is due to the vertebræ which have changed shape and will rotate, making the corresponding ribs in the curved area protrude on the convex side. It will also be

9

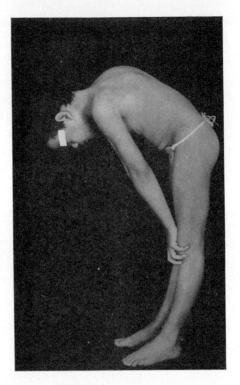

FIG. 33.—Adam's position.

noted that in the recumbent position the spine does not straighten even when stretching is applied (Fig. 34).

If this situation is found, no time should be lost in urging that the parents submit the child for examination to, preferably, an orthopedic surgeon. Undoubtedly, he would attempt to correct as far as it is possible through the use of a plaster cast or a succession of casts. To prevent the return of the scoliosis and further collapse into a more severe deformity, it may be necessary to operate and fuse or lock the corrected segments by some form of bone graft or other stiffening procedure (Fig. 35).

KYPHOSCOLIOSIS

This term is used to indicate that there is a combination of round back or "kyphosis" with a lateral curvature or "scoliosis." This is a severe problem to contend with and should always be referred to an orthopedic surgeon promptly.

PRONATED ANKLES AND FEET

When considering deviations of the ankles and feet, it is well to look critically at the knees and thighs to observe the relation to conditions below. This includes rotation outward of the thigh as

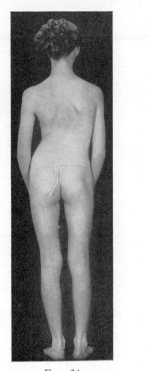 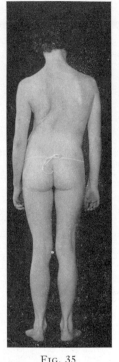

Fig. 34   Fig. 35

Fig. 34.—Structural scoliosis.
Fig. 35.—Mild structural scoliosis, body shift.

well as tibial torsion, which is often combined with pronation of the ankle and consequent flatfeet. When these combined factors are present, it may usually be assumed that the anterior tibialis and gastrocnemius muscles have shortened, which results in a stretching of the plantar muscles. This allows the scaphoid and cuboid bones to drop and produces a flatfoot. When the base of a structure is weakened, the stability of the entire framework above is thrown out of alignment. One foot may not always be considerate enough to drop an equal amount to that of the other, and hence one hip may be lower than the opposite one. Many postural deviations and functional ills may be traced to the feet and should always be checked regarding segments above (Fig. 36).

It is apparent from the description of dissimilarities in the lateral plane that such conditions are of equal importance to those of the anteroposterior plane. Differences in structure and function have a corresponding effect upon the total being. Their should be no rationalization for not doing something for incipient or serious conditions. True, heredity plays its part, but environment may likewise assume its role in overcoming such weaknesses for they are truly a handicap not only to the individual himself, but also an obligation which society may later need to assume.[11]

If parents are to bequeath to their children a better inheritance, they must assist nature to overcome frustrating situations, thus enabling their offspring to achieve a more desirable way of life.

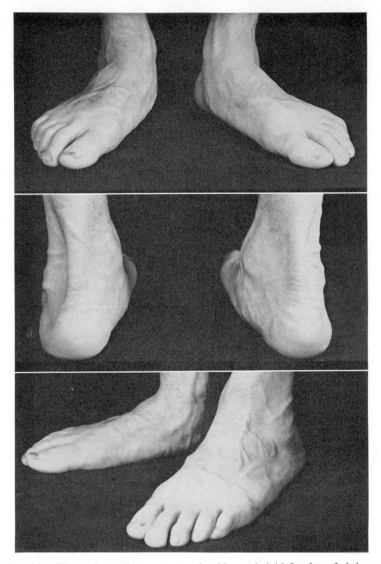

Fig. 36.—Bilateral pes planus, pronated ankles and rigid flat feet, 3rd degree.

REFERENCES

1. LOWMAN, CHARLES LEROY, COLESTOCK, CLAIRE, and COOPER, HAZEL: *Corrective Physical Education for Groups.* New York, A. S. Barnes and Company, 1928, Chapter VI.
2. V-5 ASSOCIATION OF AMERICA: *Conditioning Exercises, Games, Tests.* 3rd ed. by Karl C. H. Oermann, Carl Haven Young, *et al.* Annapolis, Maryland: United States Naval Institute, 1960, Chapter IX.
3. LOWMAN, CHARLES LEROY: Effect of Faulty Skeletal Alignment upon the Eyes, Am. J. Orthopedic Surg., *16*, 459–492, 1918.
4. ————: Heavy Breasts as a Factor in Production of Faulty Posture, J.A.M.A., *78*, 173, 1922.
5. CYRIAX, EDGAR F.: On the Anterior-Posterior Tilt of the Pelvis; Its Variations, and Their Clinical Significance in Children, Br. J. Child. Dis., *24*, 280, 1924.
6. *Ibid.*, p. 281.
7. STEINDLER, ARTHUR: *Kinesiology of the Human Body.* Springfield, Illinois, Charles C Thomas, 1955, p. 181.
8. LOWMAN, COLESTOCK and COOPER, *op. cit.*, Chapter VII.
9. *Ibid.*, Chapter VIII.
10. V-5 ASSOCIATION OF AMERICA, *loc. cit.*
11. LOWMAN, CHARLES LEROY: Feet and Body Mechanics, J. Health and Phys. Educ., *11*, 137, 1940.

The above references are not repeated in References for Extended Reading.

REFERENCES FOR EXTENDED READING

BOWEN, WILBUR P., and STONE, H. A.: *Applied Anatomy and Kinesiology.* 7th ed., Philadelphia, Lea & Febiger, 1953, 462 pp.
    Chapter XIV: Erect Posture.

COLSON, JOHN H. C.: *Postural and Relaxation Training in Physiotherapy and Physical Education.* Springfield, Illinois, Charles C Thomas, 1956, 105 pp.

DICKSON, FRANK D., and DIVELEY, REX L.: *Functional Disorders of the Foot.* Philadelphia, J. B. Lippincott Co., 1953, 345 pp.

DREW, L. C.: *Individual Gymnastics.* 5th ed., Revised and edited by Hazel Kinzley. Philadelphia, Lea & Febiger, 1949, 222 pp.
    Chapter VI: The Feet.

HAWLEY, GERTRUDE: *The Kinesiology of Corrective Exercise.* 2nd ed., Philadelphia, Lea & Febiger, 1949, 192 pp.

JONES, R. L.: The Human Foot. An Experimental Study of Its Mechanics, and the Role of Its Muscles and Ligaments in Support of the Arch, Am. J. Anat., *68*, 1–40, 1941.

KENDALL, HENRY O., KENDALL, FLORENCE P., and BOYNTON, DOROTHY A.: *Posture and Pain.* Baltimore, The Williams and Wilkins Co., 1952, 204 pp.
    Chapter II: Postural Faults.

KUHNS, J. G., KLEIN, A., REGAN, E., WILLIAMS, P. C., and CROWE, H. E.: *Posture and Its Relationship to Orthopaedic Disabilities.* Report of the Posture Committee of the American Academy of Orthopedic Surgery, Chicago, Illinois, 1947.

LEE, MABEL, and WAGNER, MIRIAM M.: *Fundamentals of Body Mechanics, and Conditioning.* Philadelphia, W. B. Saunders Co., 1949, 377 pp.

LICHT, SIDNEY, (ed.): *Therapeutic Exercise.* New Haven, Conn.: Elizabeth Licht, 1958, 893 pp.
    Chapter XVIII: Posture and Its Re-education.—Wilfred Barlow.
    Chapter XIX: Exercises for Scoliosis. Y. Le Grand-Lambling.
    Chapter XXII: Exercise in Orthopedics.—Thomas Gucker.
    Chapter XXIII: Exercise in Foot Disabilities.—Joseph H. Kite.
    Appendix Two: Other Exercises.—Sidney Licht.

LOWMAN, CHARLES LEROY: Therapeutic Use of Rocker Sole, West. J. Surg., *58*, 243–245, 1950.

McCLOY, C. H.: X-ray Studies of Innate Differences in Straight and Curved Spines, Res. Quart., *9*, 50–57, 1938.

MORTON, DUDLEY J.: *Human Locomotion and Body Form*. Baltimore, The Williams and Wilkins Co., 1952, 285 pp.

Chapter XIV: Structural Factors.

Chapter XVIII: Postural and Locomotor Habits.

————: *The Human Foot*. New York, Columbia University Press, 1935, 244 pp.

Chapter XVI: Foot Balance.

PHELPS, WINTHROP M., KIPHUTH, ROBERT J. and GOFF, CHARLES W.: *Diagnosis and Treatment of Postural Defects*. Springfield, Charles C Thomas, 1956, 190 pp.

Chapter V: Abnormal Varieties of Posture.

RASCH, PHILIP J. and BURKE, ROGER K.: *Kinesiology and Applied Anatomy*. Philadelphia, Lea & Febiger, 1959, 456 pp.

Chapter XVIII: Kinesiology of Posture.

RATHBONE, JOSEPHINE L.: *Corrective Physical Education*. 5th ed. Philadelphia, W. B. Saunders Co., 1955, 318 pp.

Chapter IV: Faulty Development.

ROYAL AIR FORCE: *Principles of Anatomy and Physiology for Physical Training Instructors*. London, His Majesty's Stationery Office, 1946, 180 pp.

SCHWARTZ, R. P.: Conservative Treatment of Functional Disorders of the Feet in the Adolescent and Adult, J. Bone and Joint Surg., *31-A*, 501–510, 1949.

STAFFORD, GEORGE T., and KELLY, ELLEN DAVIS: *Preventive and Corrective Physical Education*. 3rd ed. New York, Ronald Press Co., 1958, 395 pp.

Chapter IV: Body Mechanics of the Trunk.

Chapter V: Trunk Posture Faults and Treatment.

Chapter VI: The Feet.

STEINDLER, ARTHUR: *Kinesiology of the Human Body*. Springfield, Illinois, Charles C Thomas, 1955, 708 pp.

Parts II, III, and IV.

WELLS, KATHERINE F.: *Kinesiology*. 2nd ed. Philadelphia, W. B. Saunders Co., 1955, 516 pp.

Chapters X, XI and XII: Movements of the Upper Extremity.

Chapters XIII, XIV, and XV: The Lower Extremity.

WILES, PHILIP: *Essentials of Orthopaedics*. Boston, Little, Brown and Co., 1955, 538 pp.

Chapter I: Postural Defects.

CHAPTER 6

Examining Procedures and Cues to Observe

No advice could be more pertinent to this subject than the remark of John Benjamin Murphy, who said, "Listen, listen to the patient's story! He is telling you the diagnosis." In spite of well intentions on his part, he can only list the symptoms and these in themselves may not be accurate. Yet these cues in the hands of skilled physicians aid in the identification of bodily aberrations from the normal, and make possible comprehensive care.

The constant demands upon the time and energy of the medical profession have made necessary the educating of trained persons who are frequently in close contact with youth as well as adults. These groups include, especially, (a) health, physical, and recreation educators as well as classroom teachers who seek to inform students as to pertinent health aspects, and who are often in the most favorable position to recognize incipient conditions, and (b) particularly therapists, public health workers, nurses, and members of other allied fields who are close to those with personal health problems and who may in turn bring such cases to the attention of the physician.

For these reasons, the following recommendations as to examining techniques and observable landmarks related to postural conditions are presented. Under a preceptorship plan, students are able to utilize such theoretical information and apply it to actual laboratory situations under close supervision, for better understanding and preparation.

There are three general methods which may be used in checking postural fitness of students in schools or in similar situations where there are groups to be examined. The first technique, which is known as the gross screening test, is particularly adapted for the initial check of classes in physical education departments, to be later followed with a detailed appraisal for ascertaining more minutely the facts first discovered through group screening. Second, there is the functional test for judging efficiency in action situations. These evaluations are aside from the third method, the medical examinations by the school physicians, which should be conducted at least annually but may be given in conjunction with the previous check-ups when medical advice is available.

SCREENING TEST

It is possible at the beginning of the school year by means of the following group posture screening tests to get a rough estimate of the general fitness of those examined. Those cases warranting follow-through should be re-examined individually in order to make certain further need for follow-up attention. With experience, a competent physical educator with special training in this area, should be able to check approximately 50 students in an hour.[1,2] The following techniques are recommended as to sequential procedure:

Previous to the time of examination, a chart should be prepared which contains the desired information. Data are listed at the top of the page in vertical columns, with space for names to the left horizontally, and the names of class members are entered alphabetically prior to meeting the class. A recorder is assigned to enter the degree of severity, and letters as to either, H-high, L-low, T-tilt, F-forward, B-back, D-down, U-up, S-short, AP-anterior posterior, LA-lateral, SC-scoliosis, with c or s to designate type of curve, LO-lordosis, KY-kyphosis, KYLO-kypho-lordosis. For the feet, ankles and knees use LO AR-longitudinal arch, TR AR-transverse arch, PR AN-pronated ankles, TO-toes. Key letters are placed above the condition degree in same column according to the item listed. Use of these abbreviations saves considerable time and space in the recording of the findings.

The examiner's procedure is to arrange a class alphabetically in a group of from 20 to 30 students, equally divided into two lines a few feet apart with backs to each other. The only direction the examiner gives is in regard to the position of the line in order to avoid suggesting posture cues. One line stands in a rest position, while examiner moves down the opposing line, checking items seen from the front view, and these are entered by the recorder. This section is given at rest and the other line brought to attention, and similarly checked from this aspect.

The examiner then gives "at rest" to this group and brings the first line to attention again, and proceeds to examine from the rear view, with items being entered by the recorder. When this group is placed at rest he alerts the second line and checks in a comparable manner as to the lateral conditions.

A similar change to the original line is then made and the students face left or right, whereupon the examiner observes anterior posterior conditions from the side view which are then recorded.   Relaxing this group and facing them in their former position, he checks the students of the remaining group in a similar manner.

Reversal of alternate lines with intervening rest periods allows for relaxation and lessens tension, while the practice of always having one group with their backs to the other prevents students from noticing points being observed by the examiner and avoids their anticipating weaknesses which they may correct through conscious posing.

When gym or bathing suits are worn and without shoes and socks, it is much easier to conduct such screening tests and the data obtained are more reliable.   It is possible, however, for experienced instructors who use their hands, to detect prominent points of the body while carrying on such testing.

ANTERIOR ASPECT

Body type and alignment should be checked regarding the general classification category for clues posturally, and for guidance purposes as to activities most suitable.   Body tilts or torsions are noticeable using an imaginary vertical line, which if actually used falls between the feet, at the umbilicus, linea alba or sternum of the chest, and the tip of the nose.   It is not wise to waste time trying to decide on questionable or border line cases, since these may be later examined individually.

Head and neck adjustment is important in relation to the rest of the body, since head tilts may indicate improper balance of the segments below for re-examination.   Torticollis or wry neck may be evidenced from this view, while eye levels can be a contributory factor with posture.   Malformations of the chest are prominent from the anterior view, and are indicative of rickets which often change the rib cage.

Shoulder levels or comparative height may be observed by placing the tips of the index fingers on the acromion process or points of the shoulders, which show either a high or low level and may be either a structural or postural condition.   The relation of the arm hang in respect to the stance should also be noticed, because of the significance to functional action.   An example of a high shoulder is shown in Figure 37.

Pelvic line indicates the lateral height of the hips when the index fingers are held over the iliac crests, and the thumbs are placed horizontally, just below the anterior superior spines; then the examiner sights across the two points of reference.   The degree of tilt is recorded as L.L. $\frac{1}{2}$ inch, left low, or as L.H. $\frac{1}{2}$ inch, left high.   These are usually connected with lower segments.

Legs, knees, ankles and feet are so closely related or conjoined in significance to each other, that they ought to be examined in terms of relationship. With the feet pointed straight ahead, the knees and ankles should be touching each other. Where the ankles are touching and the knees overlapping, there is a condition of *knock knees* existing.

In *bowlegs* the ankles may touch but the knees are apart, and by placing the hand between the condyles of femora or ankle bones or internal malleoli, the amount of space for either condition may be noted. One to 3 inches apart, first degree, 3 to 5 inches, second degree, and 5 inches or more, third degree (Fig. 28, p. 125).

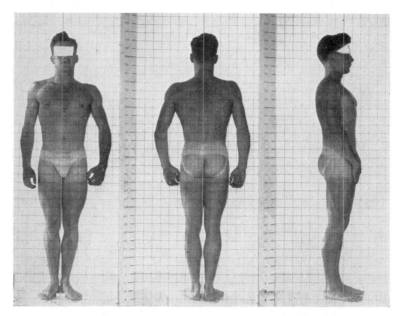

Fig. 37.—High shoulder, asymmetrical development

A condition known as *tibial torsion* is sometimes found in connection with ankle and foot conditions, and involves the twisting of the tibia in relation to the foot and knee.

When ankles are turned inward, it is known as *ankle pronation*, and usually there is a corresponding eversion of the foot in walking. There may also be an inversion in some feet which is associated with the pigeon-toed walk, and is to be preferred to that of eversion which places so much strain on the entire leg.

Weakness of the *longitudinal arch* may be determined from the amount of sag in the plantar muscles of the foot, and the degree of drop of the keystone bone known as the navicular or scaphoid, which normally has its inner margin in a line from the internal malleolus to the first metatarsal or big toe joint. This keystone of the arch is generally about the thickness of four fingers off the floor. One inch or 2 fingers below this height is called first degree, $1\frac{1}{2}$ inches or about 3 fingers from the normal position is second degree, and way down nearly to the floor is considered as third degree.

Other conditions to watch for are to be found in the arch or toes and include *pes cavus* or excessively high arching of the foot, and *hammer toes* which is a contraction of the toes and often connected with the wearing of shoes which are too short.

POSTERIOR VIEW

Shoulder and scapular deviations are apparent from this aspect and are indicative of a fatigue slump, structural or functional changes. Forward shoulders and winged scapula or angel wings are often a part of the fatigue picture and likewise may be combined with round shoulders and forward head, since the body attempts to compensate through weight distribution for unilateral alignment of segments below. Use letters in accordance with key as to items.

Back and Spinal variations are made more apparent through the use of an imaginary plumb line passing vertically between the heels, at the cleft of the buttocks, bisecting the spinous processes, and in the middle of the neck and head. Actual use of the plumb line test is generally used for individual testing purposes, since a considerable amount of time is needed. Figure 38 shows excellent alignment. Lateral curves may also be detected by tracing the fingers down both sides of the spine, thus making more visible such lateral curves as the "C" and "S" scolioses.

Pelvis variations should be checked from the rear as well as in front, since height of hips refers to both aspects. By placing of the palms of the hands flat on the buttocks with fingers extended upward, the thumbs are pressed firmly into the indentations of the posterior spines, thus making it possible to observe by sighting as to the equivalent height of the innominate bones. Particular care should be exercised to ascertain whether or not there is a rotation of the pelvic girdle which may accompany lateral curvatures.

Ankles and feet are best examined with the feet pointed in a straight line with heels slightly apart. Ankle pronation is observed from a slanting of the tendon achilles, with the os calcis or heel bone rotating inward. When the plantar muscles are weak there is usually a puffiness on the inner aspect of the foot, especially in severe third degree flatfoot conditions.

While the transverse arch weakness is clearly evident from the front view, with a slight depression at the joint of the toes, it is even more clearly seen by raising the foot to the rear by bending the knee. Callous formations are under the ball of the anterior arch when condition is severe, and slight pressure from below in this area shows how much discomfort is present. In women, whose weight is carried mainly on the front part of the foot, this trouble is all too evident.

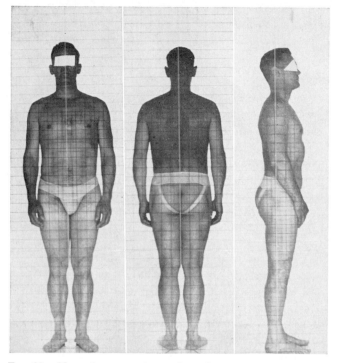

FIG. 38.—Normal posture shown through vertical alignment test

LATERAL VIEW

Body discrepancies as to the anterior posterior aspect when viewed from the side, are best determined when an imaginary line is considered to be running vertically from the external malleolus of the foot, through the middle of the knee, through the great trochanter to the acromion process or tip of the shoulder, and tragus of the ear. Variations are judged as to anterior lean, posterior lean, or body sway which are related to unequal development of the front and rear muscles. That is, the agonist and antagonist muscles are of unequal strength and the body is thrown out of balance, which causes fatigue and postural problems to accrue.

Head and neck conditions to be considered are forward head, back head, turtle neck and dowager hump in the cervical region.

Vision, hearing and occupational pursuits are all causative factors, while postural distorsions below also add to such changes in segmental balance.

Shoulder and chest changes from normal are seen as forward with matching winged scapulas, and round shoulders, actually a back condition yet related to the shoulder girdle. Chest irregularities often present are flat, hollow or funnel, and pigeon breast. They are discerned by placing the palm of the hand on the chest to determine the particular contour.

Trunk and pelvis are the crucial areas in respect to vertical alignment and refer to kyphosis or round back, lordosis or hollow back, kypholordosis or a combination of the two, and ptosis or a relaxed abdominal wall known as pot belly. Anterior posterior pelvic tilts are usually associated with the previous factors, while there may be a forward rotation of a single innominate bone in the presence of a short leg. By placing one hand on the abdomen and the other on the gluteals, the pelvis may be rotated in the form of a tuck, making possible a decision as to whether the condition is structural or functional and can be corrected.

Knee weaknesses found to be most prevalent are the forward or hyperflexed knee, and backward or hyperextended knee. In the latter instance, this situation may throw all the segments above out of proportion. Sometimes, backknees are a secondary result of faulty weight distribution above, in an attempt to secure proper balance.

It should be appreciated that the screening test is only a rough estimate of conditions, and when more than one severe deviation is present the student should be referred for further examination. Those with the most serious malalignments should be given precedence in assignment to adapted or developmental classes, or individual examinations. The normal or nearly normal may then proceed with regular classes, with the information obtained being used for guidance in choosing proper activities in keeping with his particular needs.

INDIVIDUAL EXAMINATION

The preliminary record card reveals the need for further investigation of various students. A school program is not complete unless provision is made for the identification of those who may already be handicapped, and the adaptation of school programs to meet their needs or prevent further impairment by neglect. All too few schools in the nation offer classes in adapted or developmental physical education, so that in many instances the entire burden falls upon the school physician and may result in a rather cursory inspection.

Teachers of special classes need to have a ready record of the various cases and conditions for constant referral. Therefore, in spite of the time involved, permanent card forms should be devised for the recording of all pertinent items, and preferably filed in a visible Kardex file. By means of this reference, any data are readily available and results of progress are easily ascertained. Such a record is shown in Figures 39A and 39B.

NOTE: This section of card should be folded down when it is placed in the permanent file. Keep straight for Kardex.

UNIVERSITY OF CALIFORNIA, LOS ANGELES
Department of Physical Education   •   Developmental Division
CASE ANALYSIS

Disability..

....

Physician's Recommendations..

.... Code Classification 1 2 3 4 5 6 7 8 9 0
(Health Service)

Other conditions..

.... Duplicate conditions: 1 2 3 4

RESULTS AND DISPOSITION

Date entered Developmental.......................... Date discharged..........................

Results by semesters:	1	2	3	4	Other
Disability corrected......					
Disability improved......					
Preventive program......					
To Reg. Phys. Educ......					
Temporary assignment...					
Left school......					
Remarks......					

NUTRITIONAL STATUS	Freshman		Sophomore		Junior		Senior		Other
Semester	1	2	1	2	1	2	1	2	
Age (Yrs.–Mos.)......									
Height (Inches)......									
Pelvic (Width cm.)......									
Chest (Width cm.)......									
Weight (Normal)......									
Weight (Actual)......									
Weight (Variation)±									

FOLLOW UP EXAMS	DATES CHECKED	* RESULTS	EXAMINATION	DATES CHECKED	* RESULTS
Blood Pressure......			Spine......		
Heart......			Tracings......		
Cardiogram......			Flexible Rule......		
Others......			Anthropometric (Specify)......		
X-ray......			1.		
Photography......			2.		
Posture......			3.		
Special......			4.		
Foot......			Nutritional......		
Tracings......			Diet Analysis......		
Pedograph......			Basal Metab......		
Others......			Others......		
Joint Measurements......					
Calipers......					
Goniometer......					
Tracings......					

CODE USED ON CARD
1° = Noticeable—Slight—(Brown tab)   1st Exam = Black
2° = Moderate—(Blue tab)   2nd Exam = Orange
3° = Severe—(Red tab)   3rd Exam = Green
* Results of Follow-up examinations.   4th Exam = Purple

FIG. 39A.—Case analysis.

Admittedly, the physician is the responsible and qualified person who makes the physical examination, and the postural aspects are an integral part of such checking. This is not always possible because of the time element, and physicians often utilize medically trained personnel, when delegating this responsibility, to assist in conducting the postural phase of the appraisal, given either in conjunction with the medical examination or otherwise. Those who have been prepared to recognize important postural diver-

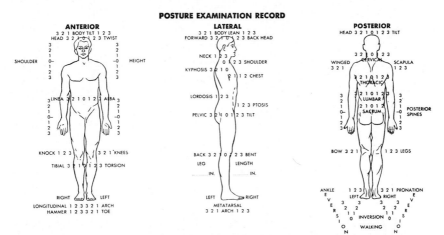

FIG. 39B.—Posture examination record.

gencies from the normal should be capable of aiding the physician in this respect, never presuming to have too much knowledge nor overstepping the bounds of professional ethics.[3]

EVALUATION OF INDIVIDUAL POSTURE

In making an individual examination as a part of the follow-through procedure in schools, the specially trained adapted physical educator may make the initial postural check. He may well profit through the use of a posture screen, where a student stands behind a frame which is bisected equally, both vertically and horizontally, into segments of 2-inch squares. Proper lighting is necessary to avoid the presence of shadows which may divert or change apparent contours of the body.[4,5,]

When using this device, the student first faces straight ahead so that from the anterior aspect, lateral deviations are apparent. He then turns to the right in order that anteroposterior changes may be seen from the lateral plane, and finally, again rotating to the right, the lateral divergencies are made evident from the posterior view. Sequential photographs taken with this device are useful for motivational and record purposes. All disorders previously described can be observed in the same manner, and a more accurate measure using the guide lines can be obtained.

An excellent reference source is available in the Master's thesis of Walter Campbell Crowe in which all known instruments, devices, and techniques are described. These are useful in conducting an adapted physical education program, and suggestions together with photographs are included which may be used in making examinations.[6]

Following this manner of judging, it is often essential that further appraisal be made. Since there are innumerable processes for determining more specifically as to items indicated, only a few are described. Nutritional and Exercise Prescription Record Cards are shown in Figures 40 and 41.

A 2-inch piece of adhesive tape is placed on the back, so that *"C" and "S" curvatures* become more evident and a permanent record is available. While holding a plumb line vertically, the examiner places the middle of the tape at the center of the sacrum. He then locates the center top of the tape where the line will bisect this point, and makes a dot for reference. Starting from the lowest center dot, he uses the index and middle finger of one hand to locate the spinous processes on either side of the spine, and makes a dot between the two fingers at each vertebra until the entire back has been checked. He then removes the tape, draws a vertical line from top to bottom dot to indicate proper alignment, and then connects the dots, whereupon the line of the curve is apparent. This method is particularly valuable in showing the student his back condition, and offers a record which may again be made to indicate amount of correction or progress accomplished.

An architect's flexible steel rule provides an excellent device for obtaining the *anterior posterior alignment* of the neck, back and

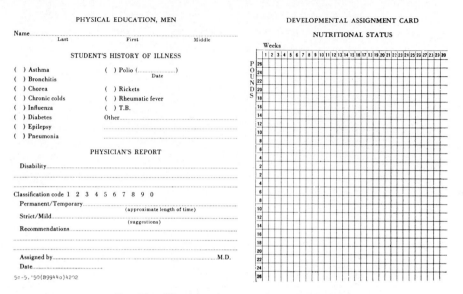

FIG. 40:—Nutritional status sequential record.

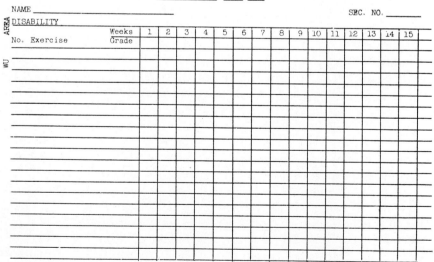

FIG. 41—Exercise prescription record card.

10

spine. Starting from the head and progressing downward, press the instrument firmly against the back surface. When the instrument is removed, the outline of the posterior curves are retained and may be traced upon a piece of paper. Subsequent tracings should be made periodically to show the amount of improvement.

Structural conditions in the *lateral plane of the spine*, as differentiated from functional divergencies, may be ascertained through the use of the *Adam's position*. From a standing posture, the student slowly bends first the head forward, then the shoulders, and on down the back until in a complete relaxed position. By tracing the spine with the index and middle finger on each side, the actual line of the vertebra is located. Then if the scoliosis or curve becomes straight, it is said to be a functional curvature and may be amenable to correction. If the curve remains approximately the same as in the vertical position, it is considered of a structural nature and should be referred to a physician, for exercise may be harmful if corrections are attempted.

There are a great many additional instruments and techniques which may be helpful in checking upon the posture. Reference to these procedures are to be found in the literature, from lectures and demonstrations, from instructional classes in colleges and universities, as well as from personal experience. Only those who are willing to invest of their time and energy in the search for knowledge, will become adequate to conduct such examinations. Preparation is a continuous task and yet a privilege, for the opportunity to help others to a fruitful life is granted to all too few persons.

PHYSICIAN'S FOLLOW-THROUGH

Upon selection, those cases chosen for further judgment are brought to the attention of the physician for his opinion as to final treatment. To enumerate all the items which he looks for would seem unnecessary, but suffice it to say that he is concerned with all medical factors which are pertinent to the particular case.

Naturally, he will review the symptoms and conditions first discovered to either verify those of concern or reject others as being relatively unimportant. In those cases of a questionable nature, and after a detailed examination, he may wish to call upon an orthopedist or a pediatrician specializing in such conditions.

After reviewing all available data, he will undoubtedly check the *physiological factors* and adequacy of the student's nutritional status, powers of coordination, body balance, skin color, and other such items. He will casually note the appearance of the student in respect to the prepubertal stage of beginning secondary sex characteristics, axillary and pubic hair, voice changes, breast changes, and genital development.

The physician is especially alert as to any evidence of developmental retardation, direct or indirect, such as malnutrition or obesity, history of amenorrhea or dysmenorrhea, headaches, nosebleeds, childish demeanor, bashfulness, easy embarrassment, efforts at concealment, skin conditions such as acne, and all other signs by the student's actions.

A more detailed analysis is then conducted to observe the *neural factors* in relation to the condition for which the student is being checked. The following are of special pertinence to structural and functional conditions and are listed in detail for this reason.

The *equilibrium* is tested, with first the eyes open and then closed and both feet together, then right and left eye closed alternately for balance. The physician will note the result as steady, uncertain, or poor, and may add toe pointing to the side, then forward, and crossing the foot over as in the Romberg test. An additional check may be made through placing a short board between two balance scales with the student standing in the center, noting the difference in weight distribution on the respective scales as a check on the lateral balance. This technique may also be used in a similar manner for anterior posterior determination.

Reflexes are made evident with a slight quick tap on the joint of the elbow, knee or ankle, noting the amount of jerk as normal, increased, dull or absent. Such reaction is important as an indication of nerve reaction.

When the arms and hands are extended with the fingers spread apart, abnormal *tremors* or movements may be seen as fine or coarse. Nervous conditions may be recognized in this manner.

In making the *hand coordination* test, the student's arms are extended sideways, and while his eyes are closed he attempts to touch his index finger tips in front of his face. If successful the action is recorded as normal, or pass pointing if finger tips miss. With the arms down at sides and index fingers extended, the student attempts to touch his nose with both fingers while his eyes are closed. If the fingers miss each other and the nose is touched the action is normal, otherwise it is recorded as pass pointing.

Observations of the *sensory reaction* should be noted as tactile or touch, or checked by having the student closing his eyes and make a fist. The examiner then gently touches the hair of the student's fingers or even toes to see if the finger extends or reacts. Thermal reactions or sensitivity to hot or cold pressure are likewise important clues of nerve damage.

It is possible to observe unobtrusively *muscular twitching*, either local or general, and regular *tic or spasm* noting the area involved. In this respect any suspected *hypo- or hyperactivity* should be entered on the record for possible future reference.

During this personal examination every effort should be made to develop good rapport between the student, physician, and teacher of physical education or school nurse. In this way the student gains confidence and special trust in these persons as his friend, and brings personal problems to such individuals with friendliness and confidence.

FUNCTIONAL TEST

The two previous testing procedures described were mainly of a static nature, and by themselves cannot be considered as adequate. How an individual moves and acts is the significant point if purposeful activity is to result. Whether the movement is of a locomotive type in which the lower extremities are mainly involved, or implicates the upper extremities or appendages in actions of strength or dexterity skills, or includes movements of the total body, the kinesthetic response must be inextricably synchronized if effective movement is to take place.

Neuromuscular function or motor skills play a predominant part in survival, for without emotion there is no motion, and without motion life departs. Test items which are proposed in this section are within the jurisdiction and capability of the well-trained physical educator, therapist or nurse, since the background of experience in their educational preparation qualifies them to understand the dynamics of activity.

In presenting elements for inclusion in a functional test, no effort is made to make such a listing all inclusive, but merely to alert the tester as to actions in daily living which may indicate weaknesses. It is well to remember that subjective judgment in the hands of experts tends to become objective in nature. The physical educator who sees youth in play is favorably situated to pass judgment concerning effective dynamic function.

Either during the screening or individual test, students should be expected (*a*) to walk and jog a short distance in order that gait, stride, balance, use of arms in relation to the body, and coordination in general may be observed, (*b*) to climb a short flight of stairs to discern difficulty, (*c*) to lift an object from the floor to discover whether the knees are bent and used rather than placing the entire burden on the back muscles, (*d*) to throw a ball with either hand to see if more than only the arm and shoulder is involved in the action, (*e*) to strike a ball with a bat, racket, golf club or other implement to check hand eye coordination, and (*f*) to jump over a low height or project the body a short distance or jump-reach toward a mark or goal.

Those who are capable of performing such skills, ordinarily would be considered to have normal range of motion, native capacity in respect to spring, and coordination of all parts of the body demanded for life functions. Numerous research studies have been conducted as to *reflex action*, such as the tossing of a ball to a person and noting his response. Investigators have tested *reaction time* through the medium of starts in track meets. All too often, many activities of research workers have as their immediate purpose the determination of what is, or what has been, rather than what should be.

As a means of stressing the importance of having the feet point straight ahead, place a student without shoes or socks with heels resting on a line marked on the floor. Evert the feet, if a student is not available who normally walks in such a manner, and make a mark at the farthest point of each great toe. Correct this stance pointing feet straight, and again mark the farthest reach of each toe. By placing a ruler on the marks for each position, measure the difference in distance between the two methods of walking or running. It will be observed that there is a variation of from 1 to 2 inches saved through the latter manner, which amounts to a considerable saving in distance, energy and improved gait. Such minor adjustments may make the difference between mediocrity and world records.

The above example has been cited to aid in pointing out the reason to young people for making such tests. There are of course many other approaches but the following poem exemplifies the importance of function to the older person.

> When I was young, my slippers were red,
> And I could kick as high as my head.
> As older I grew, my slippers were blue,
> Couldn't kick as high as I used to do.
> Now I am old, my slippers are black,
> I walk to the corner and slowly drag back.
> How do I know that my youth is spent,
> My get-up-and-go has got-up-and-went.
> But I waste not a tear when I think with a grin,
> Of all the grand places my "get-up" has been.[7]

OBSERVABLE CUES

Those who work with young people or adults have the chance to detect the beginning of deviations. If they are interested and know what to look for, they are able to accomplish much good.

An example of third degree knock knees and surgical correction is shown in Figure 42. Habits assumed unknowingly suggest clues, and even the spoken word may do much in avoiding further difficulties.

Prevalent today among students is the tendency to become fatigued quickly. This is a red signal calling for attention, for often this condition is related to the nutritional status, the attempt to return to vigorous activity too soon after illness, or an indication

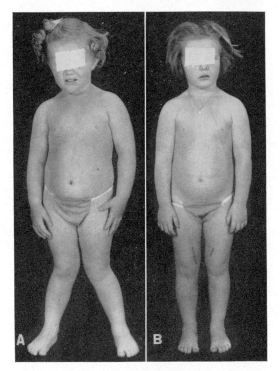

Fig. 42.—*A*, Third degree knock knees. *B*, Correction by surgery. Note marked improvement in leg alignment, hence re-establishment of muscle balance throughout legs and feet 10 months later.

of debilitation. It is possible that the personal program is over-crowded and that these individuals are expected to do too many things in a day. There are instances in which young boys are play-ing basketball with as many as six and eight different teams, so is it any wonder that they are not able to keep up.

Newspaper boys, golfers and tennis players are prone to have a low shoulder. In view of this it is easy to explain the need to change weight carrying to the opposite shoulder occasionally. The tennis player, other athletes and dentists who are active in one-sided activities should cultivate means for overcoming imbalance.

Youngsters are seen every day riding bicycles improperly with the arch of the foot on the pedal, thus favoring active pronation, and generally wearing tennis shoes which offer little support. The practice of using soft soled shoes throughout the day should be eliminated by those parents who are responsible and concerned about their child's welfare.

Too few opportunities are presented for participation in rhythmical activities, for on every hand people are seen who have little grace of movement and where every action is an effort. The cultivation of this type of activity is not for the sake of the performance, but rather for the sake of the performer.

During physical education class periods, students are seen in their natural state, unconscious of the requisites of society. The shower room and dressing stage offers a time to check on standing position, bulging of inner ankles, soft flaccid or even flabby muscle texture, structural make-up, kinds of shoes being worn, muscle development, in fact almost all bodily conditions.

Parents should be asked to assist in this "Sherlocking," for it is not a one man job, and should include the student or person himself. As the ancient Chinese philosopher Emperor Shi Hwang-ti once remarked, "He who squanders today talking of yesterday's triumph, will have nothing to boast of tomorrow."

REFERENCES

1. LOWMAN, CHARLES LeROY, COLESTOCK, CLAIRE and COOPER, HAZEL: *Corrective Physical Education for Groups.* New York: A. S. Barnes and Co., 1928, Chapter V and Chapter XXI.
2. V-5 ASSOCATION OF AMERICA: *Conditioning Exercises, Games, Tests.* 3rd ed. by Karl C. H. Oermann, Carl Haven Young, *et al.* Annapolis, Maryland: United States Naval Institute, 1960, Chapter VI.
3. LOWMAN, CHARLES LeROY: Orthopedic Problems: Responsibility of School Physicians. Health Educ. J., *14:* 3–4, 1951.
4. LOWMAN, COLESTOCK and COOPER, *loc. cit.*
5. V-5 ASSOCIATION OF AMERICA, *loc. cit.*
6. CROWE, WALTER CAMPBELL: The Use of Audio-Visual Materials in Developmental (Corrective) Physical Education. Unpublished Master's thesis, The University of California, Los Angeles, 1950, 219 pp.
7. "Slippers," Senior Citizen, November, 1956, p. 48.

The above references are not repeated in References for Extended Reading.

REFERENCES FOR EXTENDED READING

BLESH, T. ERWIN, MEYERS, CARLTON R. and KIPHUTH, OSCAR: *Photometric Photography in Posture Evaluation of Yale University Freshmen.* New Haven: Yale University Press, 1954, 17 pp.

CLARKE, HENRY HARRISON: *Application of Measurement to Health and Physical Education.* 2nd ed. New York: Prentice-Hall, 1950, 493 pp.
    Chapter VII: Posture and Foot Measurement.

CONANT, RICHARD D.: The Utilization of Photographic Techniques in Adapted Physical Education. Unpublished Master's thesis, The University of California, Los Angeles, 1956, 113 pp.

DANIELS, L., WILLIAMS, M. and WORTHINGHAM, CATHERINE: *Muscle Testing.* Philadelphia: W. B. Saunders Co., 1956, 176 pp.

DREW, L. C.: *Individual Gymnastics.* 5th ed. Rev. and edited by Hazel Kinzley, Philadelphia: Lea & Febiger, 1949, 222 pp.
    Chapter IX: Examinations.

KELLY, ELLEN D.: *Teaching Posture and Body Mechanics.* New York: A. S. Barnes and Co., 1949, 212 pp.
    Chapter VI: Posture Examinations, Records and Grading.

KENDALL, HENRY O., KENDALL, FLORENCE P. and BOYNTON, DOROTHY A.: *Posture and Pain.* Baltimore, The Williams and Wilkins Co., 1952, 204 pp.
    Chapter VI: Procedure for Postural Examination.

LICHT, SIDNEY, (ed.): *Therapeutic Exercise.* New Haven, Conn.: Elizabeth Licht, 1958, 893 pp.
    Chapter VII: Muscle and Joint Measurement.—Nancy Salter.
    Chapter VIII: Manual Muscle Examination.—Thomas F. Hines.
    Chapter XVII: Principles of Therapeutic Exercise.—Robert L. Bennett.

LOS ANGELES CITY SCHOOLS: *Corrective Physical Education.* Los Angeles: Los Angeles Board of Education, 1958, 400 pp.
    Chapter V: Posture Analysis.
    Chapter VI: Suggested Group Tests for Selecting Exercises for Pupils in the
                Corrective Physical Education Class.

McCLOY, C. H.: *Tests and Measurements in Health and Physical Education.* New York: F. S. Crofts and Co., 1944, 412 pp.

MORRISON, W. R., and CHENOWETH, LAURENCE B.: *Normal and Elementary Physical Diagnosis.* 4th ed. Philadelphia: Lea & Febiger, 1947, 373 pp.
    Chapter IV: General Appearance, Height and Weight.
    Chapter V: Nutrition.
    Chapter VII: Posture.
    Chapter VIII: The Feet.

PHELPS, WINTHROP M., KIPHUTH, ROBERT and GOFF, CHARLES W.: *Diagnosis and Treatment of Postural Defects.* Springfield: Charles C Thomas, 1956, 190 pp.
    Chapter VI: Postural Examination.

PRESCOTT, DANIEL ALFRED: *Emotion and the Educative Process.* Washington, D.C.: American Council on Education, 1938, 323 pp.
    Chapter VI: Basic Personality Needs and Conditions Which Frustrate Them.

YOUNG, CARL HAVEN: A Procedure in the Organizing of a Corrective Physical Education Program for High School Boys. Unpublished Master's thesis, The University of Southern California, Los Angeles, 1935, 150 pp.

CHAPTER 7

Dynamics of Exercise

It is essential to recognize that there is a very important relationship between spinal alignment and the function of the organs attached to the vertebral column. Such integration of function involves the framework of spine and thorax, the heart, great vessels and lungs, and neuromuscular apparatus involved in their activity.

The genesis of this statement is to be found in that the failure of the parts to mesh properly can bring catastrophic results. Basically, the pertinence of the muscle fibers and tissues directs the attention to deriving all possible knowledge as to how to make more effective organic functioning. Since the anatomical structure is involved, an operational analysis demonstrates a discrepancy between the theoretical and actual performance of some individuals who are handicapped by their poor body mechanics. Therefore, it becomes essential to understand, conclusively, such interrelationships and their control.[1,2]

BIOMECHANICS OF RESPIRATION

Exercise of all the muscles and organs of the body requires oxygen to be brought to them through the capillaries, and the toxins or carbon dioxide to be taken away by the venous system and returned to the heart and lungs to be purified or oxygenated. For this reason, teachers and students should have at least a nominal understanding of the dynamics of this process.

Respiration in this sense consists of action in the peripheral capillary beds of allowing passage or interchange of oxygen and CO_2 from the muscle cells. It also includes a similar interchange in the alveolar portion of the lungs, plus the neuromuscular action of the respiratory muscles. The latter process is discussed because of the importance and relationship of postural alignment, which has so much to do with the efficiency of breathing.

The principle muscles involved in inspiration are controlled by the respiratory center in the medulla of the spinal cord, which is composed of a specialized group of cells that send out motor impulses in rhythmic fashion to these muscles. These cells are organized for the control of inspiration and expiration and maintain the function of the diaphragm and ribs as well as the accessory muscles. It is believed by some authorities that expiration is taken care of through the elasticity of the lungs, weight of the chest walls, elevation of the diaphragm, and in particular the muscles of the abdominal wall and transversus thoracic.

Action of the diaphragm as the active element in a pump should be considered from the dynamic standpoint. When the diaphragm goes down in inspiration, it forces the ribs outward, forward, and upward, thus increasing the actual ventilation capacity of the thorax. It also affects the shape of the ribs, and their spring-like action causes elastic tension to be built up in the thoracic cage, which action on the opposite stroke is one factor in expiration.

In order to be effective, a pump must have a compression chamber in which to work, and in this instance it is the abdominal cavity. The downward pressure of the diaphragm is resisted by the musculature of the abdominal wall which causes some of this pressure to compress the visceral organs. This affects the movement of the venous flow of the blood and the lymphatic return, and the rest of the pressure is stored up in the muscles which elastically return to their normal tension on the opposite stroke of the pump.

Faulty posture, therefore, very directly affects the integrity of the breathing process, for when the dorsal spine droops into a rounded or kyphotic position the ribs are lowered, the diameters of the chest decrease, and normal tension cannot be built up in them. Anteriorly, as the ribs and sternum sag, the abdominal wall relaxes since these muscles cannot store up tension. Furthermore, the large suspensory ligament or the cervical fascia from the base of the neck which helps to hold the heart and lungs will sag. Thus, their position is lowered and the general slump of the upper trunk will reduce the efficiency of the whole respiratory action.

CARDIO-RESPIRATORY MECHANISM

There is a definite reason for starting weak posture cases in the fundamental recumbent position, since breathing as such is not given as a separate exercise, for it is felt that the oxygen carbon dioxide interchange will be taken care of reflexly in connection with other exercises. Physiologically, the respiratory process is complicated and for better understanding requires a technical knowledge of the neural and chemical factors involved. Such information may be readily found in recent texts dealing with the physiology of exercise.

There is a general tendency to teach that the effort at correcting trunk posture is connected with breathing. The prevailing practice is to raise the chest, throw back the shoulders, take a deep breath, and contract the abdominal muscles. It is sometimes difficult to teach the student to breathe naturally and at the same time alter his alignment.

Since the skeletal faults are eliminated in recumbency, it is often advisable to use this position while teaching normal breathing. This permits emphasis on the proper tensing of the back and pelvic muscles without interfering with free respiratory movements. A word of caution is advisable in relation to holding the breath as a part of the fixation effort, while raising the legs or trunk from the recumbent position. It is always wise to do exercise with the throat open, because the closing of the glottis and forcing down on the diaphragm, while the abdominal stabilizers are acting, tends to invite a rupture or hernia.

SEGMENTAL CONTROL

The type of approach used in remedying postural deviations or developing exercises for any activity, depends upon the analytical ability of the teacher, who knows that time must be spent on the unit parts before the whole body can be brought to a proper position. The dynamics of the body must be related to the framework and the muscles controlling the segments. Beginning at the base of the body, they are considered in sequence from the feet and legs, pelvis and abdomen, trunk, shoulder girdle and chest, head and neck.

Correct unilateral balance between the opposing muscle groups must be obtained to maintain the body balance and the pull against gravity in the optimum position. After the physical educator has motivated the student toward the idea of wanting a more efficient, graceful, and beautiful body, he should be aided in gaining insight as to how each part or segment should be held, and helped to visualize what he should want to look like.

Later, in an effort to obtain a total motor pattern of performance, refinement of the actions controlling each segment receive attention. Specific exercises or activities must be selected which will be beneficial in such adjustments.

LOCALIZATION

A person with some postural fault ordinarily does not feel any different from the person who is straight. His sensory mechanism registers his position as natural, unless after too much tension or activity he feels pain or discomfort which makes him want to stretch or change position to get relief. When he attempts to assume the correct position which the teacher describes, he may say that it doesn't feel natural, but when he looks in the mirror or watches the teacher demonstrate, he may see and feel what must be done and become segmentally conscious.

This centering of the attention on the segment, and the effort required of certain muscles which act to assume and maintain the right position is spoken of as *localization of effort*.

It is essential that there be a mental effort as well as a physical participation in conscious performance. By repetition and improvement of control, a freer and more easily obtained correction is gradually evolved and the action becomes automatic. Gradually, when sufficient muscle strength is built, a good habit supplants the bad habit and good position no longer feels unnaturall The sensory registration of the improved posture becomes norma. and reflex action habitual.

ANTAGONISM AND SYNERGISM

Sensory-motor factors in altering the position of body segments which are out of normal alignment have been discussed. Usually the muscles on the flexor side are adaptively shortened, and the opponent antigravity ones on the extensor side are stretched and weaker. This is well illustrated in the shoulder girdle segment in the fatigue slump, for the pectorals are shortened from over-activity and favored by gravity, while the rhomboids and lower trapezii or scapular adductors are stretched.

These muscles are antagonists, and it is important to understand that the agonist muscle or group which initiates a movement, is controlled by an opponent muscle or group which is the antagonist. Just as it is indispensable to establish balance between them to obtain proper alignment of body segments and joints, so is it essential to know that through the action of reciprocal innervation, which is called Sherrington's Law, the development of skilled movements takes place. The antagonists control the speed, range and force of agonist action.

Consequently, in order to get finer coordinative adjustments, it is essential to develop the strength of the opponents of the acting agonists. This point is commonly overlooked by teachers and coaches who are interested in developing skills. They usually attempt to perfect a technique in gymnastics and sports by a repetitious trial and error method. The student should be taught that in order to get a complete range of movement of his joints, he should work hard to build up the weaker, stretched out antagonists so that they become sufficiently shortened to balance the tight and overactive opponents.

In attempting to correct faulty posture by therapeutic or developmental exercise, this muscle balancing of adversaries, as well as joint and segment position, will automatically become the soundest base by which plans for fostering skill can be derived. More specifically, all who come in contact with those who have such troubles should take an active interest in basic postural correction and not sidestep the issue by saying, "Let the adapted or developmental classes take care of these cases, its their job."

As soon as this adjustment and improvement in strength of opposite groups has become reflexly habitual, it will be noted that fatigue generates more slowly. The synergists are helper muscles and act when greater strength and control are needed. They may also act to control the direction of movements and force necessary to apply by either the agonists or the antagonists.

As an illustration, in leg raising the thigh flexors or iliopsoas are the agonists, but in order to keep the leg being lifted from going outward, the adductors of the thigh act and their opponents, the thigh abductors, likewise act to prevent it from going inward and to keep the leg straight in a rotatory plane, while the rotators similarly act to keep the foot pointed straight forward.

KINETICS OF BALANCE

When body balance is thought of, the spatial relationship or connection to its environment is usually considered. Nevertheless, two other relationships immediately claim the attention from an exercise standpoint, (1) the balance of the various body segments, and (2) the balance of opponent muscles in their relation to the control of joint action. These two elements are closely related because, when poor body mechanics exists, the various segments list or sag so that the bony columns that should support the weight with a minimal expenditure of energy, fail to do so. This places undue strain on ligaments and muscles requiring them to take on an extra burden.[3]

When competing muscle groups are already in a state of imbalance from faulty posture, they tend to become so, habitually. As has been pointed out, if the joints are used in improper alignment or through a working range shorter than their full limits of action, the stabilizing ligaments and muscles which control their performance become stretched on one side, while the antagonist opponents are shortened. Hence, they are not in balance.[4]

In relation to balance of joints and muscles and their related body segments, it is hard to say which is cause and which is effect. The flexors, having a position of advantage, are stronger than the extensors. They are favored by acting with and not against gravity as their opponents must do. Consequently, static or postural strain increases in proportion to the weakness of the antigravity muscles and the quantity of divergence which must be controlled.

As imbalance increases, excess work is required of the central mechanism because incoordination results more quickly and is a definite indication of the start of fatigue. Therefore, both rest and activity must be carefully related, and exercises graded or modified to meet the neuromuscular needs.

The maintenance of tonus in the muscles is, according to the English physiologist Sherrington, to a large extent and particularly in relating to gravitational forces, controlled by the labyrinthine mechanism in the inner ear and acts as man's gyroscope. The posturing reflexes established by most physical activities from infancy on become habitual and automatic and are evidence of the neural aspect. The degree of ease with which the balancing muscles act is influenced by the state of their structural and physioological status in nutritional states, fatigue, insufficiency of strength from over stretching, and faulty alignment of joints upon which they act.

A question often arises as to how a high degree of coordinative skill in students may be obtained unless a state of balanced action is developed. Training for such action should start in the simplest and easiest positions of the parts involved. Too often the malaligned student is urged toward a goal of exactness and good form which requires continuous repetition on a trial and error basis.

From the sensori motor standpoint, this is a slow, wasteful and inefficient method of obtaining skilled movements in a body that is in a poor state to develop them. As every movement of the body and its parts is registered in the sensory area of the brain, the habit pattern of the registration of such movements will be just as imperfect as the motor elements that execute it.

Body parts, that are habitually malaligned under the control of muscles which are not balanced or properly opposed, cannot develop as high a degree of skill or as correct a pattern of total performance as would occur in the person whose body segments, joints, and muscles were all in balance.

Making muscles work is not the main end in view, but, rather, the *building up of neural stability and control should be the aim.* That is the chief measure of endurance for which all strive, and *neural capacity is the chief determinant of accomplishment.*

In order to graduate the stresses on the equilibrating mechanism, fundamental exercises in the recumbent and procumbent positions should first be used. Sitting, kneeling, and standing positions should follow, and after a period of activity in the standing position, the recumbent position should again be resumed for localized muscle work so that ligaments and muscles involved in balancing obtain needed rest.

BALANCE EXERCISE

It is axiomatic that all remedial exercises should be carried on from a basically correct position due to the prevalence of faulty foot and leg positions. Walking on a straight, narrow beam as on the Swedish board or even on the flat floor, places undue stress on groups of balance muscles that are asymmetrically developed.

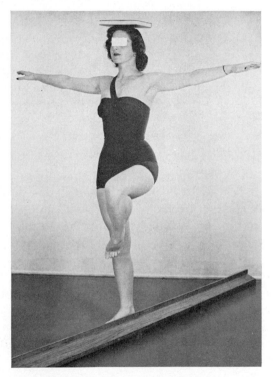

Fig. 43.—Centralized push-up on tilted balance board

For this reason the Lowman tilted balance board[5] was devised in which the treads are slanted outward and downward at about 15 degrees. Standing on these treads, the leg is rotated outward and the feet are thrown into a mild varus or inversion state, which corrects the pronation and valgus which are so common. In this position there is a taking up of the slack of the stretched muscles and a lengthening of the shortened muscles every time one foot is raised (Fig. 43).

The effort to "keep the balance" or to maintain stability, while the opposite leg, body or arms are doing something else, gives a powerful stimulus to all the equilibrators. Consequently, a double action is involved in such exercises, with a passive holding or stabilizing effort for certain muscles, and an active effort on the part of others that are executing some other movements.

Motor skill patterns involved in keeping the balance are begun as soon as the child begins to stand and walk, and as a result the muscles involved must adapt themselves in length and tension to maintain all joints in controlled positions. If faulty alignment exists at any of the joints implicated, the muscular adjustment of control tends to become habitual. In this way, early fixed faults of posture evolve which, during growth, may influence structural skeletal development or even lead to deformities of varying grades.

Tactile kinesthetic mechanism then works at a disadvantage in forming coordinative skills when faulty alignment exists. This means decreased efficiency of movement, use of a greater amount of energy than necessary if joints are not in line, and early onset of fatigue.

VALUE OF TILTED BALANCE BOARDS

Aside from the therapeutic effect on muscular and ligamentous imbalance in working from a fundamental position, there is the psycho-physiological stimulus of doing something that is challenging. The monotony of ordinary floor work becomes boresome to many children, while exercises and games on the balance boards require skill and coordinative effort (Fig. 44).

Children enjoy exhibiting their skill, and teachers realize how hard it is to maintain concentrated effort because of a shortened span of attention. Such a condition is often provoked or prolonged because of a lack of interest or challenge which, through the use of such boards, offers something different and serves as a motivating influence.

THERAPEUTIC MERITS

Briefly recapitulating, the principle remedial values in using the balance boards are described in the following context. There is a wider base than the Swedish beam, while the "tracker board" centered between the treads, guides the placement of the feet and helps develop the sensory pattern regarding position. All efforts are made in relation to the center line which aids the feet in feeling the central push up, and if exercises are done before a mirror the visual image is also of help.

Such a device furnishes maximal interest because of its challenge to skill, assists in the creating of attention and concentration, aids in developing opponent muscle balance, especially in the feet and legs, while reducing tension on stretched ligaments of the feet, legs and pelvis.

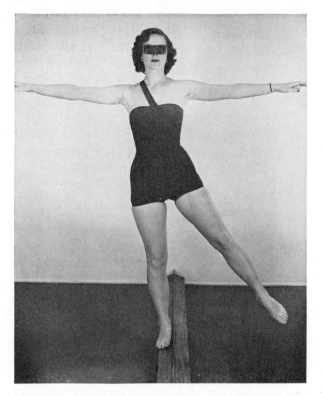

FIG. 44.—Use of tilted balance board in foot exercise.

The use of such boards tend to correct pronated ankles, knock-knees, inward rotation of leg, and hollow back. In the latter it decreases the pull on the piriformis muscle which is the chief outward rotator of the thigh. Since this muscle attaches to the front of the sacrum, the drag of its upper end into a forward tilt produces lordosis.

Without doubt the principle advantage in recommending its use is that it develops the mechanism of equilibration in relation to spatial orientation and to the environment. Likewise, it offers a medium which presents variation in the approach to improvement of balance.

11

SUGGESTIONS FOR USING

When the balance board is raised to varying levels above the floor, or when it is raised at one end to form an incline, or when it is supported in the middle and used as a teeter, the degree of stress on the whole neuromuscular mechanism is increased. Such activity should be as a progression from the simpler starting exercises, which require chiefly large muscle work, to the more finite or difficult exercises requiring use of the more delicate muscles.

Complicated balance work should be of short duration because the more exacting demands of complex skilled execution produces early fatigue. It is a good policy to follow balance board drills with exercises in recumbency or sitting position.

POSITIONAL SIGNIFICANCE

In using activity as a vehicle for changing divergent conditions, many factors must be considered, a task requiring diagnostic ability, sound judgment and analytical tact. Not only must the condition be known regarding its effect on the being, but there needs to be comphrension as to the type of exercise from a kinesiological and anatomical standpoint which is most suitable, motivational possibilities and time elements needed to accomplish desired results, and sequential order and degree of difficulty inherent in the exercise.

Of paramount importance is knowledge concerning the most favorable position in which the activity may operate, for there are many extenuating circumstances to consider from a functional approach and some are more conducive to success than others. In addition to these positive essentials, there are likewise certain admonitions to appreciate which may negate any amount of effort. With this background understood, the subsequent presentation of recommended positions is suggested.

RECUMBENCY POSITION

Recumbent or procumbent positions are commended as the primary base for beginning developmental exercises. It makes little difference whether the older and more commonly formalized procedures are used or not in this regard. The important thing is that all exercises must be given from basic positions for efficient dynamic action. A controlled base of action requires a static or stabilizing force.

In recent years, there seems to be a tendency to over emphasize dynamism in an effort to get away from the older and more formalized procedures in which posture was thought of as a rigid, fixed state. There has been, however, insufficient attention to the

relationship between static and dynamic elements in all performance.

Modifying the dosage of dynamic action and controlling the
basic fundamentals of position from which action takes place
should be stressed, for exercises in recumbency lessen the work
load on the whole balancing mechanism, and alignment of body
segments are thus improved. The position is fundamentally sound
and a safe one from which to start in regard to cardiovascular
action, convalescent period following illness, helping to slow down
the overactive high tensioned lithe type individual, considerably
lessening fatigue, and allowing valuable conditioning of both
skeletal and organic body elements for lengthened periods before
fatigue ensues.

In the overcoming of fatigue, it is important to get rid of the
causative toxins, and in the recumbent position, the dorsal spinal
curve is flattened and the rib cage raised forward. This increases
the diameter of the thorax, makes more ventilating area, and
enables the diaphragm to step up its function. Because the diaphragm is pulled up taut and has a wider stroke between inspiration
and expiration, there is faster expulsion of the CO_2.

Consequent improvement of body position also makes for a
more desirable position of the abdominal organs, so that they can
function to better advantage. The massaging effect of the dia-
phragmatic thrust in breathing improves circulatory action.
Through this compression, the movement of the lymphatic flow
is similarly affected.

A frequent objection to recumbency exercises is insufficient
floor area, especially where there is no gymnasium and little floor
space. In many places, such work can be conducted out-of-doors
with a paper towel being used to protect the head and hair.

SITTING POSITION

Next of value in respect to the decrease of load during exercise
is the sitting position, which has similar value to that of recumbency in reducing musculo-ligamentous stress while being a
progression from the lying state. It takes advantage of many of
the factors represented in the margin of safety, especially in relation to heart action and flattening of low back.

Thus, the sitting position becomes a fundamental one from which
upper trunk, shoulder girdle, head and neck, as well as the arms
may be given corrective movements. Some of these are push-ups
of the spine with hands in a neck firm position, stretching tight
pectorals, shortening stretched rhomboids and lower trapezius,
thus raising the rib cage and consequently increasing respiratory
function.

The pelvis is held in a fixed position in relation to the spine when sitting. There is less strain on the sacro-iliac joint ligaments than in standing, and of course, none on the feet and legs. When combined with a cross-leg position, sitting is considered a completely safe and fundamentally correct position for exercise.

STANDING POSITION

Increment in terms of weight load during exercise is assumed to be the next step possible in the standing posture. This position must naturally be a step in the sequential process for increasing postural tone, and many resistive exercises may be given which are directly related to all segments.

Standing position exercises cannot be overlooked as an essential part of the definite effort to encompass totality in balance design. Venous flow of the blood is stimulated to a greater extent, neuro-muscular action increases, and organic demands are made more constant.

Even from a standing position, a gradual increase in degree of intensity is prescribed, proceeding from gross movements to finer and more intricate patterns. Care should be taken to avoid tension situations which, through improper concern for compensating force, place abnormal burden upon contradicting actions.

For such reasons, the standing position is considered a definite phase in sequence as a part of any developmental program. Wisely used, this procedure may be employed to advantage for a majority of conditions.

ACTION SITUATIONS

Integrated movements found in games of skill or other physical activities are the ultimate objective as a means of decision as to the completely synchronized function. Here are evidenced in the physically fit, such desirable elements as strength, endurance, speed, skill, reaction, spring, control, coordination, poise, grace, relaxation, and all the other factors essential in the gamut of movement.

Weaknesses are also apparent in the sluggish performance of those who, in spite of extreme desire to excel, are handicapped in various ways. These restrictions do not lessen the obligation of society to provide an opportunity for participation within the limits of the participant. The many advantages of such situations are an activating force in the amelioration of difficulties with the added stimulus of enjoyment and companionship.

It is necessary to warn against too great resistance in the under-par, for too much load on the intrinsic actors must be balanced in proportion to the extrinsic fixators. Other strains may result than those of structure, for stress has no regard for segments or locale.

The body in action may be likened to an orchestration by skilled musicians, blending with practiced artistry the variable ingredients into a symphony of rhythm and motion.

Increasing regard for the use of activities for developmental and rehabilitative purposes, demands intelligent application of the principles of dynamics.

It should, therefore, be meaningful to have reviewed together the intricate composition of the body germinated in nature. Only when people in positions of guidance apply these facts to the solving of personal needs will fullest benefits be achieved.

REFERENCES

1. LOWMAN, CHARLES LEROY: The Importance of Stabilization, Physiotherapy Rev., *29*, 253–255, 1949.
2. LOWMAN, CHARLES LEROY, COLESTOCK, CLAIRE, and COOPER, HAZEL: *Corrective Physical Education for Groups*. New York, A. S. Barnes and Co., 1928, Chapter XII.
3. LOWMAN, CHARLES LEROY: *Balance Skills in Physical Education*. Ann Arbor, Michigan, Edwards Brothers, 1935, 42 pp.
4. LOWMAN, COLESTOCK and COOPER, *op. cit.*, Chapter XI.
5. LOWMAN, *loc. cit.*

The above references are not repeated in References for Extended Reading.

REFERENCES FOR EXTENDED READING

HAWLEY, GERTRUDE: *The Kinesiology of Corrective Exercise*. 2nd ed. Philadelphia Lea & Febiger, 194 , 192 pp.
 Chapter X: Proper Use of the Body in Standing, Sitting, Lying and Walking.
HOWARTH, M. B.:   Dynamic Posture, Hygiea, *25*, 198, 1947.
HOWARTH, M. BECKETT, *et al.*:   *A Text-book of Orthopedics*. Philadelphia, W. B. Saunders Co., 1952, 1110 pp.
 Section on Neurology.
LICHT, SIDNEY, (ed.):   *Therapeutic Exercise*. New Haven, Conn., Elizabeth Licht, 1958, 893 pp.
 Chapter VI: Vicarious Motions.—C. B. Wynn-Parry.
 Chapter XXX: Exercise in Pulmonary Disease.—J. D. Sinclair.
PHELPS, WINTHROP M., KIPHUTH, ROBERT J. and GOFF, CHARLES W.:   *Diagnosis and Treatment of Postural Defects*. Springfield, Illinois, Charles C Thomas, 1956, 190 pp.
 Chapter VII: Posture in Physical Education.
STEINDLER, ARTHUR: *Kinesiology of the Human Body*. Springfield, Illinois, Charles C Thomas, 1955, 708 pp.
 Lecture VII: On Body Balance and Body Equilibrium.
 Lecture IX: The Mechanics of the Spinal Column.
WELLS, KATHERINE F.:   *Kinesiology*. 2nd ed. Philadelphia, W. B. Saunders Co., 1955, 516 pp.
 Chapter VI: The Muscular System.
 Chapter VIII: The Spinal Column.
 Chapter IX: The Movements of the Thorax in Respiration.
 Chapter XVI: The Characteristics of Skillful Performance in Motor Skills.
 Chapter XVII: Postural Skills.
 Chapter XVIII: Locomotion: Walking and Running.
WELLS, K. F.:   Practical Body Mechanics, J. Health and Phys. Educ., *19*, 591, 1948.
WILLIAMS, M., and WORTHINGHAM, CATHERINE: *Therapeutic Exercise for Body Alignment and Function*. Philadelphia, W. B. Saunders Co., 1957, 127 pp.
 Chapter I: Introduction: Standing Posture.
 Chapter II: Analysis of Body Alignment.
 Chapter V: Positions of the Body in Activity and Rest.

CHAPTER 8

Basis for Individual Activity Planning

PLANS for developmental physical exercises, leading to the mastery of skilled movements intended for the amelioration and improvement in terms of body education, must be based on a sound comprehension of anatomy and kinesiology. It is not sufficient to know the names of all the muscles and their relation to the framework, and where they arise and are attached, but also how they function and the part each individual muscle plays in the total combination of movements which produce a purposeful performance.

Because of the multitude of motor acts and the complexity of the neuromuscular response to stimuli, it is necessary to recognize that physical education encompasses the sequential development of muscular actions. These progress from the earliest undirected movements of infancy to the most complicated, highly coordinated acts of maturity.

It is valuable in planning for a progressive exercise program to begin with simple movements of large masses, thence proceed to the more highly coordinated action of lighter or intrinsic muscles, which carry out the expression of the will through what is known as skill.

PROGRESSIVE GROWTH FACTORS

As the prenatal position is one of flexion, the earliest movements are those of unfolding, and require extension movements of the body and extremities. The infant's earliest activities are apparrently aimless movements of the arms and kicking of the legs, pulling them up and forcefully extending them, rolling over, bending and twisting the trunk and arching the back, all of which are large muscle activities.

After anywhere from 10 months to a year the child stands and balances, and then begins to walk with a continuous day after day repetition. He sits down and rises, falls and gets up, in other words, fighting against gravity is his major activity.

Holding up the head and grasping with the hands are among the first activities of a child, and together with sucking and crying, are instinctive physiological responses. Meanwhile, the legs are being conditioned to move the body from place to place. Grasping, holding and pulling serve to bring objects to the body, hold it in position in relation to the environment, or pull the body toward the object that is heavier than itself.

That situation from which the extremities work is known as body position. Intrinsic movements act from a fixed base whose stability must be maintained by trunk musculature which fixes the base of support. Before a child can begin to develop coordinated skilled action of the intrinsic muscles, he must first build up strength and control of the muscles to maintain position.

Because the base of action requires training of the muscles of the abdomen, pelvis, trunk and shoulder girdle, these segments for effective extremity action, must be related to each other in optimum positions. For instance, since crawling is needed for the building up of muscles that later maintain the body in the erect position over the legs for standing and walking, it is the next step in the sequence which starts with trunk movements in lying. There is a logical basis for the emphasis which is placed on the major thesis, that antigravity muscles should receive more attention than is usually given in the planning of individual activities.

ACTIVITY PATTERNS

It is granted that running, jumping, climbing, throwing, and lifting are natural in play and are essential to a child's physical development. However, if a child has not yet built up his antigravity muscles so that his various body segments are not stabilized or cannot be held in proper relation to each other, and if he cannot hold the whole structure in proper balance for the static need of maintaining a continuous holding position and moving the body from place to place, basic postural changes will develop despite play or work activities.[1]

There should be balanced plans for early physical education, by which is meant alteration of emphasis in accordance with individual needs. The process of throwing everyone into the same hopper and expecting to care for differences is really absurd.

Children, who are developing normally with good spinal alignment and trunk control, may well have the emphasis placed on recreation aspects for the promotion of skills, endurance, and the satisfaction of participation. Adults may also utilize such media for maintenance purposes, yet ordinarily a play program alone is not adequate for best physical fitness.

The less well-developed children, and they are in the majority, who have not yet built up the power of basic trunk control against gravity, should receive more attention to trunk control as their fundamental need. It is obvious that attempting to force improved performance from an automobile whose essential parts are out of alignment, by increased performance without first correcting its faults, is a foolish approach just as it is with human beings.

Attention should be directed in exercise planning, to the basic essential need of doing sufficient big muscle work from positions which will facilitate the improvement of alignment, in order to prepare the less well-developed children for later life activities. Since all individuals have to fight gravity, it is essential that carry-over values be kept in mind in this phase as well as in other educational fields.

Properly devised plans for progressive development by whatever system chosen will use, as previously explained, certain working positions from which the sequence of exercises may move from the simple to the complex acts. The same principle holds good for both intrinsic and extrinsic muscle development. It is not wise to give a preponderance of exercises for intrinsic extremity muscles without sufficient emphasis on the stabilizers of their action in the body through their base fixators.

This is a sound engineering policy and if carried out, will not only produce improvement in execution of movements of skill, but also the proper maintenance of fundamental skeletal positions. Following out these principles upon which to build specific plans, it is necessary to make use of a variety of body positions from which to work, taking advantage of the main starting or base positions.

For the posturally needy who are in the majority, exercises should be used in order of difficulty. For those who tire easily, it is desirable to change back from the more complicated movements to those in a sitting or lying posture. This will reduce the stress on the whole neuro-motor mechanism from highly coordinated movements, to easier big muscle work in more favorable positions. In this way the greatest amount of activity may be obtained, in the prescribed time allotment, and without danger of injury.

PRECAUTIONARY MEASURES

In the administering of remedial activities, many different types of conditions are found which demand modification of programs. Students may be broadly classified as (a) those capable of indulging in a wide range of activities, yet refraining from certain forms of participation unsuitable to their condition in such adapted sections, (b) those who because of the nature of the case are assigned work with a developmental class, and (c) those others with conditions of a more severe or restricted form who are relegated to a rehabilitation program.

Many such classes are composed of all three types of sections within a single grouping, with attention being personalized as a part of the group. Assignments are designated to make necessary adjustments, but require alertness on the instructor's part to avoid any shifting by students who should refrain from some forms of activities which might be harmful by inclusion in sections outside their sanctioned sphere of action.

This sub grouping eliminates one of the arguments against separating such students from regular classes, which causes them to lose social contacts with others. Under such a plan it is possible to take advantage of all play values, offer companionship, furnish an invigorating competitive element, feel the association of team work, and achieve the sense of accomplishment in doing together technically difficult movements.

On the other hand, the degree of excitement, amount of stimulation, quality and quantity of effort may suffer through such a scheme, unless definite control is maintained. However, as a whole, the benefits far outweigh the unfavorable aspects with such class organization.

MODIFIED SPORTS ACTIVITIES

The use and adaptation of regular physical education class activities such as games, stunts and relays, rhythmical forms and mimetics are advisable whenever possible. Many of these elements of the program may be adjusted and adapted to the level of ability of special students, and are temporary substitutes for the more strenuous regular game. Skills of throwing, catching, batting, bouncing objects and other intricate movements can be developed as preparation for later use, while their immediate purpose and use serve to aid in overcoming students' present conditions.[2,3]

Research analysis of activities which will show the implications for usefulness in specific conditions is greatly needed. Data of this nature are already enlarging the scope of influence in developmental classes, making possible an expanded program of activities which may be adapted for a particular purpose. In spite of some progress in determining definite uses for modified sports activities, an opportunity exists for further investigation which may open new avenues of approach.

EXERCISE ADJUSTMENT

In many instances there are individuals incapable of participating in certain activities due to physical limitations, while others require very specific adaptation for their particular condition. It is difficult to visualize generalized movements being used to correct scoliosis, funnel chest, or flatfeet, unless definite exercises are fitted to the necessary action for correction.

Each divergency has a requirement of its own as far as development or correction is concerned. The procedure sometimes used, whereby all class members are given similar exercises whether the particular movements are individually indicated or not is unwise, and will accomplish little real good specifically. In the main, classes conducted in such a way have value to the total fitness, but there must also be additional applications particular to certain differences in needs.

Each distinguishing characteristic of the limiting circumstance must be established, while the essential muscle demand as well as the explicit origin, insertion, and action of each muscle needs to be determined. Information of this nature is indispensable in all instances, thus permitting exercise adjustment to the limiting state.

CRITICAL ANALYSIS OF COMMON EXERCISES

Cautionary judgment is advised in respect to several generally accepted practices in connection with many traditional exercises, such as the dips, sit ups, leg raising, deep knee bends, and questionable foot practices. The mechanical execution of such movements is contraindicated for the intended purpose, since other problems arise in this reference than are immediately obvious.[4] It is imperative that exercises be used as replacements in which the hazards or kinetic faults are removed.

Any exercise which is to be employed for a test, strengthener, or on a therapeutic basis should be evaluated most carefully from the dynamic angle. Numerous activities may be perfectly proper when available to those persons whose body segments are in balance and correctly aligned. However, when scrutinized as to their application for the average student, there is much to question. The following examples are cited to show why some exercises should be eliminated or modified.

DIPS OR PUSH-UPS

Primary actors in this movement are the serratus magnus and pectorals, teres major and minor, and latissimus dorsi, in addition to the arm muscles. The weight of gravity in this movement pulls down on the head, requiring tension of the extensors or erector spinal and cervical vertebral muscles to hold it stable, causing the back and abdomen to sag. This necessitates strong flexion of the lumbar spine and hips with some contraction of the extensors of the pelvis. The action of the arms is similar to that of pushing, and it should be realized that flexion and extension of the arms is strenuous effort against weight resistance.

It is well known that gravity and rapid growth account for drooped shoulders, round shoulders, or round back in approximately 80 or 90 per cent of all cases. In these instances the rhomboids and trapezii are relaxed and there is an imbalance in the shoulder girdle, while their antagonists, the pectorals and serrati, tend to become shortened. These muscles in general get much more action than do the rhomboids.

In the immature overgrown individuals of the stout type or in rapidly growing lanky youngsters who have muscle insufficiency, the body weight in this prone position will be held by the sling action of the shortened serrati and pectorals. Consequently, they become further developed and shortened, tending to perpetuate the deviation and stretching the abdominal wall.

In a high proportion of students with compensatory or actual hollow back in which there is a tilted pelvis and tight psoas, the weight of the body against the fixation of the lower extremities is held by the tight psoas which pulls the spine further forward.

When a hollow back prevails, the abdominals are too long and the lower back muscles too short, which rotates the pelvis forward. This load results in a sag in the abdomen allowing the visceral organs to become displaced. The use of dips should be reserved for that time when segmental alignment and balance have been accomplished, and there is sufficient strength to execute them properly, otherwise the postural deviation may become habitual and hence cause much harm.

Care and discrimination should be used in giving this exercise to girls and women because of its effect on the pelvic joint ligaments, which in older girls tend to be relaxed normally just before and during the menstrual period.

Alternate exercises to use instead of the dips and push-ups to develop the same general areas are described in the last chapter, page 209, dealing with exercises for specific conditions.[5]

SIT-UPS

Although there are many variations used in doing the sit-ups, the most common techniques are of three types, descriptions of which were forwarded to a prominent orthopedist for the purpose of obtaining an opinion as to their effectiveness.

1. From a back lying position with the feet spread about 2 feet apart and with the fingers interlocked behind the head, the subject raises to a sitting position and touches his elbow to the

opposite knee in alternate order. The movement is continued and the score is represented by the total number of sit-ups made. The feet are held down by inserting under a supporting object or by a partner. No bouncing or rolling over on the elbow is permitted.

2. The same exercise as above is performed while sitting on a low bench with the feet placed under a stall bar if available. A check is advised for the instructor, who palpates the interspace between the upper portions of the abdominal recti to see if there is a widening of the interspace which is called a diastasis, because there have been cases of ventral hernias at this location occurring from this exercise. The throat should be kept open to avoid downward pressure by the diaphragm.

3. A further variation starts from the bench with the fingers touching but not interlocked behind the head, or may be modified by using the fist clenched above the shoulders to avoid the tendency to push the head forward. With foot support, and knees slightly flexed, the trunk is lowered in a hyperextension of the back until a point 3 or 4 inches from the floor is reached, then returning to the upright position.

The request for information was directed toward securing judgment regarding two major points through use of these exercises; namely, as a method of developing the abdominals, and as a means of testing the strength of the abdominal musculature. The returned opinion stated that:

In order to do this the abdominal musculature has to contract, but only on the basis of fixation. The actual work is being done by the psoas. In all three of the movements you describe, it is the chief muscle involved as the intrinsic flexor. There is a fair activation of the adductor longus and the muscles fastened to the anterior spine which control inward and outward deviation when the legs are raised or which are activated when the legs are held fixed. They help in pulling the pelvis forward on the leg and the psoas raises the body forward on the pelvis. The insertion of the adductor longus is high up on the symphysis—consequently, it is an opponent to the rectus abdominus.

A high percentage of individuals have either a normal lumbar curve or an exaggeration of it up to a lordosis, in which case the pelvis is in a position of flexion in relation to the leg. Consequently the psoas, adductor longus, sartorius and tensor fascia are all in a shortened position. Why one should wish to develop them to shorten them still further is hard to understand. I will agree that if you have strong enough abdominal muscles to keep your back flattened while you do these exercises, you may develop both abdominals and psoas but if the majority of individuals examined have a forward inclination of the pelvis then it would seem to me that it is not a good exercise.[6]

Quoting further from the reply, the following exercise is recommended as a substitute for both strengthening and testing of the abdominal muscles:

In regard to testing the strength of the abdominal musculature, the pulling up movements from the supine lying position, bending the head forward and then gradually raising the chest and legs at the same time decreases any pull on the psoas and forces the load on the abdominals. In this way a fairly localized effort can be estimated.

I would say that these exercises are harmful and should be discontinued because I believe the basic effort should be put on fundamental exercises and not upon those which tend to accentuate segmental deviations.[7]

Again caution must be given regarding the danger of provoking a hernia when the glottis is closed during all such strenuous exercises of a similar nature, as well as from the downward thrust of the diaphragm against the fixed abdominal wall.

SUPINE LEG RAISING

Far too often, it has been customary to use leg raising in back lying as an abdominal strengthener, perhaps due to the fact that the abdominal muscles tense during its execution as a defense reaction. The psoas magnus and all other hip joint flexors and directional control muscles are actuated to accomplish the leg raising, either when lifted singly or both legs at a time. Before such action can take place, the weight of the legs must be overcome and unless the abdominals act to hold the pelvis still, this load will tip the pelvis forward into further flexion at the hip joints.

Because such a high percentage of all students have some degree of lordosis in which there is an imbalance between lower trunk muscles, or shortened sacrospinalis and lengthened abdominals, and since the pelvis is flexed on the thighs with the psoas magnus adaptively shortened, this exercise only tends to make the hip flexors even shorter and to increase the segmental imbalance.

Although the muscles may become more powerful, intrinsically it is not sensible to habituate faults in alignment by further shortening muscles that are already too short. This is especially true of the flexor aspect because in growing youngsters, structural changes will tend to perpetuate such skeletal imbalances.

DEEP KNEE BEND

A variety of the ordinary deep knee bend is the pose attained in the full squat position, duck waddle, and the Russian bounce. These exercises should be avoided as they contribute to the production of chronic synovitis, similar to but more exaggerated than the condition known as a football knee. Such exercises place undue stress upon the joints and ligaments of the knee, and subject them to accidental twists and strains.

Whereas, the knees take sufficient beating during life to call for special care and protection, faulty use and activities that have potentials for the early onset of arthritic changes should be avoided. When the subject is in a full bend position, the anterior portion of the joint is pushed forward and the extensors stretched, while the posterior aspect must support the entire body weight with the flexors tensed.

If the object is to stabalize the entire knee, the internal rotators especially must also be strengthened, which is possible through the use of exaggerated pigeon-toed walking for short distances, when supplemented with stair or hill climbing. The desired purpose may also be assisted by (a) bicycle riding, either actually, or using the movement in back lying, (b) stepping over low objects which necessitate lifting of the entire leg, or (c) running with high knee action.

IMPROPER FOOT PRACTICES

Because of the high ratio of foot and leg deviations, it is advisable to consider some of the wise as well as unsound practices. Every effort should be directed to establishing the best structural support with exercise aimed at remedying faults in alignment for standing and walking, in order that the weight may be largely borne on the bony framework, and stress on ligaments and muscles may be decreased to a minimum.

Feet should be used in a position approaching the parallel rather than the old *toe out* stance. When the feet are straight ahead, the knees are slightly rotated outward, thus raising the arch and throwing the weight on the outer borders. This position will assist in correcting pronation and reduce the tendency for lengthening and flattening of the long arches. It will also aid in prevention of eversion and abduction which are elements in flat-feet or factors in reducing the potentiality toward such divergencies. Therefore, instructors should seek to avoid positions that are conducive to toeing out action in activities, for it is a known fact, that, if for no other reason, performance is improved through proper foot position which allows the muscles and joints to function correctly.

A questionable exercise, which will not stand up under kinetic analysis in relation to the corrections for which they are ordinarily given, is the *rising on the toes*. This movement is used to develop the gastrocnemius and soleus, or calf muscles, and further strengthening only shortens them more and throws additional stress on the balls of the feet. In consequence, the elongated plantar structures tend to stretch further and allow the arch to fall. Whenever the movement is used, the feet should be in the inverted position to prevent such stretching.

It is quite common practice in cases of flexible flatfeet to add *rising on the heels* as well, which activates the anterior tibial, dorsal toe extensors and the peroneus tertius. In such flatfeet the falling of the middle of the foot means that the front and back abutments of the arches are lifted, and the gastrocnemii behind and anterior tibials in front have had to become adaptively shortened. Since they must carry more load because the bony arches do not do so, they become overdeveloped. Therefore, they do not need more exercise which would tend to habituate the deviation. Thus, it may be seen how easy it is for such conditions to be made worse and perpetuated by the very exercises which are so thoughtlessly used for correction purposes.

Care must also be used in giving the *curl toes* exercises in flexible feet because the action of the big toe flexors will cause an upward thrust on the distal end of the first metatarsal, which should remain down in a depressed position as the front bony support. If the exercise of inversion is used to cause development of the posterior tibials, the anterior tibial which is a synergist and also acts in inversion may be made stronger, so that its supinating action further flattens the arch.

The best exercise to maintain the inverted position and throw the weight on the border of the feet is outward thigh rotation, for when the arch is down and the feet pronate, the outer rotators of the leg are stretched. Hence, they should receive special attention and the antigravity thigh rotation exercise is indicated.

As pointed out many years ago, the fact that special emphasis in development of outward thigh rotators tends to aid in preventing and correcting valgus ankles and pronated flexible flatfeet, has now been accepted.

In this action the mortise of the ankle joint grips the astragalus or ankle bone, so when the rotators of the upper end of the leg act, there is a corresponding effect at the lower end and the foot is twisted outward just as though a socket wrench had been applied to it. Note that the big toe joint should be held down strongly on the floor, so that the action of the anterior tibial mentioned above does not lift it off the floor by its supinating movement. This action will actuate the peroneus longus, the chief pronator of the forefoot.

Another fact to remember is that the *improper carrying of the body weight produces foot faults*. First, the pelvic segment is too far forward and causes pressure on the forefoot that then tends to put too much stress on the plantar structures, and secondly, because of the rotatory thrust inward due to muscular laxity which is further accentuated in the presence of knock knee, bowlegs or tibial torsion.[8]

The major muscle of importance in relation to the leg rotation is the pyriformis, which is attached to the front of the upper portion of the sacrum and passes out through the sciatic notches to fasten to the hip bones and great trochanters. Because of its attachment the sagging of the feet inward will rotate the leg in and tend to pull the upper end of the sacrum downward and forward.

Outward thigh rotation is of benefit to the *sacro-iliac* area as well as to the feet. This is due to the fact that the pyriformis muscle is the only one that crosses the sacro-iliac joint. Since this joint is under great stress from weight bearing, it is essential to keep it in good alignment and to reduce the ligamentous stress. As already mentioned, it is wise for older girls and women to avoid all heavy or asymmetrical exercises just before and during the menstrual period because of the laxity of the pelvic ligaments.

FURTHER DEBATABLE EXERCISES

The continuing practice of using exercises about which there is some question or without thorough appreciation as to their real applicability is to be frowned upon. Many of these calisthenics have been accepted as remedial exercises when they were originally intended for other purposes, such as development of strength, grace of form and movement, skill in action, and rhythm. For this reason, all exercises should be analyzed as to their benefits and possible dangers before attempting to apply their use to those persons who have existing weaknesses.

LUNGING

Weak feet may be easily injured rather than aided through an exercise such as lunging with the toes out and coming down hard on a flat floor. The movement in itself can accomplish little real good in terms of development, and when utilized should be carried on with the use of a mat to eliminate the jar. Skipping rope likewise causes considerable pounding and mats should also be used in this case.

BACKWARD BEND

Due to the large number of students who already have varying degrees of hollow back with stretched or relaxed abdomens, the assigning of back bending exercises should be of concern. This exercise tends to develop further the extensors of the low back, that are already too short, and to increase the flexion of the pelvis on the legs. It thereby pulls the shortened hip flexors or iliopsoas, which, being attached to the front of the lumbar spinal vertebræ, only drags it further forward. It is suggested that this movement be eliminated.

OVERDEVELOPMENT OF PECTORALS

There is a tendency to overdevelop muscles that are already too short in the upper trunk and shoulder girdle. Dips or push-ups have already been dealt with previously, but there are other activities which contribute to this condition. It should be realized that when the pectoral muscles have become habitually shortened, the shoulders are drawn forward and the scapulæ spread apart. This shifts the arm weight forward of the lateral gravity line and requires a compensatory increase of the dorsal curve of the spine backward.

In the presence of a fatigue slump, this only tends to perpetuate a malposture common to 90 per cent of the people, and against which these persons must fight all their lives, since it ages the vertebral joints more rapidly than would otherwise be the case.

Too often, coaches overlook the need for developing posterior muscle groups as a means of increasing efficiency in athletics. When such essential means are recognized and put into practice, present records in which the upper segments of the body are involved should increase accordingly. The same principle applies to all other portions of the body and may well provide the answer to even greater athletic achievements.

CHINNING

In connection with overaction of the pectorals, a word regarding the hand hold for chinning is advisable. When the hands are clasped with fingers toward the face, greater pectoral action is involved, whereas in palms facing outward the directional pull is changed and greater activation takes place in the brachioradialis. With hands facing inward so that they are closer together and the arms in inward rotation, there is insufficient action of the antagonists of the pectoral, for example, the scapular adductors and outward rotators of the arms.

TUMBLING AND PYRAMID BUILDING

It is believed that these activities are ill advised for the elementary and junior high ages, because the stresses on the growth centers and joints are likely to provoke actual or potential injury. This is especially true in case there is a discrepancy between the chronological and the physiological ages or in weight and height

12

differences. Special care must be used in all handling of stout type boys and girls in this connection.

ILLUSTRATIONS THROUGH CASE STUDIES

A few instances of injuries caused or accentuated by ill-advised use of certain activities or exercises may be instructive, as shown through the following case studies.[9]

Case 1.—A young man, 18 years of age of medium build, wished to do some hard exercising to prepare himself for probable military service. He came for advice because in early childhood he had played competitive tennis and basketball and admitted having some low backache after a game. X-ray pictures of the lower spine and pelvis showed that his last lumbar vertebra had slipped forward on the sacrum about ½ inch, causing a luxation called spondylolisthesis.

He might have easily developed a complete dislocation with possible paralysis from weight lifting, pyramid building, a twist in wrestling or other torsion movement, or in jumping from a height, in which instance he might well have injured one or more of the nerve roots where they exit from the spinal canal. He was advised and accepted an operation for correction of the defect.

Case 2.—This university student 20 years of age, complained of shin splints. Running, jumping, skipping rope and other similar activities in a physical fitness course produced pain over the shin. Examination showed acute inflammation of the periostium or covering of the bone, evoked by the jerk on the anterior tibial muscle attachments incident to relaxed flatfeet.

Such incidents or symptoms from exercising in uncorrected positions in the presence of static faults is common. If they occur after structural maturity, what will happen to the immature skeleton of the teen-ager?

Case 3.—This boy of early high school age, came to the hospital with severe sciatic pain with absence of patellar and ankle reflexes. He had been injured in football 1 week prior to admission. He was of slight build and weighed 132 pounds. Upon operation, the cartilaginous disk, between the fourth and fifth lumbar vertebræ was found crushed and the nerve caught. Atrophy of the leg had been present for a long time, and with the release of the nerve and repair of the vertebræ, recovery was then possible.

Case 4.—This 15-year-old boy, with mild knock knees and weak feet, came in because of pain over the tibial tubercles just where the anterior thigh muscles attach. Pain resulted after playing competitive basketball in which the sudden starting and stopping, pivoting, shifting and jumping, imposed too much stress on the growth cartilage which was nearly pulled apart at the knee. This resulted in an osteochondritis or the so-called Schlatter-Osgood disease. Weeks in casts were required to allay the symptoms and allow nature to correct the condition.

Case 5.—In this case, a 13-year-old lad of stout type, weighing 166 pounds, and nearly 6 feet tall, was used as base man in a pyramid team in junior high school. His instructor was located in one of the best known schools, but being ignorant of the potential for injury had not recognized the possible danger to the boy. He was a glandular case and was already too heavy to carry his own weight to say nothing of holding several times that amount.

The results were tragic. He was injured for life from having the growth caps or epiphyses crushed off both femora. There were, at one time, five different teen-age boys in adjoining beds of the hospital for this condition known as slipped epiphysis; all in traction and some of them awaiting surgery.

Case 6.—A tall lanky university student, reported complaining of pain in the right shoulder which came after practicing the javelin throw. The diagnosis was obviously inflammation of the attachment of the pectoralis muscle on the humerus. This illustrates what has been mentioned previously under tight pectorals.

Every time he drew his arm back, the short pectoral would jerk on its attachment, and since it was the chief agonist in hurling the spear forward it would jerk again. If he had had complete range of backward motion with ample strength of control in the scapular adductors, he would not have developed the painful shoulder.

Case 7.—The physician called to see a muscular boy of 11 years of age, regarding pain in the upper abdominal wall. Inquiry elicited that this condition had developed a few days previous in a gym class at the junior high school. He said that the instructor made the class do dips 25 times in succession, and being a gritty lad had kept it up even after he felt soreness.

Examination showed that the fascia between the upper recti abdominals had been stretched and separated in what is called diastasis, and why he did not develop an abdominal hernia is not known. Such a procedure at this age showed little if any knowledge of the dynamics involved in this exercise on the part of the physical education instructor.

Excessive strain of the stretched abdominal wall, as has been explained under dips, could have caused one of three or four types of rupture. This boy called attention to an easily overlooked fact, that on the slippery gym floor his feet would slip and let him down with a jerk, thus causing even greater strain.

Case 8.—A lad of 12 years of age complained one day that his knees hurt. When his father inquired about his limp, the answer was, "I just can't take the exercises they give at our junior high school." In taking a history of the injury, he stated, "they had to do a duck waddle for a whole period." What resulted was a very acute traumatic synovitis of both knees from the successive pinching of the synovial folds under the tension of the tightened quadriceps over the patella.

The pinching caused swelling so that the lining became congested. Hence, the lining got in the way and was pinched more and more, producing an acute inflammation which caused the increase of joint fluid. This position was stretching the joint capsule until the youngster could hardly walk. His knees had to be aspirated to draw off the excess fluid and tied up on splints until the inflammation subsided.

As a result, two weeks attendance was lost from school plus the actual average daily attendance cost amounting to a loss of $35.00

to the taxpayers, to say nothing of the medical costs to the family and discomfort and loss of time to the boy. Is such a loss justified? Are the taxpayers carrying an indirect load because of the lack of training of teachers and coaches? Or does their lack of interest in the health aspect and failure to share responsibility for some portion of this load discredit them as teachers?

In conclusion may it be said a strong feeling prevails that more attention and heed should be given by all physical education instructors and coaches to the major premises brought out in this chapter, not only to make their work safer, but also to give them protection from criticism. By failing to understand or apply the basic fundamentals from a sound kinesiological standpoint, or to appreciate the fact that by repeating certain traditional exercises which they have either learned or observed that are illogical and unsound, they may be doing actual harm. True, these exercises may still be used by the armed forces or taught by other physical and recreation directors and yet be unwise. It is also possible that they are retarding the form and development which they wish to attain for the student.

There is widespread concern over the fact that so many leaders are satisfied with conducting a lot of reruns in relation to exercises, rather than endeavoring to face the problems confronting them in an intelligent manner. Many believe that the schools must help in meeting changing conditions, questioning the *status quo*, and reflecting a favorable attitude toward experimentation which may furnish some of the answers.

It is a travesty that physical education does not stress even more greatly the education aspect than it sometimes does, for the two are conjoined, and what is done with youth in turn reflects as to how they will be when they are older.

Our nation must depend for its future not only on those who are healthy or able, but upon all its citizens including the underpar who likewise have a contribution to offer. Since this nation cannot afford to carry them as mere substitutes, the talents of each child and adult must be sought out and developed to the highest level of which he is capable. One can no longer be satisfied with good enough, and as leaders all must be dedicated to the tasks ahead.

REFERENCES

1. LOWMAN, CHARLES LeROY: Faulty Posture in Relation to Performance, J. Health, Phys. Educ., Recreation, *29*, 14–15, 1958.
2. V-5 ASSOCIATION OF AMERICA: *Conditioning Exercises, Games, Tests.* 3rd ed. by Karl C. H. Oermann, Carl Haven Young, *et al.*, Annapolis, Maryland, United States Naval Institute, 1960, pp. 73–118.
3. LOWMAN, CHARLES LeROY, COLESTOCK, CLAIRE, and COOPER, HAZEL: *Corrective Physical Education for Groups.* New York, A. S. Barnes and Co., 1928, Chapters XXIX and XXX.

4. *Ibid.*, Chapter XIII.
5. *Cf.* post, p. 209
6. STEINDLER, ARTHUR: (Personal communication to Charles LeRoy Lowman).
7. *Ibid.*
8. LOWMAN, CHARLES LEROY: Feet and Body Mechanics, J. Health and Phys. Educ., *11*, 137, 1940.
9. Case Studies from personal files of Dr. Charles LeRoy Lowman and from the files of the Orthopedic Hospital, Los Angeles, California, where Dr. Lowman has been associated for many years.

The above references are not included in References for Extended Reading.

REFERENCES FOR EXTENDED READING

AINSWORTH, D. and EVANS, RUTH: *Basic Rhythms.* New York, Charwell House, Inc., 1955, 200 pp.

AMERICAN ASSOCIATION FOR HEALTH, PHYSICAL EDUCATION AND RECREATION: *Physical Education for High School Students.* Washington: Amer. Ass'n Health, Physical Education and Recreation, 1955. 406 pp.

BANCROFT, JESSIE H.: *Games for Playground, Home, School and Gymnasium.* New York, The Macmillan Co., 1937, 685 pp.

DANIELS, ARTHUR S.: *Adapted Physical Education.* New York, Harper Bros., 1954, 538 pp.
    Chapter IV: Principles of Organization and Administration.

EDWARDS, LINDEN FOREST: *Concise Anatomy.* 2nd ed., New York, McGraw-Hill Book Co., Inc., 1956, 502 pp.
    Chapter IV: General Myology.

EWERHARDT, F. H., and RIDDLE, GERTRUCE F.: *Therapeutic Exercise.* Philadelphia, Lea & Febiger, 1947, 152 pp.
    Chapter VII: Special Applications of Therapeutic Exercise.

GOFF, C. W.: Posture in Children, Clin. Orthop., *1*, 66–79, 1953.

HALE, C. J.: Changing Growth Patterns of the American Child, Education, *78*, 467–470, 1958.

HUNT, VALERIE V.: *Recreation for the Handicapped.* New York, Prentice-Hall, Inc., 1955, 340 pp.

JONES, EDWINA, MORGAN, EDNA and STEVENS, GLADYS: *Methods and Materials in Elementary Physical Education.* New York, World Book Co., 1957, 432 pp.

KRAUS, RICHARD: *Play Activities for Boys and Girls.* New York, McGraw-Hill Book Co., 1957, 236 pp.

LA SALLE, DOROTHY: *Rhythms and Dances for Elementary Schools.* New York, A. S. Barnes & Co., 1951, 201 pp.

LICHT, SIDNEY, (ed.): *Therapeutic Exercise.* New Haven, Conn.: Elizabeth Licht, 1958, 893 pp.
    Chapter XXXI: Exercise in Heart Disease.

LOS ANGELES CITY SCHOOLS: *Corrective Physical Education.* Los Angeles: Los Angeles Board of Education, 1958, 400 pp.
    Chapter VIII: Rhythms, Games, Stunts and Relays for Pupils in the
                Corrective Physical Education Class.

MASON, BERNARD, and MITCHELL, ELMER D.: *Social Games for Recreation.* New York, A. S. Barnes & Co., 1935, 421 pp.

MITCHELL, ELMER D.: *Sports for Recreation.* New York, A. S. Barnes & Co., 1952, 522 pp.

NEILSON, N. P., and VAN HAGEN, WINIFRED: *Physical Education for Elementary Schools.* New York, A. S. Barnes & Co., 1954, 552 pp.

OBERTEUFFER, DELBERT: *Physical Education.* Rev. ed., New York, Harper & Bros., 1956, 479 pp.
    Chapter VI: Physical Education and Organic Development.

SONTAG, L. W., and REYNOLDS, E. L.: The Fels Composite Sheet: I. A Practical Method for Analyzing Growth Progress, II. Variations in Growth Patterns in Health and Disease, J. Pediat., *5*, 194, 1934.

STAFFORD, GEORGE T.: *Exercise During Convalescence.* New York, Prentice-Hall Inc., 1947. 334 pp.

————: *Sports for the Handicapped.* New York, Prentice-Hall, Inc., 1947, 334 pp.

THOMPSON, GEORGE G.: *Child Psychology, Growth Trends in Psychological Adjustment,* Boston, Houghton Mifflin Co., 1952, 667 pp.

Chapter VII: The Development of Motor Abilities.

VAN HAGEN, WINIFRED, DEXTER, GENEVIEVE, and WILLIAMS, JESSE FEIRING: *Physical Education in the Elementary Schools.* Sacramento, California State Dept. of Education, 1951, 1004 pp.

Chapters VII–XXI: Games and Activities.

CHAPTER 9

Procedural Specifications

BEFORE accepting a bid for any form of construction work, an architect must inform himself as to what the client's desires or aims may be. Then after surveying the site, he prepares a blueprint and specification with requisites or objectives for accomplishing the aim or purpose. Another way of expressing such an undertaking is in terms of mission and tasks.

In this instance the *mission* of the developmental or adapted physical education classes may be stated as preventive, developmental, adaptive, habilitative, restrictive and rehabilitative. Student or even adult needs generally fall within one of these categories, and the purpose of such programs, whether they be in school, recreation, clinic or hospital situations must be directed toward the solution of these problems and meeting the blueprint specifications.

Characteristic of best programs and what makes them click is attention to the elements which constitute essentials. This requires delving into the *tasks* confronting the instructor, and attempting to anticipate the minutiæ on every hand to assure preparedness. Succinctly stated, these include such items as survey of situation, selection and assigning of students, class procedure, motivational techniques and evaluation. Readiness for these responsibilities enables one to plan his work and then work his plan.

Space does not permit extensive delineation of every phase of possible procedure, and although those means which are described cover the background for the picture, the artist himself must supply the colors and form which best project the particular painting. To best determine the authenticity and practicability of past and present practices demands utilization of all available resources including research, extensive use of reference materials, visitations, observations and experimentation. From all these sources it is then possible to deduce ideas from others, incorporate these with personal experiences, and blend them into a working unit.

Rather than making the attempt to segregate the approach to application of these principles in conformability with various ages and grade levels, the eclectic concordance approach is followed. That is, the basic fundamental doctrines or tenets are considered to be significant in guiding the conduct in all situations. It is in the degree of emphasis and restraint that such differences in applicability must be made.

If this be so, visual perception is indicated in evolving constructive and purposeful programs that incorporate all possible desirable features, yet establish safeguards contingent with known facts. Thus, wise counsel of physicians and qualified instructors working as a team together, will not condone mediocrity nor countenance incidents which are not conducive to the furtherance of the mission. Those who are in such positions of trust must be hand picked on the basis of their breadth of experience, knowledge of the subject matter, and desirable attitudes, all of which enable them to work for and with people.

CLARIFICATION OF THE MISSION

Within the statement of the mission are found several premises which call for clarification regarding the job to be done. Each concept in itself deals with the nature of the work to be undertaken rather than the condition or manner of treatment. What is done in behalf of one phase may well have reciprocal value in another, but neither is considered as having distinctive functions. A description of the terminology of reference cited below, seeks to delineate as to the separate differences in the nature of the work.

PREVENTION

Students who are found to have incipient or potential weaknesses which may result in future maladjustment, are considered to be in need of preventive work. This may be in the form of referral to a physician, assignment to rest, adjustment of program, providing counsel, or in conjunction with the parents striving to eliminate all possible causes. When certain activities are indicated, it is important to make them available and suitable to the occasion.

DEVELOPMENT

Many students are weak because they lack the tools to carry out the job, which calls for developmental emphasis to bring them up to par. Conditions may be present merely because some portion of the balance mechanism is not carrying out its share of the load in counterbalancing the structure. In this case the class exercises for the individual are directed to equalizing the agonists' and antagonists' relationships for better stabilization against gravitational strain. In a large proportion of instances the greatest need is for all round development and improvement of muscle tone, which may call for close cooperation with the health instruction classes, school nurse, classroom teachers, parents and physician in order to make more certain that nutritional status is satisfactory, health habits sound, and organic functioning properly adjusted.

ADAPTATION

Conditions which exist when students are recovering from accidents, convalescing from illness, or have modifying circumstances which make it inadvisable to partake in strenuous endeavors, make it necessary for adaptive planning. Some activities may be suitable and these must be determined, while other cases might best be served through rest and relaxation. Heart cases, nervous circumstances, hernias, asthma, loss of limbs and similar limitations will prescribe the form of activity, so that the program is adapted rather than the student making the adjustment.

HABILITATION

People must learn to live with certain disorders, including not only those who are handicapped, but also those subject to particular restraints. The anemic person or diabetic patient, also those with organic malfunctions of an hereditary or environmental nature, must understand what they can and cannot do safely. They must also be taught how best to maintain a state of fitness in spite of their condition, which oftentimes calls for an intertherapy approach with all other resources being used. This is habilitation or maintenance.

RESTRICTION

There are those who are definitely restricted as to many forms of activity due to their condition, where taking part in class activities might be dangerous. Participation must be limited to competition against themselves, the socializing values being derived from companionship with those in comparable situations or circumstances. There are the blind who are capable of skills and contests of strength such as wrestling, the rheumatic fever cases whose prescription makes no reference to taking any exercise, or in fact warns against its use, and the individuals with rheumatoid arthritis who must be closely guarded. All are examples of restricted cases for which provision must be made.

REHABILITATION

A major portion of those referred to classes for special attention are students who need to have specific work which will help in restoring or reestablishing them, or correct handicapping conditions. Of this type are those with poliomyelitis, cerebral palsy, congenital cases, pre- and post-operative needs, convalescent neuromuscular reeducation, and a great many others of similar seriousness which fall within this purview. When working with those in this area, close contact and interrelationships must be maintained with the physician, developmental instructor, therapist, school nurse, and classroom teachers.

It is easily seen that there are many ramifications to prepare for in such classes. A fairly large amount of the effort in working with the elementary and junior high school ages demands that greatest endeavor be directed toward the first five aspects, although rehabilitation may also require considerable attention. In high school and college greater stress needs to be placed upon the latter four phases, since prevention and development should have already been cared for in the earlier years.

That these elements are so closely related as to make difficult any segregation by types is accepted, although an appreciable amount of adjustment in class procedure would be required to care adequately for the many variations.

AGE VARIATIONS IN FUNDAMENTAL NEEDS

From the teachers' standpoint, technical differences naturally exist in elementary, junior high school, senior high school, and college levels of practice, because of the dissimilarities in age levels, individual needs, facilities, and the activities involved. However, from the pedagogical viewpoint the know how or tricks of the trade which is the art or practice of teaching technique, is more or less alike throughout these school ages.

Some disparities in degree, from the standpoint of immaturity and maturity and the psychological variants, due to such phases of development are found which may demand special consideration. In spite of these variations, there are still some common practices that make for sequential progression toward the desired goal. Herein are presented basic differences in emphasis and needs as to the two broad categories, remembering that there are in turn levels in these respects between the elementary and junior high school, and the senior and college groups.

ELEMENTARY AND JUNIOR HIGH SCHOOL

The importance of child development in the years spent in the elementary schools is becoming increasingly recognized as the most important time in the entire school life of the child. Elementary school education reaches the largest number of boys and girls and furnishes the background for their entire life, while the pre-elementary and junior high school age as well can not be over-estimated.

These stages in the child's life are the foundation upon which the present and later structure must be built. They are the periods of greatest growth, the formative period for habit and judgment, and the period for fundamental training in mental, social and psychological reactions. Too much time, money and effort cannot be spent in these important years, for the development of the child should receive primary consideration in every school system.[1]

Generally speaking the child *needs* a maximum opportunity to grow, for growth is a characteristic of life, and education is intended to assist in the process. The ability to grow depends upon supplying basic needs which are most demanding during these periods. In order to cultivate growth there should be an increase all along the line in terms of activity, and the organism must have an appetite for work which physical fitness and interest require.

When a child understands his environment in relation to his present and future, he develops habits which give him control over environment and the ability to utilize this power to his personal advantage. Contacts and responsibilities inherent in group activity from the altruistic and egoistic standpoint help in character development.

Big muscle activity supplies a stimulus to growth and may be found in play or recreational activities, while health instruction and rest are likewise factors in developing a strong physical background. Thus, desirable hereditary traits and powers are developed which make for social usefulness and individual happiness, and programs must have sufficient interest to influence the child both while in or out of school.

Inherent in the programs should be consideration for (*a*) the total health, nutrition, fatigability, endurance, and malposture, (*b*) promotion of physiological improvement without added strain, (*c*) receiving of therapeutic values found in recreational activities which enable the student to better handle his school work and outside program, and (*d*) development in fundamental skills commensurate with his ability, which will be therapeutic rather than deleterious.

Students should not be deprived of group activities with their resulting development of the sense of fair play, courtesy, justice and honor, but the activities may need to be modified as to the character, forcefulness, range or frequency of participation, in order to obtain these values without endangering the child.

HIGH SCHOOL AND COLLEGE

Therapeutic considerations at this age level differ somewhat from those of the elementary and junior high school, although the basic fundamentals are largely the same. The chief differences are those of growth as related to physical deviations, those of skills, activities and postural faults as referring to the more mature skeletal and organic capacities of the post adolescent age. There is, however, no sharp dividing line, for the period of pubesence is quite variable and in many instances may extend into the late teens. Sexual and skeletal maturation are often delayed well into the high school or college age, although some precocious youngsters may be well advanced in this respect at 13 or 14 years of age.

Likewise, there may be marked irregularities in physiological age, chronological age, mental and social levels. For example, a girl 12 years old and as tall as an 18 year old had physiological development equal to most high school girls, well established menses, secondary sex changes well advanced, and an intelligence quotient of 128. Her skeletal age was so delayed that she had developed a marked round back from delayed development of vertebral growth centers. This resulted in a severe kyphosis, and a social behavior of a youngster of 10 years of age. In fact she had little sense of right and wrong and would appropriate small belongings of her classmates without the slightest idea that she was stealing. She was amoral but not immoral.

As previously indicated, the major *need* in these years is to seek improved body mechanics. This is considered as segmental consciousness, the vision and feeling of proper posture of the body parts and a kinesthetic sense within the muscles as to development of their relationship to the environment.

This position sensing, or kinesthetic tactile mechanism, and the sensory registration of the position of the joints and the degrees of tension in ligaments and muscles controlling them, requires education or reeducation in altering faulty postural habits and building new and more correct habit patterns. As the development of coordination and strength in the antigravity muscles is basic in maintaining posture, both statically and dynamically, it is wise that all students understand the importance of antigravity exercises. They should also realize that the condition of these muscles, and the discipline needed to keep the body in the best position for all movements of skill, aid in the development of endurance and the maintenance of an attractive personality throughout life.

There is little question that more severe conditions may be found in these age brackets, for many young people have either neglected or considered these divergencies as immaterial, whereas in reality they are really serious.   For this reason there may be a greater preponderance of rehabilitation work necessary, for unless something is done at this time, little correction may be made.

IMPLICATIONS OF THE TASKS

Constituents of the program vary somewhat in respect to the nature of the particular state of affairs or locale.   Yet within the declaration of tasks are set forth the procedural steps necessary for administrative organization in nearly any circumstance. Successful completion of the following tasks are at least some assurance that the mission may be accomplished.[2]

Achievement in the performance and use of these tools rests mainly upon the comprehension and experience of the operator. At this stage the construction engineer takes over from the architect and interprets the specification, surveys the site, prepares for the equipment and supplies, selects and assigns his workers, plans for and proceeds with actual construction.   Upon completion of the structure, it must successfully pass an inspector's check.

Developmental or adapted physical education instructors are serving in a similar capacity, for without foresight something is bound to be overlooked.   To capably carry out such an important assignment requires even more than the equivalent training compared to that of the clinical technicians, for the lives of human beings are involved.   Insight and tact as well as ingenuity and dedication are requisites which must characterize these leaders, and the greater the breadth and depth of their thinking the greater the length of influence to be derived from such programs.

SURVEY OF SITUATION

Before a definite program can be settled upon, it is necessary to know what there is to work with as far as facilities and equipment are concerned, as well as the conditions and needs of the particular situation.   All possible resources need to be ascertained and the potential assistance and support available be discovered. The information sought must oftentimes be subtly gathered in order to prevent misunderstanding and the creation of the idea that the instructor may believe in any divine rights of his own. He should emphasize the desire to be of assistance to the other instructors and classroom teachers, as well as coaches, in the solution of many common problems, thus inspiring confidence and cooperation on the part of the entire school membership.

Every attempt needs to be made to obtain a separate space from the regular classes in a portion of the gymnasium or special room, where interruptions are kept to a minimum, selective equipment may be reserved for the use of those who require it, and within which the climate may be such that ideas are caught and not taught, with a chance to germinate.

Some estimate of needs must be made as to the number of students to expect for enrollment in these classes, remembering that it will be possible in most instances to provide for only the third and second degree cases and those requiring rest facilities. Such data may be obtained in many schools from information supplied by the school nurse, prior to the postural or body mechanics screening which may at least show the students with medical conditions.

In case there are deficiencies apparent regarding facilities, equipment, supplies, overload for instructors, or possible gaps in service resources, the proper administrative authorities should be informed in order that they may make necessary adjustments or at least be cognizant of the situation. A condensed report in an easily perused form is more apt to be read and offers definite proof as to potential needs.

Presenting of such findings to the school health council is likewise a beneficial procedure, which may result in cooperation and participation by all those concerned with the solution of such problems.

SELECTING AND ASSIGNING OF STUDENTS

A detailed description of the various procedures used in the selection of students has previously been presented in Chapter 6, page 135. It may be advisable to conduct at some time during the term a follow-up appraisal of those students where doubt existed as to need. It is also to be expected that there will be students who, because of extenuating circumstances, should be chosen throughout the school year for inclusion in the special classes.

Assignment to developmental classes should if possible be made with the full consent of the student and parents. It has been found that when time is taken to inform them as to the needs and benefits possible, better cooperation accrues and the student will work for dear life to overcome his difficulties.

In some cases it may be best to assign certain students for only a portion of the class period for special work, returning them to their regular physical education class upon completion of the necessary exercise program. This dual plan is an excellent method of stimulating real interest on the part of the individual, but there must be close cooperation between the special and regular class teachers to make such coordination possible.

Continuous reappraisal is essential to avoid having students feel that once assigned to such classes, they are "stuck" there for an indefinite time. Whenever it is possible to return them to their regular classes, this should be done at any time in the semester. This means added incentive to get busy and correct the divergency and is a motivational influence to others in the class.

CLASS PROCEDURE

An extremely flexible schedule and not too heavy program should be arranged for the teacher assigned to such classes, for his responsibilities are many with the arranging of all exercise plans, examinations, consultations and record keeping. Classes must also be kept within bounds as to numbers if best results are to be expected, with a recommended class size ranging from 12 to 20 students. When facilities are adequate it is often possible to care for an even greater number, or by means of home assignments, to have students report weekly for check-ups and reassignment of exercises.

In large cities or in case programs have been in existence for some time, the class procedure may already be defined. Naturally there is always a chance for changes which may be beneficial in better handling of the work, but when supervisors are made responsible throughout a city their suggestions must be followed. Should a better plan be proposed by an instructor, most supervisors are amenable to changes which make for improved handling of classes.

Classes may be conducted in many ways, as for instance there are instructors who prefer (a) to group all students together according to various conditions supervising these groups at different times during the period, (b) to work with groups as a whole irrespective of their divergencies, with all students doing each exercise whether there be need for the movement or not, believing that at least no harm and possible benefit may result, and (c) to work individually with students within a group, each carrying on his own exercises according to individual requirements. The latter method would seem to be more applicable and make for specific correction in accordance with personal needs.

Certain students may require activity for a portion of the period and then make use of the balance of the class time in resting. Generally this type of individual belongs to the semi-restricted or nutritional classification, and may profit from a combination of activities of this nature.

Exercises are grouped according to type into passive, assistive, active, and resistive, with the purpose being two-fold—habit-freeing and habit-forming. In addition to the prescribed exercise phase, there is the emphasis on play activities which may be a part of the regular program or a supplemental portion in the latter part of the period. Where two teachers are working together in the same class, one instructor may supervise the play, while the other instructs in the exercises, or they may combine handling the exercises first, then supervise recreational activity later.

In clinics and hospitals it is customary to treat the cases one at a time. This is obligatory because of the severity of most of their conditions. The strength of the patient, number of exercises to be done, pace of the exercise, when to rest, mental attitude toward the activity, and his reaction to treatment are all necessarily important points to consider.

No matter what method of class organization may be followed, some variety should be arranged to make more interesting programs for students. Classes may start with a warm-up period, to be followed by the specific assignments, and then a recreational time in which all may join. Such a variety offers stimulation and pleasure, yet accomplishes the purpose for which the program is intended, causing students to seek enrollment rather than having to be pressurized to do something about their conditions. This is the attitude which is sought and when found is a worthy adjunct to the total physical education program offering.

MOTIVATIONAL TECHNIQUES

Motivating enthusiasm is the mainspring of education and is essential in the achieving of results with any form of program, but especially so with classes for the underpar. An indifferent student may be carried along by the enthusiasm of other teammates in some games or classwork, but improvement of one's posture or condition is an individual's own problem, and can be achieved only by his voluntary effort.

It is of consequence that the pupil's interest and responsibility be aroused, and that he participate in a cooperative frame of mind because he desires to improve. It is the task of the instructor to inspire, direct, explain, and sell the student as to the immediate and remote benefits resulting from careful application.

Attention to public relations is a form of motivation and the instructor must consider its importance not only from the standpoint of the student, but from the angle of the school, parents, physicians, and community as well. To meet the many diverse situations manifold ways and means must be employed including lectures or talks, newspaper articles, personal letters, visits to parents or family physician, exhibits and demonstrations, as well as visiting days.

An attractive atmosphere, acquaintance with the cause of his condition, and the possible means for correction becomes a real challenge to most students. Encouragement can frequently do more than any amount of "know how" by the instructor, and the presence of sincerity as well is soon reflected in the efforts of the student.

The use of numerous devices and techniques are of immeasurable value as motivational tools. The rapport between student and examiner offers the first contact for reaching the person, while use of the scales, photographs, silhouetteographs, schematographs, pedographs, tracings, charts and measurements also assist in the desired process.[3]

Various pieces of apparatus become added incentives, and games, stunts and relays have a certain lure for most young people when there is an element of competitive spirit present. The posting of sequential measurements and photographs, where others may see them, furnish enticement to still others to do something about their conditions, and the assistance to athletes has great meaning in that a satisfied customer is your best advertisement.

Service personnel found that cadets and young men with difficulties were most receptive to efforts at correction, and waiting lists were not unusual with these men requesting assignment. In large measure this was owing to the opporunity to see pictures of those who had taken such work, as well as being due to the passing around by word of mouth of good reports by those who had benefited through developmental or remedial measures.

Bulletin boards are an excellent medium for reaching students in the schools, with slogans and mottoes being displayed. Posture contests, tag days, skits, radio and television programs have been most effective in many situations. If an individual has the desire to participate in certain activities, a little explanation on the part of the teacher, parent, and particularly the physician, will do more than most any other thing to motivate student's interest in his own behalf.

Every means must be made use of in an effort to reach not only the young person, but the older people as well. Here is a chance for the community to become an active participant through clubs and other organizations, by sponsoring contests or projects to further such programs. Newspapers are especially effective through publication of articles, photographs, illustrations, and findings resulting from examinations and evaluation of the results of such classes.

Particular stress has been paid to the aspect of motivation, for all too few communities offer the opportunity for people who need such attention. If you have a worthwhile product to sell, which

13

you do, the entire community and nation should understand its worth in order that they too may include developmental or adapted physical education as a part of the regular school offering.

EVALUATION

Record keeping is a chore which all too few enjoy or will do, and yet, every bit of data collected from the initial contact to the final results should be entered. Such records are the only evidence of the findings, recorded schedule of activities or treatment given, and the results of the individual's progress. Every visual or manual device, which is used for appraisal purposes, is likewise useful for the motivation and evaluation of these persons.

The placing of mirrors in strategic spots is helpful, the keeping of weight charts serve their purpose, and x-ray pictures are further evaluative means. Students are smart enough to see for themselves objective evidence, and everyone is thrilled when needed adjustments are made. Most people have visions which they would like to achieve, and when they see with their own eyes their accomplishments, they are doubly fortunate.

The lack of scientific follow-up information and convincing evidence of results are the greatest drawbacks when submitting definite proof of progress. Presentation of reliable data must be offered to substantiate the claims so often made. Every administrator should require that at least an annual report be presented for his own and the school board's benefit. It is amazing how sparse and scattered are reports as to conditions found among students and adults in this nation. When research findings pertaining to the fitness of youth are published, the public become greatly concerned. Would they not be similarly upset if they were to be made acquainted with the facts in regard to the number of young people with handicapping conditions of posture?

There is no better method for presenting such data than through the compilation and publishing of such evaluations. An appraisal takes on new meaning and purpose when something is done about the situation. Such problems are not new but have been with us for many ages, and it is time that the entire nation realize that they are being shortchanged in many schools within their communities.

Pointing out procedural specifications should make more clear that for effective administration of a department like any business, standardization of practices, which still retain flexibility, is the fundamental basis for success. Knowing how to begin and what to do, are coordinate parts, and the preparation of plans on paper as to the program being conducted, forces the instructor to analyze and arrange procedures. Yes, a paper program is necessary just as is a blueprint and specifications, for without it too frequently the mission and tasks are not clear and, at least, such a plan gives direction toward a purpose.

REFERENCES

1. LOWMAN, CHARLES LEROY, COLESTOCK, CLAIRE, and COOPER, HAZEL: *Corrective Physical Education for Groups.* New York, A. S. Barnes and Co., 1928, Chapter XVII.
2. YOUNG, CARL HAVEN: A Procedure in the Organizing of a Corrective Physical Education Program for High School Boys. Unpublished Master's thesis, The University of Southern California, Los Angeles, 1935, 150 pp.
3. CROWE, WALTER CAMPBELL: The Use of Audio-Visual Materials in Developmental (Corrective) Physical Education. Unpublished Master's thesis, The University of California, Los Angeles, 1950, 219 pp.

The Above references are not repeated in References for Extended Reading.

REFERENCES FOR EXTENDED READING

HAWLEY, GERTRUDE: *The Kinesiology of Corrective Exercise.* 2nd ed., Philadelphia, Lea & Febiger, 1949, 192 pp.
    Chapter IX: Suggestion Relating to Practical Procedure in the Conduct of
           Remedial Exercise Classes.

HAYES, ASAHEL E.: Determination of Bases for Developmental Physical Education in the Public Schools. Unpublished Master's thesis, The University of California, Los Angeles, 1950, 109 pp.

KELLY, ELLEN D.: *Teaching Posture and Body Mechanics.* New York, A. S. Barnes & Co., 1949, 212 pp.
    Chapter IX: Teaching Fundamental Skills.

LOS ANGELES CITY SCHOOLS: *Corrective Physical Education.* Los Angeles, Los Angeles Board of Education, 1958, 400 pp.
    Chapter II: Organization and Administration.
    Chapter IV: Programs for Pupils with Specific Disabilities, Malformations,
           or Growth and Development Problems.

POLEY, M. S.: The Adapted Physical Education Program at the University of Oregon, J. Ass'n. Phys. & Ment. Rehabilitation, *11,* 81–84, 1957.

RAND, WINIFRED, SWEENEY, MARY E., and VINCENT, E. LEE: *Growth and Development of the Young Child.* 6th ed., edited by Marian E. Breckenridge and Margaret Nesbitt Murphy. Philadelphia, W. B. Saunders, Co., 1958, 548 pp.
    Chapter IV: The Child's Physical Equipment for Growth
               Development and Functioning.
    Chapter VIII: Aspects of Behavior and Their Development:
               Motor Development.

RATHBONE, JOSEPHINE L.: *Corrective Physical Education.* 5th ed., Philadelphia, W. B. Saunders Co., 1955, 318 pp.
    Chapter VII: An Exercise Program for Physical Education in Rehabilitation.
    Chapter IX: Administrative Problems.

SODEN, WILLIAM H.: *Rehabilitation of the Handicapped.* New York, Ronald Press Co., 1949, 399 pp.

STAFFORD, GEORGE T., and KELLY, ELLEN DAVIS: *Preventive and Corrective Physical Education.* 5th ed., New York, Ronald Press Co., 1958, 395 pp.
    Chapter X: Organization of Programs.

VAN HAGEN, WINIFRED, DEXTER, GENEVIEVE, and WILLIAMS, JESSE FEIRING: *Physical Education in the Elementary Schools.* Sacramento, Calif. State Dept. of Education, 1951, 1004 pp.
    Chapter II: The Elementary School Child.

YOUNG, CARL H., and CRAIG, ROBERT E.: "Control Objectives in Adapted Physical Education," *College Physical Education Association, 61st Annual Proceedings.* 1958, pp. 244–250.

CHAPTER 10

Exercise Precepts

SPECIFIC exercises and carefully chosen activities in the hands of specialists may well be delicate instruments of purpose, whereas when unwisely selected and administered they become unwieldy and harmful practices of doubt. Knowing how to use these tools to advantage and in an expert manner requires knowledge of their potential, understanding of their dangers, and skill in using them.

Caution is urged in such applications for it is not enough to have a set of prescriptions for promiscuous indulgence. This is the easy way and a fallacy which young teachers often believe sound, that for this condition you do *this* or that, never stopping to realize that *this* is not enough. They must know (when selecting an exercise) *what* indicates advisability for its use, *where* to avoid using it, *when* it applies, *how* to use it best, *why* it is being used, and *who* is competent to use it with advantage, for improper exercise and too strenuous activity may be as dangerous as penicillin to those who are allergic.

The human body will not change in our lifetime. The movements of the body's bones by the muscle motors will not vary no matter who classifies or describes them. Probably every possible combination of coordinated, skilled movements has been described by someone. The important thing for workers in the physical education and therapy fields is to *know* those joints and muscles, use this knowledge with imagination and resourcefulness, and apply it for the purpose needed.

Work of the developmental department may be a near failure if the instructor lacks ingenuity and tries to use routine formula exercises, learned at school or taken verbatim from someone's system of exercises. Too much statics and not enough dynamics become a deadly bore. The student cannot be blamed for feeling that he is wasting time in attending such classes, unless everything offered him has real significance to his life and needs. He must not be disappointed by a drab, dull, unvarying schedule, but must be able to accept readily and to put into daily practice what is being proposed.

It should always be remembered that whether it be for the mind or the body that exercises are given, they are one and inseparable and a part of the total educative process. Whatever the system followed, the major premise must not be lost sight of and the learning procedure should retain the elements of education.

PURPOSES OF EXERCISE PROGRAMS

Any exercise program whether it be intended for use in the home, school, hospital or any other situation, needs to be directed to the benefit of the individual. What may be sound for one may be detrimental to another, while action in one segment may have reciprocal involvement of other parts, so that it is impossible to say that specific exercises for a condition, without reference to other relations, will by themselves correct or rectify the divergency. Mere exercises are no panacea for all troubles, for when an adult says that he would like to get some exercises for his ptosis condition, there are other aspects involved such as glandular and nutrition checks, in other words interrelationships must be considered.

Generally, the purposes of exercises should include such points as:
(a) all-round development as well as specific muscle groups,
(b) adaptation to the needs of the individual, group, and particular situations,
(c) being physiologically, anatomically, biologically, dynamically and kinesthetically sound,
(d) serving to prevent divergencies and aiding in correction of minor weaknesses,
(e) improvement of definite muscle inadequacies through exercises which lend themselves to prevention of possible injuries,
(f) acting as preparation for strenuous participation in activities,
(g) increasing the postural stability through improvement of muscle tone and organic efficiency,
(h) providing activities which may be used by the individual in maintaining fitness.

FUNDAMENTAL PRINCIPLES

Of necessity, principles must be established to act as guide lines for reaching the purposes intended, and these are often diversified and complex. Among the several items are those which should:
(a) foster mental and physical stimulation, preferably requiring sufficient activity to arouse perspiration or for a work-out,
(b) employ exercises of a resistive nature for those able to indulge and modified for others,
(c) seek to involve the poorly developed and physically illiterate individual in suitable strenuous skill movements,

(*d*) consider the importance of sequence in the person's schedule, proceeding from the slower and easier movements to the more rapid tempo and vigorous actions, then returning to the decreased or relaxing forms or from complex to simple movements for change of pace instead of rest, yet endeavoring gradually to build up rather than to overload,

(*e*) select exercises which will involve all segments concerned, and various fundamental positions from which they are to be carried on.

REPRESENTATIVE EXERCISES FOR SPECIFIC CONDITIONS

Many kinds of exercises or activities are feasible for use in dealing with specific conditions, although only a sample of such are presented as representative suggestions which may be performed in a variety of ways. While being directed to explicit needs they in turn reflect implications for the total being, and in many instances over-lap in application. Only broad areas of emphasis are being considered at this time. Figure 45 shows a condition of post fracture with open reduction followed by a long period of convalescence, using walking cast: right leg one inch shorter, anterior superior crest of ilia uneven, pelvic torsion, scoliosis functional, and other postural divergencies. Figure 46 illustrates utilization of neuro-muscular reeducation, showing that stretching of heel cord has nearly corrected leg length, torsion is considerably improved, scoliosis is now minor, atrophy of calf has started to recover, body tilt and low shoulder nearly normal.

FITNESS COMPONENTS OF POSTURE

A great many constituents go together to make possible best postural stability and it is impossible to segregate any one element as being more important than another. Whenever the term fitness is used the question should be asked, fitness for what? In reference to posture it might well be assumed to mean, the most efficient structural and functional alignment which assures effective action in supplying all bodily needs. Among the components for which exercises might be prescribed are the following, although a particular activity described for use in one instance may have equivalent value in each of the others.

Muscle tone is a condition of partial muscle contraction with certain physical properties such as elasticity, irritability and contractility characterizing this state. Bechtol defines muscle tone "as the resistance of a muscle to passive movements of its joints."[1]

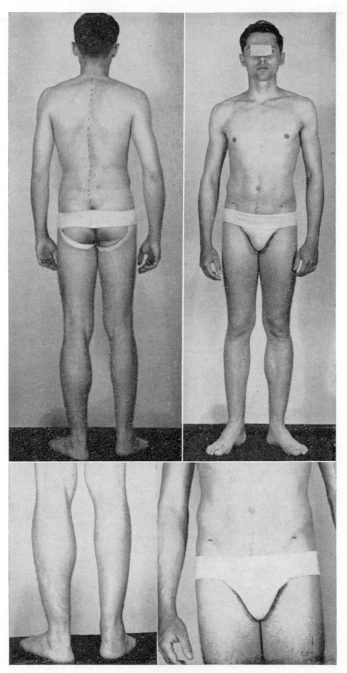

FIG. 45.—Result of walking cast after fracture.

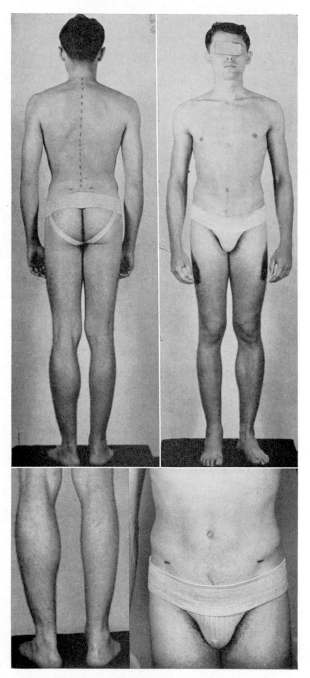

Fig. 46.—Result of 9 days' specific exercise program.

When a segment of the body is moved, a muscle or muscles are shortened dynamically, while in the stabilizing or holding of a segment in any position, the muscle maintains a length tonically. The contraction and recovery aids in the strengthening of muscle fiber.

Circulation, respiration and metabolism are so closely integrated in response to activity that stimulation of one brings a corresponding increase in activation of the others, depending upon the intensity of demands. It is possible to improve the circulation and increase the metabolism merely through respiratory effort, so that exercise which forces an involvement of energy expenditure summons greater requirements and participation in all three components. With obesity cases strong and increasingly active exercises may be appropriate, whereas in conditions of malnutrition the slower and less vigorus forms with lesser demands are more fitting.

Organic fitness is in large measure dependent upon the three previous factors plus muscle tonicity, and has considerable real effect in postural fitness. Weakness in any of the internal organs brings a corresponding lassitude, early fatigue, and a psychosomatic influence if not real inability to maintain posture. Stamina or endurance, and strength or energy are marks of organic fitness, and strenuous activity is the means for acquiring this coveted state.

One of the most comprehensive and *all-inclusive exercises* is the *sit-up*, which although specific for ptosis, is likewise beneficial in: contributing to muscular fitness of neck, shoulders, chest, and legs, correcting lordosis, and improving general muscle tone.

Starting Position.—Hook lying with knees bent, and toes under a fixture for support, arms placed at side and palms down (Fig. 47).

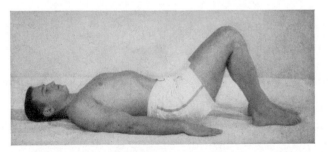

Fig. 47.—Hook lying.

1. Raise to sitting position, keeping head well back, arms extended shoulder height,
2. Sitting tall, flex fists and arms, keep chin in, inhale vigorously and hold for a four count,

3. Exhale and extend the arms to shoulder height, slowly lowering to back lying position and relax.

Caution.—Avoid using in any questionable cases, and remember to keep the knees bent throughout the exercise. Use a maximum of 5 times.

A more *intensive activity* and one which includes a great variety of different muscle actions is that of *skipping rope.* Through an alternation of routines it is possible to localize the actions to specific segments of the body, perhaps in a more varied manner than nearly any other form of movements. When combined with proper attention to correct structural alignment, it offers a medium for all of the afore-mentioned components of postural fitness to be implicated, since it is a strenuous activity.

Pattern Routine.—Start with the simple and lead into complex stunts.

1. With head and neck erect while stretching to full extension, swing rope forward while alternating the feet as in running, which through the arm action stresses the anterior aspect of the entire upper segments of the body;
2. For counter balancing purposes, then swing the rope backward with the same foot action, thus making greater use of the posterior muscle groups and segments of the upper portion of the body;
3. Repeat the same arm actions as in the swing of the rope, changing from use of first one foot and then the other to both feet leaving the floor at the same time;
4. While swinging the rope in the same manner, swing the feet alternately from side to side, then both feet at a time to first one side and then the other;
5. As skill develops along with stamina, the cross over of hands may be utilized in both the forward swinging of the rope as well as in the backward swing, varying use of the feet as has been described.
6. There are a great diversity of routines which may be utilized such as the tilting of head and shoulders in relation to the pelvis while carrying on the above movements, double swings of the rope while in the air, and adapting to music for rhythm.

Caution.—Extreme care should be exercised to increase gradually the vigor and duration of the exercise, and to eliminate completely when conditions exist which make the activity contraindicated.

A *less strenuous exercise or activity* is that of *rowing* and one that includes the entire gamut of muscular action. This may be carried on either in a simulated manner or when possible through use of a rowing machine. When not available, the lower weights on a triplicate wall machine may be used for the arm action with a sliding seat resting on guides for the leg action. The exercise is primarily for development of the posterior portions of the neck, shoulders and back, together with the muscles of the legs. When inhalation and expiration are included as a part of the action, the entire thorax especially takes an active part, while with the proper feathering of the oars and the forward lean, the anterior musculature is involved.

Starting Position.—*Sit erect on floor* with chin well in and eyes straight ahead, arms extended and knees bent.

1. With elbows level with hands on oars, pull back toward the chest and inhale strenuously, straightening the legs to full extension, thus forcing the hips and body away from the feet,
2. Flex the legs and slide the hips forward while exhaling, reaching ahead to full extension, yet keeping the upper back flat,
3. Execute the movement rhythmically, increasing the resistance either imaginatively or through tightening of tension screws on rowing machine. Considerable grace in movement is possible, for the purpose of increasing speed of actions, less resistance should be used.

Caution.—Maintenance of proper body position is extremely important, while the amount of stress will determine organic involvement.

In connection with organic fitness are the tonic effects of *constipation* and poor elimination, and the means for the assisting in the correction through exercises involving the abdominal wall and trunk. The compressive action of the diaphragm on the hollow viscera on inspiration when resisted by the abdominal muscles, and the importance of building up their tone and maintaining good alignment, so that they do not sag or become lax and weakened, are paramount.

There are two principal actions whereby the blood is returned to the heart. Namely, the *squeezing of the muscles* in the leg against each other, forces the lymph and venous blood into the abdominal cavity, from whence it is driven on up into the heart and thence to the lungs by *action of the diaphragm* against a resistant abdominal wall. The blood and chyle contains the energy producing food that all the body needs, and is a result of the digestive processes of the internal organs.

Following are a few movements upon which to pattern others for those who suffer from the toxic factors incident to poor bowel functions.

Starting Position.—Prone lying face down, place arms under the abdomen (Fig. 48).
1. Roll the body over onto the forearm, right side,
2. Return to first position,
3. Rotate to opposite or left side,
4. Return again to starting position.

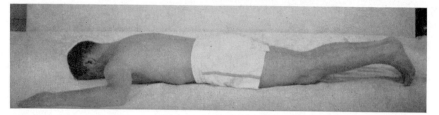

FIG. 48.—Prone lying.

From the same position with hands under abdomen, palms down.
1. Press fingers straight against floor, raising knuckles,
2. Tense muscles humping up the low back,
3. Relax. Repeat 5 times.
Caution.—Do not raise the pelvis, only flatten or curve lumbar spine. The action of the hands has a massaging effect.

Starting Position.—Hook lying on the back with knees bent, separate them widely and keep back flat.
1. Raise knees to the chest after taking a deep breath,
2. Grasp thighs back of knees, and pull down to chest while exhaling,
3. Return to starting position by dropping the heels to floor and sliding to extension, while thighs are widely abducted.
Note.—This is a modification of the old fashioned liver squeezer, exhaling as legs are raised, while low back is flattened which produces a powerful action of the abdominal muscles. It is the localization which would precede or initiate trunk flexion, the pressure of the thickness of the thigh adding a passive compression to the abdomen.

Starting Position.—Kneeling on both knees, place hands well forward.
1. Raise right knee forward, with full weight on same,
2. Bend forward right side, twisting trunk so knee presses abdomen,
3. Return to position and straighten back flat,
4. Change to left leg and repeat action. 5 times.

Starting Position.—Kneeling on all fours, hands and arms extended.

1. Extend left leg backward and stretch,
2. Lower the body supporting knee flexor until abdomen makes firm pressure on the opposite thigh,
3. Return to starting position,
4. Change extension of right leg backward and repeat 5 times.

*Caution.—*This exercise should be done with care, and for girls must not be given near or during the menstrual period as the torque on the pelvis might strain the sacro-iliac ligaments. If pain or cramps are present, omit the exercise.

CONVALESCENCE

Within the framework of this category many ramifications as to types of conditions are found, each one necessitating different procedures for recovery. Naturally, caution must be shown to prevent any delay in gaining permanent adjustment and recuperation. Broadly speaking, the subsequent major groupings are used to illustrate general areas requiring special attention.

Debilitating illness may be found in a multiplicity of forms resulting in a run-down condition which are too numerous to mention, as would be the listing of every form of activity for each illness. Therefore, selection as to exercise is based upon the broadest possible use and a sequence of progression, with relaxation techniques and light exercises leading to the complete restoration of normal physical condition. All medical aspects fall within the jurisdiction of the physician, who further supplements his services with careful supervision as to activity.

A particularly *mild form of exercise*, especially safe to start with, is known as the Mosher exercise. This is specific for improving the circulation, increasing respiration and general tone of anterior muscle groups of the abdomen and chest.

Starting Position.—Supine lying with knees slightly bent and hands resting lightly on the abdomen (Fig. 49).

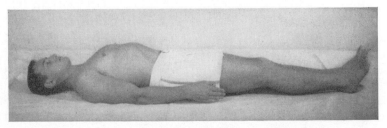

Fig. 49.—Supine lying.

1. Pressing gently upward with the palms of the hands on the abdomen, inhale and force the inspiration from the lower diaphragm to the upper thorax,
2. Hold the chin well in and flatten the shoulders and neck, while retaining breath and tensing the abdominal muscles,
3. Slowly exhale and return the hands to former position, fully relaxing for a short space of time and then repeating as the condition indicates. A maximum of 5 times is adequate.

Another *recumbent position* exercise of a mild form, which is of benefit in strengthening the abdominal muscles and those of the neck, is actually a follow-up of the former one described.

Starting Position.—Hook lying position, with palms of hands and elbows flat on the floor close to the side of the body.
1. Slowly raise the head and neck forward to chest, maintaining the shoulders and back flat while exhaling,
2. Return to position of rest and inhale normally,
3. Using the hands and elbows as levers, raise the head and shoulders off the floor about a foot, keeping the head in line with the shoulders throughout,
4. Slowly lower to rest position and relax completely. Increase the number to a maximum of 5 times.

*Caution.—*Do not inhale and hold breath while doing this exercise.

As a variation and executed from the *procumbent position* is the *swan dive* exercise, which is specific for strengthening the posterior muscles of the back, shoulders and neck and also assisting in stretching of the thorax and general muscle tone.

Starting Position.—Prone lying, face down, extend the arms to shoulder height and supinate the palms as far as possible,
1. Raise the entire upper portion of the body from above the hips, maintaining the head, shoulders and hands in original position,
2. Inhale deeply and hold for a short period,
3. Return to face position and relax.

*Caution.—*Do not attempt to raise the body more than 6 inches from the floor, emphasizing proper stabilizing position.

A definite part of the convalescent process is an assigned *rest period* following these exercises, especially when activity is first started. Following the initial period of adjustment, *short walks* may be added, changing the exercise schedule gradually, to *sitting* and *standing positions*. As condition justifies, *light games* may be included such as horseshoes, shuffle board, and table tennis, supplementing further with assignments for use of such *apparatus or equipment* as punching the light bag, pulling triplicate wall weights, using the rowing machine, and riding the stationary bicycle.

Specific attention to personal needs soon justifies inclusion of more strenuous activity, and every effort should be made to make the period of convalescence as short as possible. No attempt is made to give detailed description of each of the above activities, since in most instances they are self explanatory.

Caution must be exercised to conform carefully with the physician's recommendations, keeping him informed at all times as to the progress or changes in condition while seeking his counsel as to best procedure.

Pre and Post Operative Cases are likewise composed of diverse yet distinctive types of conditions, which call for individual care and scheduling. Generally, the previously recommended program might well be followed if sufficient caution is exercised in keeping with the physician's orders. While it is impossible to specify all feasible procedures there are general patterns which should be followed.

In all instances it is safe to say that there are recommended practices to follow. These include (*a*) *complete understanding* of the particular case and what is or is not safe to do, (*b*) making certain that all *precautionary measures* are taken to avoid over fatigue and assure adequate rest or relaxation as needed, (*c*) when specified giving necessary *stretching work* prior to surgery *or neuromuscular reeducation* following operations, and (*d*) *adaptation of program* to aid in complete recovery.

Caution.—It is impossible to emphasize too greatly the need to exercise judgment in all such cases, making certain that if no good can be accomplished at least no harm will be done. Following instructions of the physician explicitly is the most important factor in all such conditions.

RESTRICTED

It is possible to list only a few of the most common types of cases which require restriction of particular exercises classified as suitable. However, there are many such that may be used as long as the individual's condition is protected from possible danger. In most instances, such persons are referred for follow-through by a physician who either confirms or rejects the proposed movements, or suggests other forms of activity, thus assuring satisfactory care and favorable treatment.

Cardiac cases under proper guidance may profit from selected forms of activity as long as problems of over-stress are avoided. Instructors should be alert to signs of cardiac insufficiency as shown through shortness of breath, easy fatigue, swelling of the ankles, pain or feeling of restriction in the chest, color of the lips, or other indications of distress. These clues offer suggestions as to best positions for reducing possible stress, although other circulatory diseases are associated with similar symptoms which require a physician's diagnosis to determine.

Such exercises as those suggested for convalescent conditions in the beginning stage are beneficial, especially where large movements with little resistance are used. Unusually important is the developing of the abdominals, which must be carried on without possible strain. The fostering of improved postural alignment likewise makes for better circulation and improved heart action.

Starting Position.—While *lying* in a *supine* position with legs extended, place arms at the side and endeavor to flatten the back.
1. Raise arms alternately over the head until the hand touches the floor, slowly moving forward, with hand in a supinated position until it returns to the starting position,
2. Bend the knee by dragging the foot on the floor until the thigh is flexed, alternating the feet,
3. Combine these movements using the right arm and the left leg, which causes a rotary motion of the upper body, then change to opposite use of limbs, this results in stimulation of alternating reciprocal reflexes,
4. Raise both hands at the same time over the head and complete circular movement of the arms, inhaling with the upward move and exhaling as arms are lowered,
5. When the arms are being extended to the stretch, draw both knees to chest while inhaling, then slowly exhale and lower the arms and legs to their former position.

Caution.—It may be advisable to complete only the first portion of the movement when starting the exercise, carefully observing any reaction. Later, when no signs of distress are shown, the additional steps may be included.

Asthmatic conditions are frequently amenable to activity which improves the respiration and circulatory response, as long as the exercise is progressively increased and no signs of difficulty in breathing are apparent, at the same time guarding against fatigue. Since there are numerous causes and forms of this condition, it is often necessary to try out exercises as a means of amelioration, desisting when no results are accomplished and seeking further assistance of a physician for other corrective means.

Several of the previous exercises may be used to advantage at the start, in a recumbent position, then proceeding to those in a sitting position, and finally to those from a standing position, such as the following example of a *swan dive* from a standing position.

Starting Position.—*Rest standing* position with finger tips touching behind the head, with chin and elbows held well back, and feet pointed straight ahead (Fig. 50).

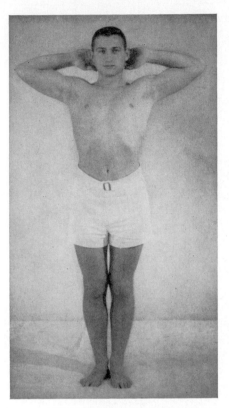

FIG. 50.—Rest standing.

1. Bend the trunk forward, holding hands, shoulders and head in original starting posture,
2. While maintaining the same body position, extend the arms to the side shoulder height and level, with palms supinated,
3. Raise the body to the erect stature, rotate the hips, tighten the fists and bend the elbows against simulated resistance while inhaling vigorously and drawing the abdomen in and upward,
4. Return the arms to the side and relax without losing the erect posture position attained.   Repeat a maximum of 5 times.

Caution.—Since the assuming of proper position, attaining of maximum tension of arms and shoulder muscles, as well as expansion of the chest is the main object, every effort should be directed toward this goal. In asthmatics emphasis should be given to slow

expiration with lips pursed or hissing, which dilates the walls of
the bronchi.

Rheumatic fever is inextricably involved with potential heart
lesions and offers a challenge to the instructor to best determine
what is and is not feasible as far as activity is concerned.   It is
somewhat similar in respect to treatment of heart and neurasthenia
cases, which require protection from exposure, fatigue and especially nervous tension.   The person who has faced this dilemma is
often completely restricted as to activity, and as a result worries,
loses sleep, and meets with many bitter disappointments because
of such restraints and the monotony of daily routine tasks which
offer little outlet for his expression of desires.

In all instances, such cases must be under the direct supervision
of the physician, since a total reeducative process is made necessary
in order that the individual may revise his way of life.   Rather
than prescribe exercise, which has a place in the complete readjustment, greater emphasis should be directed to relaxation techniques.   Lessening of residual tensions in turn frequently causes a
subsidence of symptoms which are harmful to the recovery, and
when available, instruction can be utilized preferably to any
amount of complete rest alone.

Work schedules must be in keeping with the individual's condition and abilities, seeking very gradual increase of his work tolerance.   Every effort should be made to maintain joint range,
muscle power to a degree, as well as sound body mechanics.
Above all else, he must be enabled to find a place for himself with
companionship, enjoyment, and a sense of belonging.

Since it is impossible to delimit the description of broad relaxation techniques to any specific condition, it would seem best to
urge complete perusal of authorities who have made careful
studies of the scientific approach as to the most effective forms.
Should it seem beyond the reach of those responsible for class
situations, it might be appreciated to know that during World
War II, United States Naval officers were trained by Edmund
Jacobson, M.D., author of *Progressive Relaxation*, for the instruction of all Pre-Flight School cadets.[2]   In many situations well over
300 at a time were taught the advantages and ways of learning
to relax, and over 15,000 profited from such training.

Individuals who have been subjected to rheumatic fever do not
appreciate being placed on the shelf, and those who are working
for and with such persons should remember that all such cases are
not necessarily beyond help, often achieving complete recovery.
An instance may be recalled of a high school student who, under
the close scrutiny of his family physician over a period of years,
made such progress from the early incident of this illness, that he

was urged to participate in track. Strange to behold, he became a quarter miler of some note, both in high school and later in college. This example has been cited to illustrate possibilities.

Comment.—The use of musical rhythms maintains a high degree of interest and requires the flow and range of movement so desirable in this type of condition.

REHABILITATION

A major part of every hospital, clinic or school program must include attention to rehabilitation cases of a wide scope. The treatment consists of such a complex variety of procedures that it is beyond the purview of this source to direct attention to definite specifics. An example of the need for such follow-through is evident

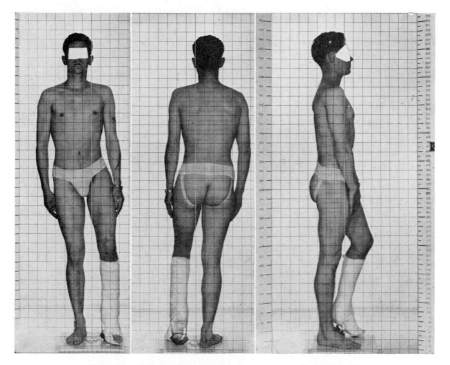

Fig. 51.—Effect of walking cast on postural alignment.

in Figure 51 following the use of a walking cast. It is not amiss, however, to reemphasize the fact that work of this nature must be carried on in complete accordance and under the direction of physicians. Too often, some persons in positions of trust presume too far as to their competence and qualifications, and every effort needs to be made to avoid such practices.

Hernias are many times considered to be due to (*a*) a weakness of the abdominal muscles and fascia, caused by the lack of exericise, poor body mechanics, and general weakness, (*b*) relaxing of the abdominal rings, internal pressure, or gravitational stress which cause a protrusion of abdominal parts into the scrotum, and (*c*) coughing, sneezing, vomiting, or lifting accompanied by corresponding weakness. Since weakness of abdominal areas is receptive to less tolerance in sudden pressure, it is reasonable to expect that in such cases where surgery is not indicated, they may be amenable to specific exercises.

It is usually safe to say that exercises given in the *supine position* are advisable to begin with, thence proceeding to the standing position. The lying exercises which have been previously presented may be used in the starting of the program, then moving to those such as the following to gain tone and poise as well as good body mechanics. Twisting movements are beneficial for tensing of the abdominal oblique muscles, hence influencing inguinal rings.

Starting Position.—While *stride standing* erect with feet spread slightly, raise arms to shoulder height with palms, flat against the neck (Fig. 52).
1. Trunk twisting, bring right hand to left foot with left hand held vertically, directly above opposite hand on same side, face eyes straight ahead,
2. Raise trunk upward, returning arms to horizontal plane and stand tall while retracting abdomen,
3. Twist trunk to opposite side with forward bending and left hand to right toe,
4. Return to initial starting position, and lower hands to side and relax.

Caution.—Maintain hips well forward, turning head and forcing top shoulder well back, resting after each complete sequence.

Pertinent to the problems of rehabilitation, are those associated with immobilization of some type. Unless volitional control of the unaffected parts are reestablished particularly, there is bound to be regression taking hold which delays the eventual recovery. Ordinarily physicians are not opposed, in fact they encourage the practice of early mobilization as long as it is wisely conducted.

Elucidation of the basic aperceptive background of what is known as *cross education*, and the influence of unilateral exercise on contralateral parts are necessarily brief, yet particularly significant in rehabilitation exercises. The essential principle is that when an unaffected limb or part of the body is exercised, there is a reciprocal response in an affected part. Application of this theory demonstrates that there is a proportionate relationship between the amount of effort expended and the extent and quality of transfer to be educed.

The importance of this belief as shown by scientific research cannot fail to be appreciated as an advantageous technique which may be used to great purpose. Practitioners of physical medicine have recognized the possibilities of this phenomenon, and extensive utilization appears imminent in the treatment and rehabilitation of many conditions.

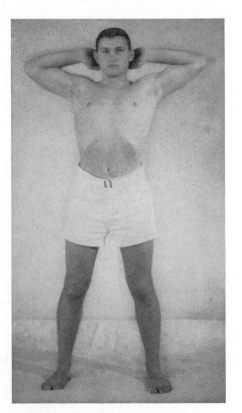

Fig. 52.—Stride standing.

While only a single analogy of progressive application of scientific principles for exercise use has been suggested, there are many additional similar approaches within the reach of those who are willing to search the literature for other such methods. Experimentation and an inquiring mind are requistes of those who work in the area of rehabilitation, and all about us today is found evidence of new techniques of promise, available for those who seek them.

STRETCHING EXERCISES

A question which comes to mind is whether exercise promiscuously used in all its ramifications should be indulged in or prescribed. The answer is definitely, "No, not to be used without discretion." For instance a word of caution needs to be given regarding the use of stretching exercises, in order that there may be better understanding of their application in athletics and physical education as well as in specific treatment of various conditions.

It has been mentioned that when the body parts or segments sag and slump, the muscles and ligaments of necessity become adaptively shortened on one side and elongated and weakened on the other. When activities are indulged in by the individual with this correction in view, they usually succeed in building up such strength, but unless guided by an intelligent instructor malalignment not only will not be corrected, but may become more fixed. Observe effect of such application in Figures 53*A* and 53*B*.

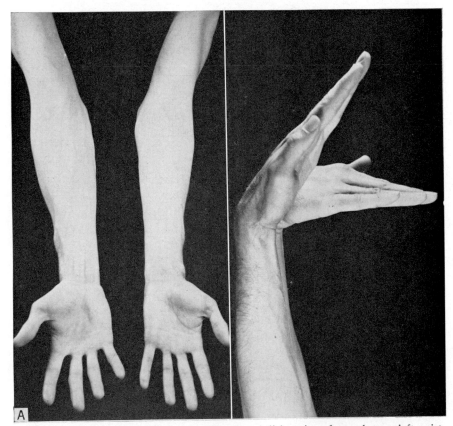

Fig. 53.—*A*, Pre-exercise—fractured scaphoid and dislocation of carpal row—left wrist.

As an illustration, consider exercises such as hanging on rings, overhead ladder, or stall bars, in case there exists the ordinary fatigue slump or habitual round shoulders. In such a person the pectorals and serrati as well as the arm adductors have become shortened. Consequently these over-active shortened muscles will be stimulated by the stretch reflex incidental to the function of hanging, with the result that the already stretched rhomboids and trapezii become further elongated and the scapulæ spread further apart (Fig. 54).

Consequently the idea of stretching as an exercise should not be done passively, unless the opponents of the shortened muscles are actively contracted to build up their strength for balance. Proper body position may determine their worth in this regard as shown in the following illustration.

In hanging from the stall bars have *back toward the bars*, with arms spread wide and hands grasping bars palms out. Then

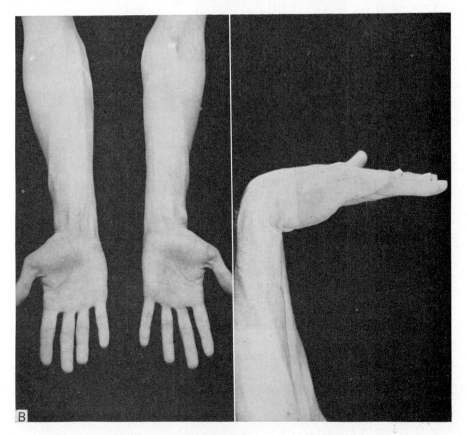

Fig. 53.—*B*, Post-exercise, illustration of correction.

flatten the neck and low back, plus a strong scapular pinch. Hold for a count of 5 and slowly and smoothly relax. Example of *opposite* position in active hanging Figure 55.

The positive impulse to the scapular adductors, rhomboids and trapezius, is accompanied by a similar impulse to their opponents, the shortened anterior scapular abductors, pectorals and teres

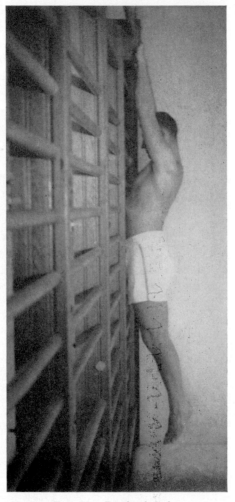

FIG. 54.—Passive hanging.

serrati. The patient or student should be told that to increase the range of his arm and shoulder action in any performance, he must elongate these shortened muscles in order to obtain full physiological range of his shoulder joints. This will be done better if he stretches his short muscle groups by building up their weak opponents.

It is admitted that a good morning stretch of all joints and muscles is a beneficial way to maintain the elasticity of the fascial sheaths, and hastens the circulation. Giving limbering up exercises as they are commonly spoken of are therefore known to be sound.

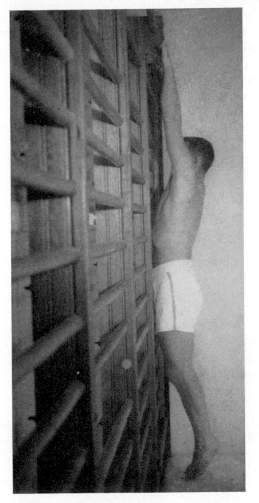

FIG. 55.—Active hanging.

Thus it is obvious that it will be necessary to stretch restricting forces before an improved alignment can be obtained. The weakened antagonists on the convex side of a curve cannot be expected to take up the slack fast enough to accomplish the desired end without continuous active effort aided by sufficient rest, a constant motivation to maintain the better position, and a corresponding improvement of all metabolic processes.

The idea of passive stretching is likely to have a negative effect and even by making the body more flexible, promote worse deviations than originally existed. Many scoliosis cases, especially when structural and adaptive changes have taken place, have been made decidedly worse and injured by the ignorance of some who have had insufficient insight into the orthopedic needs of such cases.

Stretching exercises then are valuable when properly used, but should be most carefully directed and prescribed if there are to be beneficial results obtained from their use. It is known that in certain conditions there are found contractures which must be released, but these are cases for the physician to decide (Figs. 56A and 56B).

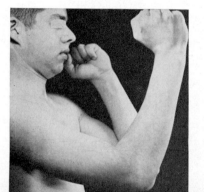

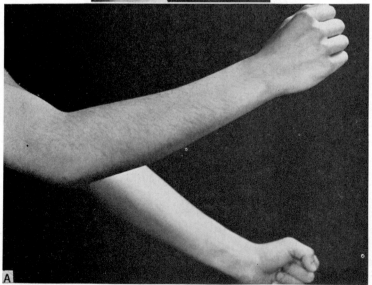

FIG. 56.—A, Fracture and dislocated elbow, condition previous to specific exercise program.

Pertinent to athletic situations is the common practice of forcible stretching *per se*, which may, through the stretch reflex, stimulate the shorter muscles to further tighten. Whereas, as stated above, more attention to activation of their weaker opponents will increase the range of movement, avoid possible injury, and more definitely assist in the improvement of performance. This principle should attract the attention of every coach, for all too often the only stress is paid to the actual movements essential to the particular skill.

As has been shown through the cautionary measures relating to stretching exercises, there are many other general practices which need reviewing. Those who understand body mechanics and appreciate the liabilities which some coaches subject themselves to, as well as their players, shudder at the stunts which are used to improve performance. Naturally, not all coaches should be

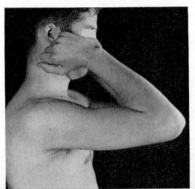
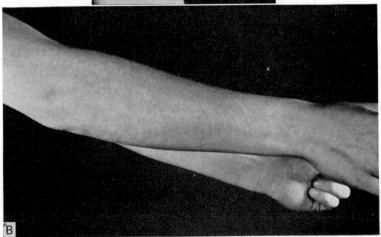

Fig. 56.—*B*, Progressive effect of exercise.

subjected to such criticism, for there are many real students now coaching who make it their business to learn what is best to achieve the desired results, but there are all too few of this type at present.

TYPICAL EXERCISES FOR SEGMENTAL ALIGNMENT

The importance of segmental alignment cannot be underestimated when it is realized that each segment below that which is being considered is the determiner of those above. The relationship of one to another must be taken into the perspective in presenting typical exercises, since a single movement is not isolated by itself in regard to the segment being activated but must be viewed *in toto*.

Exercises must therefore be evaluated in terms of equivalent action elsewhere than merely within the area of specificity. Body position may well be the determinable factor which decides the effect and involvement of other segments, and when isolated action is desired in a single part or segment, the starting position may well serve as the control.

In the descriptions which follow, segments which are closely related have been grouped as a means whereby certain exercises, intended as specific, may likewise serve as beneficial in other areas. Therefore, every condition by itself is not listed, nor are exercises suggested for each, but rather as a composite means or aggregate attack on the problem.[3,4]

HEAD, NECK AND SHOULDERS

The most common deviation at the top of the structure is spoken of as *forward head*, and is usually an attitudinal shift related to work, use of eyes, and hands, where the activities of the person are chiefly in the area in front of the body. The head may be likened to a terminal vertebra, very aptly characterized by the Scotch definition of the spine as, "Your spine is a wavy bone, your head sits on one end and you sit on the other." Consequently its weight shifts in compensation to the position of the segments below.

Lateral changes for instance may be induced by a tilted pelvis caused by a short leg or low arch, corresponding with a trunk shift and change of head posture. Similarly the *shoulder girdle* position alters when there is laxity of musculature posteriorly, especially in the rhomboids and lower trapezius, allowing the arm weight to pull the shoulders forward. Thus *round shoulders* are developed with adaptive shortening of the pectoral muscles.

Consequently shifting of the head and arm weight forward necessitates an increase of the dorsal spinal curve backward. The major indications for correction of the above faults are strengthening of the scapular adductors and stretching of their abductors or pectorals, plus retraction of the chin and flattening of the forward cervical curve. Just as in correction of all spinal deviations, it is wise to start from the recumbent and procumbent positions, progressing to sitting and standing positions. The following exercises are examples which may be modified and expanded in complexity.

Starting Position.—Hook lying with knees and hips flexed, and hands behind the head.
1. Flatten neck, and force elbows back while holding chin in,
2. Hold the position and inhale,
3. Exhale and return to original position. Repeat 5 times.

Starting Position.—Prone lying with legs straight and feet inverted, hands behind the neck, fingers touching.
1. Flatten neck with chin tucked in,
2. Force elbows well back and inhale, hold,
3. Exhale and return to starting position.
This exercise may be modified to arms in reverse "T" position, palms down. When arms are lifted, external rotators act synergistically with scapular adductors.

Starting Position.—Sitting with feet parallel and toeing in, with feet 9 or 10 inches apart to broaden the base.
1. Hands at wing position, flatten the neck with elbows back,
2. Bend to the right side and hold,
3. Return to first position and relax,
4. Repeat with bend to opposite side left,
5. Complete same action with added trunk rotation,
6. Then same action with trunk twist and lateral bend.

Starting Position.—Standing with feet 1 foot apart and arches lifted, hands on hips, flatten the neck with spinal push-up.
1. Elbows back, pinch scapulæ,
2. Hold the position and inhale deeply,
3. Exhale and return to starting position, repeat 5 times,
4. Repeat same action with added trunk side bend alternately,
5. Complete same movement with alternate trunk twist to side,
6. Then same action with trunk twist and side bend, maintaining elbows back and scapulæ pinched together.
There is often found a combination of conditions known as *lateral head tilt and unlevel shoulders*, which may be corrected at the same time. The following exercises are specific for same.

Starting Position.—Sitting before a mirror with plumb line in the center and hands on the hips.

1. Flatten and straighten head and neck, including spinal push-up,
2. Level eyes and shoulders and hold 3 to 5 counts,
3. Relax slowly and try to keep head and shoulders level. Repeat 5 times,
4. From same sitting position place hand on low side of head, with arm on high side down and back,
5. Push head up to mid line and level eyes, while depressing high shoulder and shifting body to mid line, level shoulders.

Starting Position.—Standing, feet 1 foot apart, hands on hips.

1. Shift head and body to mid line, level eyes and shoulders,
2. Tilt pelvis back and tighten abdomen, push up and hold 5 counts,
3. Return to starting position and relax,
4. Then raise arm on low side over head, and arm of high shoulder down to side,
5. Shift body and head to mid line and hold for count of 5,
6. Lower arm to side and relax, then repeat 5 times,
7. Using wand grasped with arms wide, hands outward,
8. Rotate wand to vertical in line with plumb line, with hand of low shoulder stretched above,
9. Level eyes and push head up, holding for 5 counts,
10. Return to position and relax. Repeat 5 times.

Simple shoulder shrugging done in conjunction with tensing of the neck muscles opposite head tilt, will accomplish much good. Be sure to keep shoulders well back at all times.

UPPER BACK

The most frequent deviation of the upper dorsal area is the increase of the posterior curve, which may be simple flexible relaxation or a more fixed rigid deviation and producing the so-called *round back*. It should be remembered that this divergency is practically always accompanied by round shoulders. However, the reverse is not true. If this simple deviation is not recognized and strenuous effort made to correct it, there will be changes in the structure and shape of the vertebrae involved in it, and a wedging of the anterior margins of the bodies which rapidly become a fixed or structural round back.

It is essential to explain to the individual that unless he consistently follows his exercises his back will get worse. If, after continued exercise prescription is carried out with good cooperation, he still does not correct the condition, he should be referred to an orthopedist for some more definite treatment.

Starting Position.—Hook lying with a pad under the dorsum, arms in a wing position.
  1. Flatten low back and neck,
  2. Press elbows to the floor and inhale,
  3. Exhale and relax. Repeat 5 times,
  4. From same position, stretch arms overhead for a count of 10, keeping low back flattened,
  5. Relax and repeat after a short rest.
This exercise adds a passive stretch to anterior vertebral ligaments.

Starting Position.—Hook Sitting with feet parallel and knees apart, arms folded behind the back (Fig. 57).

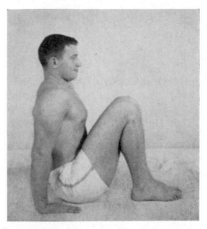

Fig. 57.—Hook sitting.

  1. Flatten the neck and do a spinal push-up,
  2. Hold a few moments, then relax and repeat 5 times,
  3. From the same position place hands on the hips with neck flat,
  4. Take moderate breath and force the ribs out laterally,
  5. Hold 3 counts, exhale and relax,
  6. Repeat same action with hands grasping wand, palms forward,
  7. Elevate arms and draw wand down as far over the scapulæ as possible,
  8. Flatten neck and raise arms overhead, relax and repeat 5 times,
  9. Using wand, elevate arms and lower left arm down back with the right arm extended overhead, return arms and relax,

10. Alternate with right arm being lowered, then relax. Repeat
    5 times.

Note that in case of a lateral curvature with round back, the
last two movements should be modified to bring the wand down
on the convex side of the curve.

CHEST CONDITIONS

Such conditions may be accompanied by round back which may
necessitate the actual changing of the rib cage for correction. This
means that considerable time may ensue in accomplishing real
results, but if persistent attention is given, desirable changes may
be achieved.

For overcoming a *pigeon breast* condition the following exercises
and positions are beneficial, and should be continued for quite
some period of time before desisting.

Starting Position.—Prone lying with arms in wing side position,
arms and hands supinated.
1. Flatten the neck with elbows back, and hands flat on the ribs,
2. Spread ribs laterally while inhaling. Body weight presses
   down on the prominent sternum, and position should be held
   for 3 to 5 counts,
3. Exhale and return to former position, then relax. Repeat
   5 times.
4. In same starting position, grasp wand over head,
5. Pull wand down over the scapulæ, inhale and hold while
   spreading the ribs laterally,
6. Return to starting position while exhaling and relax.

Starting Position.—Cross sitting with hands placed on neck,
resisting (Fig. 58).
1. Flatten neck and lean forward, pinching scapulæ,
2. Inhale and spread ribs laterally, hold,
3. Exhale and return to position, relax. Repeat 5 times.
Note.—The same type of exercises may be used in the *standing*
position.

In a *flat or funnel chest* the opposite form of correction must be
sought. That is, the rib cage must be held firmly while the
sternum is forced outward, and may be accomplished through the
use of a wide canvas band of from 4 to 6 inches wide being placed
around the chest and over the sternum while exercising.

Starting Position.—Supine lying with hands and fingers on neck.
1. Force elbows strongly back, tucking the chin well in,

2. Take a deep breath and force the sternum out strenuously, while holding the posterior fixation of the dorsal curve,
3. Exhale and return to starting position, then relax,
4. From same position, place a wide pad under the dorsal spine with knees bent, and arms in wing position,
5. Flatten the back, inhale deeply, expand sternum upward and forward and hold for 5 counts,
6. Exhale and return to position, repeating 5 times.

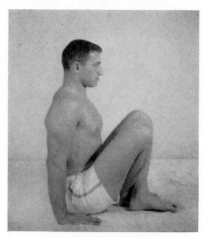

FIG. 58.—Cross sitting.

Starting Position.—Hook sitting position with hands on the ribs laterally, fingers pointing downward.

1. Press firmly on the ribs and take a big breath,
2. Flatten the neck and lift the sternum forward, then hold,
3. Exhale and relax, return to position. Repeat 5 times,
4. Same position, executing a forward body lean while stretching the sternum forward,
5. In same manner except using wand grasping, palms forward,
6. Bring wand to mid dorsum, lean back and inhale deeply, forcing sternum outward,
7. Exhale and return to starting position. Repeat 5 times.

LOW BACK AND PELVIS

One of the commonest variances is that of lordosis or hollow back which is an exaggeration of the normal anterior curve, with a compensating increase of the posterior dorsal curve or a localized lordosis below and trunk lean backward with shoulder girdle overhang.

15

The pelvic segment is a key one because of the necessity of compensatory changes above and below. Hence the importance of recognizing that its correction of position is essential to efficient use of the body. The major factor of its importance in relation to the development of antigravity musculature should be understood, explaining to the student or patient that it is the most essential segment in body development.

Any machine works more effectively when all bearings are trued up or aligned. The individual must be impressed with the fact, that all of us will be fighting the pressure of gravity all of our lives. Hence, every effort must be made to decrease the wear and tear on the body machine, and to keep it from aging too fast, a goal all should strive to attain.

Starting Position.—Hook lying with knees together and feet apart.
1. Raise the head, flatten the low back, hold for a 6 count, but do not hold the breath during exercise,
2. Relax and lower the head,
3. Same position but with hands behind the neck, elbows back,
4. Raise the head as though starting to rise, flatten low back, turn head and arms to first one side and then the other, repeat 5 times after relaxing.

Starting Position.—Hook Sitting position with knees apart, feet toeing inward, hands placed on forehead.
1. Flatten the neck and push head forward while resisting with the hands,
2. Slowly turn shoulders right then left, and return,
3. Same position with legs extended and arms reaching forward as in rowing, exert strong pull backward resistively,
4. As trunk becomes erect, add elbow flexion and scapulæ pinch with end of stroke, trunk leaning backward. May also use wand.

Starting Position.—Standing as in archery position, feet apart and bow hand down, grasping string with other hand.
1. Flatten the lower back, tilt the pelvis down behind, tensing the abdominal muscles,
2. Raise arms as in releasing the arrow with right hand to chin, left arm extended as on bow, imagining strong bow action,
3. Return to position and alternate to opposite side 5 times,
4. Trunk half bent forward, arms in wing position, flatten neck and hold back straight in lumbar area,

5. Rise to erect position, twist trunk to alternate sides, relax,
6. Same position with hands on the hips, elbows well back and pelvis tilted down, turn right and bend left as far as possible, may be done with twist rotation as well.

Note.—In all standing positions when there is a lateral pelvic tilt, the twists should be made to assist in such correction by emphasizing twist to overcome condition.

COMBINED VARIATIONS OF BACK

Quite frequently anterior posterior deviations are found to be complicated by lateral or rotational factors such as a kyphosis of the dorsal spine and may have in conjunction with it a *lateral curvature* producing a kypho-scoliosis, with or without any shoulder girdle maladjustment.

This condition when found early may not have any structural faults in the spinal column and may be amenable to exercise treatment. If, however, when checked in recumbency and the vertebral column does not completely straighten out, one should recognize that the condition may be entering a stage of structural alteration, or at least be in a transitional phase between the postural and the structural stage. If the latter condition exists, the attention of the parents and physician should be called to the situation.

Starting Position.—The exercises advised for round back are also applicable, especially the spinal push-ups with trunk shifting to the plumb line. It should be recognized that efforts to correct lateral curves, unless carefully guided, may result in producing an opposite compensatory curve. From *hook lying*, arm on concave side of curve, thrust outward and upward, opposite arm downward.
1. Flatten neck and tense the lower arm firmly while supinating hand,
2. Pinch shoulder blades, flatten lower back and hold 5 counts,
3. Return to position and relax. Repeat 5 times.

Starting Position.—From *half-side lying*, convex side of curve down (Fig. 59).
1. Extend opposite arm shoulder height to side and supinate hand, lift hip clear of floor, hold for 5 counts,
2. Lower hip to floor, turning to assume long sitting position for resting. Repeat exercise 5 times after relaxing.

Caution.—When raising hips, back must be in a straight plane with neck and head well back, chin in. Upper leg is always placed in front of supporting leg for better balance.

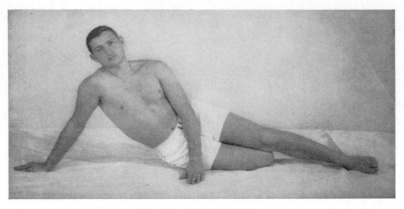

FIG. 59.—Half-side lying.

Starting Position.—From *side lying*, concave side of curve down (Fig. 60).
   1. Supinate upper arm and tense fist firmly while lower arm, palm up, is being stretched vigorously.
   2. Relax and turn on back for resting. Repeat 5 times.
Caution.—Lower leg is bent at knee for stability, with upper leg extended.

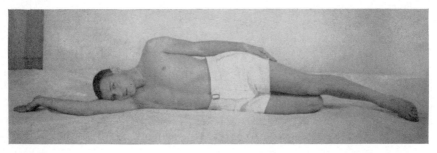

FIG. 60.—Side lying.

Starting Position.—*Prone lying*, arm on concave side over head and opposite hand placed on side above hip.
   1. Push down and in with lower hand, while tightening scapular adductors and hold, and raising extended arm and shoulders clear of floor,
   2. Return to position and repeat 5 times,
   3. Same position grasping wand, push down with wand over the scapula on high side and elevate its opposite end,
   4. Tighten lateral muscles on convex side taking a deep breath and forcing concave side outward.
   5. Hold and push spine upward, then return to position and relax. Repeat 5 times.

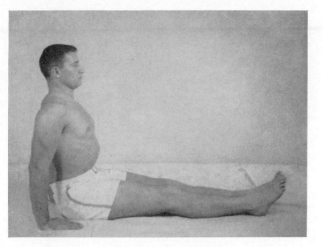

FIG. 61.—Long sitting.

Starting Position.—Long sitting with back to stall bars if possible or against a wall, with arms in wing position (Fig. 61).
1. Flatten the neck and raise the elbow of low or concave side and lower opposite arm downward,
2. Tighten lateral muscles on thorax of that side and hold,
3. Return and repeat 5 times, guarding against the bending at the waist, the force should be upward on the diagonal toward correction of concavity.
4. Same arms reverse "T", palms forward,
5. Reach out and up on side of low shoulder, down on opposite side, grasping the stall bars and holding,
6. Push up and over toward concave side, relax. Repeat 5 times.

Starting Position.—Stride standing feet apart facing stall bars or wall.
1. Climb up with fingers on concave side and down on the opposite,
2. Flatten neck and low back, pushing up and over on low shoulder side, hold 3 counts, return to position. Repeat 5 times,
3. Same position with one hand on low side of head, off hand on the chest over the high part of convexity with fingers pointing to the rear,
4. Half bend forward, pushing in on convexity and hold 3 counts, then relax and repeat 5 times.

LATERAL PELVIC TILT, LORDOSIS, LATERAL CURVE

This is a quite common deviation which is found in about 40 to 50 per cent of all individuals, with a corresponding lowering of one side of the pelvis due to several causes. Such exercises as those for lordosis and round hollow back are applicable, provided the tilt is corrected by a lift in the heel of street shoe on the low side, or, when exercising, in gym shoes. The fundamental stance should be altered by placing the foot of the high side outward to level the pelvis.

It is obvious that such exercises in a recumbent position are valuable because the deviation is corrected in lying and there is no gravity load. Hence, the strengthening of the musculature in this position will give a more symmetrical thrust as well as corrective result.

In *sitting* if the pelvis levels in this position, it shows that the fault is below the pelvis. However, because any malalignment from a developmental fault on one side of the pelvis may be present, it should always be checked because exercises over an unlevel pelvis will only tend to perpetuate the lateral spinal deviation above. Hence, it is just as important to wear a "sit pad" under the ischium of the low side as it is to have a heel correction for standing.

Such correction may be done by sewing a three-eighth or half inch felt pad into a boy's trousers, and should be about 3 by 4 inches in size. Girls can wear a pad of similar size suspended by tapes from a girdle or belt, under the buttocks with tapes fastened around the thigh so that when sitting down the pad is drawn under the ischium. If this is not possible a thin magazine placed under low side on the chair may be used instead.

This tilt in sitting is frequently overlooked and hence the hours spent in sitting in school and at home during the growing period, undoubtedly aid in the production of lateral spinal curvature. It is important to inquire if the child has a habit of sitting on one foot, a habit which is quite prevalent and one which parents of the student should be cautioned to disallow through observing the child's actions.

The major elements of value in the exercises which have been offered, should be the corrected stance for standing. Exercises plus slight rotation of the thighs outward, with a flattening of the low back and tensing of the abdominals are most meaningful. These movements together with spinal push-up and trunk shift with neck firm and shoulders level, presents a corrected standing position which all should be taught to assume.

LEGS AND FEET

It is usual to consider the legs and feet together as a segment because the supporting pillars of the body or legs end in pedestals such as the feet.   Hence the deviations of the body segments above must alter the line of gravitational stress on these supports.

Consequently from the biomechanical standpoint it should be obvious that in all developmental, therapeutic, clinical, athletic, gymnastic or recreational aspects there should be a total approach. An engineer recognizes that the weight distribution of a super-structure not only necessitates strengthening all stress joints in the structure, but the stresses on the supporting columns and their footings must be met by sufficient strength and exact alignment to withstand such stress.

This is the reason why it is essential for everyone involved in these various situations where postural fitness of the human body is concerned, to recognize that although their consideration has been centered on some particular segment of the body, either above, below, or in the middle, they must nevertheless think of the whole body.

The physician or orthopedist who treats a lame back without taking foot posture and strength into consideration, does not have the best approach to his problems.   Likewise, the physical educator or therapist is overlooking this fact, who gives major emphasis to increasing muscle size and strength of the upper trunk, without recognizing what effects will be produced if the alignment of body segments (especially the pelvis, legs and feet) is not given appro-priate attention.

Unfortunately the average school child is not a patient and may have no aches or pains, but if his physical activities of any type are continued without much regard for his postural deviations now and in the future, he may in the long run be injured permanently. For instance, running or jumping may be of great interest to a lad if he does well and he is encouraged to get on a team, but unless the slight knock knees or tibial torsion or pronation in the legs, feet or ankles are taken into consideration these may be the factors that provoke the early synovitis in the knees for which football is so often blamed.   There may also be an increased flattening of the arches from other activities, all of these conditions possibly deterring performance of students and leaving permanent struc-tural changes to handicap them.

It can readily be seen from the previous discussion that an exer-cise, which is simple and should be done many times a day, will influence the total antigravity needs of the body.   Actions which need to take place in order to prevent such changes from being harmful are rotating the thighs outward and lifting the arches of the feet, tipping the pelvis up in front and down behind by tensing the abdominal muscles and buttocks, flattening the back of the

neck and standing tall. The following exercises are for the purpose of accomplishing such improvements.

RELAXED ANTERIOR OR METATARSAL ARCHES

Starting Position.—Sitting on bench, feet resting on a block or
book with big toes touching, heels slightly apart and the metatarsal
heads at edge of the block.
  1. Depress the toes over the edge of the block, keeping the toes
     straight,
  2. Relax and repeat 5 times.
  Caution.—Do not flex the toes, flexing only at the metatarsal
     joints with toes straight.

Starting Position.—Sitting astride bench, place the right foot
forward, right heel opposite the left toe and feet parallel.
  1. Keep right heel stationary with ball of foot flat, grasp the
     surface of the floor with toes of right foot, pull ball of foot
     back along floor as in gripping an imaginary towel,
  2. Relax foot and return to former position. Alternate with the
     opposite foot. Repeat 5 times.
  Caution.—This exercise should not be used in flexible flatfeet
because the flexion of big toe will lift the front end of the first
metatarsal and tend toward supination of the front foot, not
wanted in flatfoot cases. A towel may be used if desired, and is
called building mounds. Avoid in hammer toes.
  Note.—One foot is placed in front of the other for better fixation.
Hamstrings are strongly activated, hence exercise is good for
relaxed backkness.

Starting Position.—Sitting stride position on bench.
  1. Using right foot, press big toe firmly to floor and keep the
     heel stationary on the floor,
  2. Bring left foot to right knee, avoiding the pointing of toes,
  3. Replace feet to former position and alternate feet. Repeat
     5 times.

RELAXED LONGITUDINAL FLATFEET—
FIRST AND SECOND DEGREE

Recall the discussion of the fact that gastrocnemii are short in
flat feet and also that the increased load on the anterior tibial
makes it hypertrophy and shorten.

Starting Position.—Supine lying.
  1. Grip the buttocks together and rotate the thighs outward,
  2. Relax and repeat 5 times.

Note.—The external rotators are stretched in this deviation by the sagging of the leg into internal rotation. This exercise is to tighten the external rotators, mainly the pyriformis.

Starting Position.—*Long sitting* with legs extended and back flat with hands on floor, right leg crossed over the left.
1. Describe a complete circle with right foot, starting movement out and down, then inward and upward strongly,
2. Relax and repeat 5 times. Strengthens the posterior tibial and not the gastrocnemii and peroneals,
3. Same position with knees bent and feet toeing in, lift arches, keeping heels stationary on the floor, relax and repeat 5 times.
4. Sitting on bench feet together, knees flexed and feet crossed with outer borders of feet in contact with floor, lean forward and stand keeping feet crossed and weight on outer border of feet,
5. Relax and repeat movement with alternate feet crossed 5 times.

Note.—Hands are placed in the lap to keep them from assisting in assuming standing position, necessitating all muscle work being performed by leg and trunk muscles. The shortened peroneals must lengthen while the weakened posterior tibial shortens.

Starting Position.—*Standing* toes touching, heels 3 inches apart.
1. Thigh rotation outward, turning knees out but not bending, grip buttocks together and tucked under, twisting thighs outward and keeping big toe joints on the floor,
2. Return and repeat 5 times.

Note.—Centering the attention on the buttocks emphasizes the thigh element, and activates the external rotators, chiefly the pyriformis, while tucking under of hips prevents increase of pelvic flexion on hip joints. Avoid tendency to back knees.

Starting Position.—*Standing* with feet in an exaggerated pigeon-toed position.
1. Walking in this position with feet actually crossed over and in front of the other foot alternately,
2. Change to correct walking although toeing in somewhat, placing weight bearing along outer borders of the feet with each step.

Note.—This exercise is particularly useful to athletes as a preventive measure against knee injuries, especially prevalent in football. Do not make the distance too great for such an exercise.

THIRD DEGREE LONGITUDINAL FLATFEET—FLEXIBLE

Unless steady progress can be shown toward continuous correction of skeletal faults and continued improvement of arch and foot position, these cases should have orthopedic attention because of the high percentage that have faulty physiological background or actual congenital flatfoot. A conscientious tryout of 3 to 6 months should be ample to prove this point. *Improved position only held temporarily by increase of muscle power is not sufficient to justify failure to refer the case for orthopaedic attention.* For third degree rigid flatfoot no exercises are given.

Starting Position.—Hook lying, knees flexed, arms in wing position.
1. Press big toes to floor, holding arch up, pinch buttocks,
2. Relax and repeat 5 times.
3. Same position, press big toes to floor and turn feet toward each other until toes touch with heels stationary, hold and flatten the back,
4. Assume former position, repeat 5 times and relax,
5. From similar position on back place right foot resting on left knee or alternate legs in similar position,
6. Press big toe of right foot to floor and inward,
7. Relax and alternate feet, repeat 5 times.

*Note.—*In order to adduct and invert the foot to obtain this position, posterior tibial must be strongly activated and thigh is outwardly rotated.

Starting Position.—Long sitting with legs extended, back straight with hands to rear on floor for stability.
1. Cross right foot over the left one, push down on right heel and raise leg slightly,
2. Return and repeat with other foot in similar position 5 times,
3. Same position with knees flexed and right leg crossed over the left or alternate, press big toe to floor and rotate right foot toward left against friction of the floor,
4. Relax and alternate using the opposite foot. Repeat 5 times.

EXERCISES TO STRETCH THE TENDO ACHILLIS

All exercises, as in pushing down on the heels, foot adducted press big toes to floor, are given to tighten the plantar structures and actuate peroneus longus which pronates the forefoot, to prevent its opponent, the anterior tibial, from flattening the arch by supinating the forefoot. Practically all cases of flatfoot have some degree of tightening in the calf group which may be overaction or adaptive shortening. All active and passive efforts at stretching the achillis by means of force applied to the forefoot may produce further harm by stretching plantar structures which are elongating under weight bearing. Therefore, the forefoot should be kept adducted and inverted as much as possible. In case the anterior tibial is very strong and tends to supinate the forefoot in active action upward, dorsiflexion to stretch the achillis should be ruled out or minimized.

Starting Position.—Supine lying position.
1. Push down on right heel and hold foot in inverted position,
2. Relax and repeat with other foot 5 times,
Note.—Elongates short gastrocnemius and activates both tibials in adduction.
3. Same position, knees separated and flexed to chest, straighten both legs upward while steadying thighs with hands and heels pushed upward,
4. Hold in stretch then relax. Repeat 5 times.

Starting Position.—Long sitting with legs extended, back flat and hands behind on floor, fingers pointing toward toes.
1. Extend heels in stretch, letting ankles bend toward the body,
2. Relax and repeat 5 times.
Note.—The emphasis should be on the heel push and not on the ankle flexion because this would over strengthen the anterior tibial and toe extensors.

PASSIVE MOVEMENTS TO STRETCH TENDO ACHILLIS

Starting Position.—Sitting astride bench, thighs adducted, feet toeing in, hands on knees, trunk one-half bent forward.
1. Slide the feet back as far as possible, toe in, and keep the heels firmly on the floor,
2. Resume the starting position and repeat 5 times.

Starting Position.—Standing, legs abducted, feet toed in, hands on hips.
1. Bend forward, hands to floor,
2. Return and repeat 5 times.
Note.—This is to stretch hamstrings and gastrocnemii and the toe-in prevents the pressure on the ball of the foot from breaking the arch by stretching plantar ligaments and muscles more than they are. The toe-in actuates post tibials, benefiting the arch.
3. Same position, hands on hips, right foot forward, toes in and weight to outer border, bend right knee keeping trunk straight in line with the extended rear leg whose foot also toes in,
4. Relax and repeat with opposite foot 5 times.

Note.—After assuming this stance, change position, hold, then bend knee a little more, keeping rear heel on floor and hold. Repeat again as tight calf relaxes and increase to tolerance or until heel lifts from the floor.

Starting Position.—*Standing*, hands on the wall, arms distance away, shoulder height and body width apart.

1. Keeping back flat, relax the elbows and let trunk lean forward toward the wall until the chest almost touches the wall, with body and legs in line and feet adducted,
2. Hold, then return to position and relax. Repeat 5 times.

Note.—This is a hamstring and gastrocnemius stretcher.

Starting Position.—*Standing on tilted balance board*, hands on hips.

1. Step forward, keep left leg straight, trunk leaning slightly forward with back flat,
2. Hold, return to position and repeat with opposite leg.

Note.—While the straight leg is stretching the gastrocnemius and hamstrings, the foot is held inverted by the incline of the board which, to keep balance, must take up slack of the tibials, invertors, while the tightened peronei, the evertors, relax. The opposite foot is having the same correction without the stretching at knee. If a board is not available, invert the feet as though on the peak of a roof.

3. In same position, raise the right foot and grasp the front of the foot with the left hand, turn inward holding balance on the other foot,
4. Hold to count or rhythm and replace on last count.

Note.—This exercise is quite difficult and fatiguing, hence, must be modified as to frequency of repetition and time of holding. It should not be done by hyperflexible weak types with wobbly feet until sufficient balance control has been developed.

CLAWFEET OR CONTRACTED FEET, HUMP FOOT OR PES CAVUS

This condition is usually a hereditary defect in which the arch is very high and the instep is prominent. The plantar muscles are shortened, the toes being flexed at the interphalangeal joints and extended at the metatarsophalangeal joints, assuming a hammer toe form or clawing. In such cases the person should not be given work for adduction or inversion of the feet.

Exercises for claw feet had best be restricted or eliminated except under advice of an orthopedic surgeon. The only exercises of value are those for correcting general deviations above the feet

2. Place heel of right foot pr
   foot up toward the knee a
3. Return to start, alternate

Starting Position.—Standing,
hands grasping stall bars or ba
1. Rotate the knees outward
   and raising arches of feet,
   floor,
2. Emphasize rotation which
   inward, yet resist this act
   the arches. This actuate
   and external thigh rotator
3. Relax and then repeat 5 t

Starting Position.—Standing
hand low on sacrum and righ
pubes.
1. Push pubic bones up, and
2. Then grip buttocks with be
3. Hold while pressing balls o
   the surface of balance boa
4. Relax and repeat 5 times,
   forcefully.
Note.—These exercises produ
structures and help correct the
panies knock knees.

Starting Position.—Supine ly
1. Flex the knees and hips t
   the ankles are firmly held
2. Place a pillow between th
   attached to the feet, usin
   down on the table,
3. As the legs are extended
   apart by the movement,
4. Relax and repeat 5 times.
Note.—The quadriceps perfe
movement.

BOWLEGS

Strange as it may seem, with t
and the use of the tilted balan
effective for bowlegs. Howeve

with attention to the best foot stance, which should allow more toe-out than is used for other conditions.

When accompanied by pronation and ankle valgus, the rotation of the thighs outward should be done mildly and not with force enough to tip the feet into varus. The following exercises are suggested for the milder types without obvious structural changes.

Starting Position.—Sitting on a bench, stool or chair, feet parallel.
1. Press down on the foot, and then extend the toes to make longer,
2. Relax and repeat 5 times,
3. Same position with feet resting on a block or book, with heads of metatarsals in line with the forward edge of block, and press down on the balls of the feet. Keep heels apart enough to line up all joints with the edge,
4. Relax and repeat 5 times, extending toes to stretch.
Note.—Pressure lifts the metatarsals tending to correct the cock up position of the toes, while active extension of the toes automatically tends to relax the opposing shortened toe flexors.
Caution.—Be careful to point the toes out and not raise or extend at the metatarsophalangeal joints.

Starting Position.—Sitting on bench, place the right foot on left knee.
1. Grasp the right forefoot with the left hand using the thumb in order to press the ball of the foot up, while the fingers fold around the toes, pushing the ball of the foot up and pulling toes down with an extension of the left wrist. The right hand grasps the right ankle to steady foot,
2. Relax and repeat 5 times, then reverse using opposite foot.

BACKKNEES

This deviation is compensatory to postural faults in the antero-posterior plane in the trunk, with the shifting of the pelvis forward as the dorsal spine lists back and the head forward. Likewise, in connection with the above deviations, there exists relaxed arches accompanied by tightness of the gastrocnemii.

In such cases, in addition to the previous mentioned changes, there are tight hamstrings which cause the knee to be pulled back and the posterior knee ligaments to become stretched gradually. Then the vicious circle increases the segmental shifts above, and aching legs and vague discomfort in the back may ensue. The following are a few suggested exercises.

Starting Position.—Hook :
1. Raise the right foot ar
2. Rotate the foot inwar
   outward,
3. Replace foot to startin;
4. Relax and repeat with
Note.—This actuates the i
popliteus, a short muscle be
rotators of the thigh, sartori

Starting Position.—Stand
together.
1. Squat to a half knee be:
2. Climb stairs backward,

Starting Position.—Sitting
angle.
1. Place right foot forwar(
2. Rotate foot inward to
   floor,
3. Straighten, and press b
4. Slide foot back to starti
   Repeat 5 times.
Note.—Feet being 8 inche:
knee being extended enough
tion of hamstrings against f
starting position also activa1
tion of the feet.

KNOCK KNEES

The main effect to be obt
improve the tone and streng
the inward and downward
through the shaft of the leg:
floor during the propulsive
twisting for throwing, battin;
chief effort is to develop the
thigh rotation. Exercises
follows.

Starting Position.—Long si
against a wall or supporting
back on some rest or rear of
1. Roll the legs outward, ;

that the chief effort is to correct the inward thrust of the ankle or the valgus, and pronation below and the inward rotation of the leg above. The purpose is to maintain the weight thrust on the bones of the outer borders of the feet and not on the resilient springy ligaments and muscles on the inner border.

As the growth stimulus is greater on the concavity of the curves, the physiological impact of the weight will then pass through a solid bony column, and thus the bowed tibiæ are helped to grow straight. In both knock knees and bowlegs the correction is physiological and not mechanical. This fact is important and is the reason why a wedge on the inner border of the heels is indicated for both conditions, contrary to what some people often think. The following exercise is specific for this condition in addition to those previously presented.

Starting Position.—Supine lying on plinth.
1. While the legs, near the vertex of the O bending of the legs, are held together by a belt, flex the knees and hips,
2. A pillow is placed between the ankles, and a pulley weight is attached to the feet, while a broad belt holds the waist down on the table,
3. As the legs are extended, the knees are then forced together by the movement,
4. Relax and repeat 5 times.

CONCLUSION

It is well to remember in regard to exercise that there is a time for decision, for time is precious to the individual and any usurping of energies for worthless activities of little meaning should be frowned upon by all leaders. True, everyone wants a chance to belong and should be given the opportunity, and each one of us should serve as the expediter in offering streamlined reinforcements for the improvement of personal efficiency. We must counteract the influence of commercial enterprises which exploit the human frailties of people, and offer instead sound exercise precepts which will assist in the solution of individual problems.

Exercise is no short cut but rather is hard work which requires diligent and sincere effort as well as persistence. Sometimes the area of activity has been referred to as one of the frills and fads of education, but those who have profited through wise counsel of intelligent leaders attribute much of their success in life to the development of sound physical backgrounds.

In times of stress, nations have for centuries turned to physical activity to improve the well being of their citizens. If this is important in times of war, is it not doubly so in periods of peace, when man is considered from a personal standpoint as to value? If good health is an attribute of happiness, and activity is of aid in accomplishing this goal, then we must become students of sports medicine and the various techniques that are available for our use.

It is imperative that each worker in this area, by a boot strap operation in and through his own activity, apply such recommendations as are prescribed as best he can in order that those he comes in contact with may profit from his knowledge. To better prepare himself, one might well follow this poem.

> I turn to the words of wiser men,
> That wisdom may find its way to my pen.
> The experience of sages offer untold leads,
> To inspire the mind of him who heeds.
>
> Ideas of the past show the way others have thought,
> Offer guidance and counsel worthwhile to be sought.
> So hitch up your trousers and roll up your sleeves,
> Apply all this knowledge to make life a breeze.

Seriously, in conclusion, may it be re-emphasized that within the heart of our nation are those who, because of the circumstances and fallacies of nature, have vulnerable spots in their armature which prevent complete success in many physical endeavors. Among these weaknesses are those of *postural fitness*, and many *variances* which have great *significance*, and which might well be prevented or corrected.

It is these individuals that need our trust in their inherent potentiality as valuable citizens, our respect for the dignity of each as a human being, and our effort in their behalf in making democracy a reality. All have pride, ambition and courage, yet all too often there are few chances for these attributes to be used in accomplishments. A chance to belong and a chance for dreams to come true are the right of all.

Largely through ignorance the lack of integrity and concern for those who need our help, whether they be young or old, tend to be increasing. Unless our ideals and actions cause others to say, "Here is a person who gave freely of himself, that those who came in touch with him, profited by his presence," we are remiss in our obligations.

Who knows but yourself what you have to offer, and who can say how far you can reach unless you extend your hand. Within your grasp may be untold opportunities which unless proffered, will hang idly at your side. May you lift those who need your

16

help out of the shadows and into the light. You can if you will and you will if you try.

Now if there is anything else you would like to know, we shall be glad to share our mistakes with you. Just remember, when you get to the end of your rope, to tie a knot and hang on.

REFERENCES

1. BECHTOL, CHARLES O.: Muscle Physiology, *Instructional Course Lectures—Vol. V.* The American Academy of Orthopedic Surgeons. Ann Arbor, Michigan: J. W. Edwards, 1948, p. 188.
2. JACOBSON, EDMUND: *Progressive Relaxation.* 2nd ed., Chicago, The University of Chicago Press, 1956, 493 pp.
3. LOWMAN, CHARLES LeROY, COLESTOCK, CLAIRE, and COOPER, HAZEL: *Corrective Physical Education for Groups,* New York, A. S. Barnes and Co., 1928, Chapter XXVII.
4. V-5 ASSOCIATION OF AMERICA: *Conditioning Exercises, Games, Tests,* 3rd ed. by Karl C. H. Oermann, Carl Haven Young, *et al.,* Annapolis, Maryland, United States Naval Institute, 1960, Chapter IX.

The above references are not repeated in References for Extended Reading.

REFERENCES FOR EXTENDED READING

BILLIG, HARVEY E., and LOEWENDAHL, EVELYN: *Mobilization of the Human Body.* Stanford, California, Stanford University Press, 1951, 65 pp.

BOWEN, WILBUR P., and STONE, H. A.: *Applied Anatomy and Kinesiology.* 7th ed. Philadelphia, Lea & Febiger, 1953, 462 pp.
    Chapter IX: Team Work Among Muscles.

COLSON, JOHN H. C.: *Postural and Relaxation Training in Physiotherapy and Physical Education.* Springfield, Illinois, Charles C Thomas, 1956, 105 pp.
    Part I: Re-education of Posture.
    Part II: Relaxation Training.

DANIELS, ARTHUR S.: *Adapted Physical Education.* New York, Harper Bros., 1954, 538 pp.
    Chapter IX: Body Mechanics Problems.

DREW, L. C.: *Individual Gymnastics.* 5th ed. Rev. and ed. by Hazel Kinzley, Philadelphia, Lea & Febiger, 1949, 222 pp.
    Chapter XI: Exercises.

EWERHARDT, F. H., and RIDDLE, GERTRUDE F.: *Therapeutic Exercise.* Philadelphia, Lea & Febiger, 1947, 152 pp.
    Chapter VI: Physiology of Therapeutic Exercise.
    Chapter VII: Special Applications of Therapeutic Exercise.

FINK, DAVID HAROLD: *Release from Nervous Tension.* New York, Simon and Schuster, Inc., 1943, 232 pp.

GARDINER, M. DENA: *The Principles of Exercise Therapy.* London, G. Bell & Sons ltd., 1954, 260 pp.
    Chapter XIV: Individual, Group and Mass Treatment by Exercise.

GUTHRIE-SMITH, O.: *Rehabilitation, Re-education and Remedial Exercise.* London, Bailliere, Tindall and Cox, 1949, 456 pp.

HANSSON, K. G.: Body Mechanics and Posture, J.A.M.A., *128,* 947–953, 1945.

HAWLEY, GERTRUDE: *The Kinesiology of Corrective Exercise.* 2nd ed. Philadelphia, Lea & Febiger, 1949, 192 pp.
    Chapters XI through XVII.

HAYES, SHIRLEY: The Use of Rhythmical Activities in Adapted Physical Education. Unpublished Master's thesis, The University of California, Los Angeles, 1957, 132 pp.

JACOBSON, EDMUND: *You Must Relax.* 3rd ed. New York, McGraw-Hill Book Co., Inc., 1948, 282 pp.

JOHNS, EDWARD B., SUTTON, WILFRED C., and WEBSTER, LLOYD E.: *Health for Effective Living*. New York, McGraw-Hill Book Co., Inc., 1958, 507 pp.
Chapter IX: Utilizing Opportunities for Rest and Recreation.
KELLY, ELLEN D.: *Teaching Posture and Body Mechanics*. New York, A. S. Barnes and Co., 1949, 212 pp.
Part III: Posture and Body Mechanics Activities.
KRAUS, H.: *Principles and Practice of Therapeutic Exercise*. Springfield, Illinois, Charles C Thomas, 1956, 309 pp.
LEE, MABEL, and WAGNER, MIRIAM M.: *Fundamentals of Body Mechanics and Conditioning*. Philadelphia, W. B. Saunders Co., 1949, 377 pp.
LICHT, SIDNEY, (ed.): *Therapeutic Exercise*. New Haven, Conn.: Elizabeth Licht, 1958, 893 pp.
Chapter V: Motions of the Hand and Foot.—Walter J. Treanor.
Chapter XVII: Principles of Therapeutic Exercise.—Robert L. Bennett
Chapter XIX: Exercises for Scoliosis.—Y. LeGrand-Lambling.
Chapter XXIII: Exercise in Foot Disabilities.—Joseph H. Kite.
MENSENDIECK, B. M.: *Look Better, Feel Better*. New York, Harper Bros., 1954, 276 pp.
METHENY, ELEANOR: *Body Dynamics*. New York, McGraw-Hill Book Co., Inc., 1952, 225 pp.
Chapter IV: Exercise and Relaxation.
PHELPS, WINTHROP M., KIPHUTH, ROBERT J. and GOFF, CHARLES W.: *Diagnosis and Treatment of Postural Defects*. Springfield, Charles C Thomas, 1956, 190 pp.
Chapter VIII: Corrective Exercises for Strengthening.
PHYSICAL MEDICINE AND REHABILITATION SERVICE, CORRECTIVE THERAPY SECTION. *Guide to Proper Body Mechanics and Patient Self-Care*. Los Angeles: Veterans Adm. Center, 1959. 26 pp.
Physical Reconditioning. Dept. of the Army, Tech. Manual TM8-292; Dept. of the Air Force, Manual AFM160-16, 1952, 219 pp.
Physical Training. War Department Field Manual, F.M.21-22, January, 1946, 393 pp.
RASCH, PHILIP J. and BURKE, ROGER K.: *Kinesiology and Applied Anatomy*. Philadelphia, Lea & Febiger, 1959, 456 pp.
Chapters IX through XVII.
RATHBONE, JOSEPHINE L.: *Corrective Physical Education*. 5th ed. Philadelphia, W. B. Saunders Co., 1955, 318 pp.
Chapter V: Tension, Fatigue, and Conscious Relaxation.
————: *Relaxation*. New York, Teachers College, Columbia University, 1943, 157 pp.
STAFFORD, GEORGE T.: *Preventive and Corrective Physical Education*. New York, A. S. Barnes and Co., 1950, 312 pp.
Chapter III: Preventive and Corrective Physical Education.
Chapter V: The Treatment of Faulty Body Mechanics.
Chapter VI: The Feet.
WILLIAMS, M., and WORTHINGHAM, CATHERINE: *Therapeutic Exercise for Body Alignment and Function*. Philadelphia, W. B. Saunders Co., 1957, 127 pp.
Chapter III: The Therapeutic Exercise Program.
Chapter IV: Principles of Treatment and Exercises for the Various Areas.
YOUNG, CARL HAVEN: The Construction of a Manual for Use in The Physical Appraisal and Development of Cadets in the Naval Aviation Training Program. Unpublished Doctor's thesis, Stanford University, Stanford, California, 1946, 81 pp. plus Manual of 235 pp.

Bibliography

AINSWORTH, D., and EVANS, R.: *Basic Rhythms*. New York, Charwell House, Inc., 1955, 200 pp.

ABRAMSON, ARTHUR S.: Exercise in Paraplegia, *Therapeutic Exercise*. Sidney Licht, (ed.). New Haven, Conn.: Elizabeth Licht, 1958, pp. 674–691.

ALLPORT, FLOYD HENRY: *Theories of Perception and the Concept of Structure*. New York, Wiley, 1955, 709 pp.

AMERICAN ASSOCIATION FOR HEALTH, PHYSICAL EDUCATION AND RECREATION: *Physical Education for High School Students*. Washington, Amer. Ass'n for Health, Physical Education and Recreation, 1955, 406 pp.

ANSON, BARRY J.: *Atlas of Human Anatomy*. Philadelphia, W. B. Saunders Co., 1950, 518 pp.

AUSUBEL, DAVID P.: *Theory and Problems of Adolescent Development*. New York, Grune and Stratton, 1954, 580 pp.

AVIATION TRAINING DIVISION, OFFICE OF THE CHIEF OF NAVAL OPERATIONS, U.S. NAVY: *Mass Exercise, Games, Tests*. Compiler-writer, Carl Haven Young. Annapolis, Maryland, United States Naval Institute, 1943, 235 pp.

BALDWIN, ALFRED L.: *Behavior and Development in Childhood*. New York, The Dryden Press, 1955, 619 pp.

BANCROFT, JESSIE H.: *Games for Playground, Home, School, and Gymnasium*. New York, The Macmillan Co., 1937, 685 pp.

————: *The Posture of School Children*. New York, The Macmillan Co., 1919, 327 pp.

BARLOW, WILFRED: Posture and Its Re-education, *Therapeutic Exercise*. Sidney Licht, (ed.). New Haven, Conn.: Elizabeth Licht, 1958, pp. 437–448.

BARTLEY, S. H., and CHUTE, E.: *Fatigue and Impairment in Man*. New York, McGraw-Hill Book Co., Inc., 1947, 429 pp.

BAUMGARTNER, ALBERT: *Posture Training and Remedial Gymnastics*. Minneapolis, Burgess Publishing Co., 1948, 166 pp.

BAYLEY, N.: Individual Patterns of Development, Child Development, *27*, 45–74, 1956.

BAYLEY, N., and ESPENSCHADE, A.: Motor Development and Decline, Rev. Educ. Res., *20*, 367–374, 1950.

BECHTOL, CHARLES O.: Muscle Physiology, *Instructional Course Lecture—Vol. V.* The American Academy of Orthopaedic Surgeons. Ann Arbor, Michigan, J. W. Edwards 1948, pp. 181–189.

BENNETT, ROBERT L.: Principles of Therapeutic Exercise, *Therapeutic Exercise*. Sidney Licht, (ed.). New Haven, Conn., Elizabeth Licht, 1958, pp. 423–436.

BERNARD, HAROLD W.: *Adolescent Development in American Culture*. Yonkers, N.Y., World Book Co., 1957, 644 pp.

BEST, CHARLES HERBERT, and TAYLOR, NORMAN BURKE: *Physiological Basis of Medical Practice*. 6th ed. Baltimore, The Williams and Wilkins Co., 1955, 1357 pp.

————: *The Living Body*. New York, Henry Holt and Co., 1952, 792 pp.

BETTMAN, E. H.: The Human Foot, Arch. Phys. Therapy, *25*, 13–26, 1944.

BILLIG, HARVEY E., and LOEWENDAHL, EVELYN: *Mobilization of the Human Body*. Stanford, California, Stanford University Press, 1951, 65 pp.

BLAIR, ARTHUR W., and BURTON, WILLIAM H.: *Growth and Development of the Pre-Adolescent*. New York, Appleton-Century-Crofts, Inc., 1951, 221 pp.

BLAIR, GLENN MYERS, JONES, R. STEWART, and SIMPSON, RAY H. *Educational Psychology*. New York, The Macmillan Co., 1954, 601 pp.

BLESH, T. ERWIN, MEYERS, CARLTON R., and KIPHUTH, OSCAR W.: *Photometric Photography in Posture Evaluation of Yale University Freshmen.* New Haven, Yale University Press, 1954, 17 pp.

BOGERT, L. J.: *Nutrition and Physical Fitness.* 6th ed., Philadelphia, W. B. Saunders Co., 1954, 664 pp.

BOWEN, WILBUR P., and STONE, H. A.: *Applied Anatomy and Kinesiology.* 7th ed. Philadelphia, Lea & Febiger, 1953, 462 pp.

BOWLEY, AGATHA H.: *The Natural Development of the Child.* A Guide for Parents, Teachers, Students, and Others. 4th ed. London, Livingstone, 1957, 206 pp.

BRECKENRIDGE, MARIAN E., and VINCENT, E. LEE: *Child Development.* 3rd. ed. Philadelphia, W. B. Saunders Co., 1955, 497 pp.

BRIESEN, HANS V.: A Discussion of Stress and Exhaustion as a Primary as well as a Contributing Etiologic Factor in Organic Neurological Disease. Military Surg., *101*, 286–290, 1947.

BRINLEY, ELDON D.: Interscholastic Football in the Elementary School, Texas J. Sci., *4*, 464–470, 1952.

BRITTON, EDWARD C., and WINANS, J. MERRITT: *Growing from Infancy to Adulthood.* New York, Appleton-Century-Crofts, Inc., 1958, 118 pp.

BROCH, H.: *Importance of Overweight.* New York, W. W. Norton and Co., Inc., 1957.

BROWN, LLOYD T.: A Combined Medical and Postural Examination of 746 Young Adults, Am. J. Orthopedic Surg., *15*, 774–787, 1917.

BROWN, WADE H.: Constitutional Variations and Susceptibility to Disease, *The Harvey Lectures.* Baltimore, Williams and Wilkins Co., 1930.

CAILLIET, RENE: Exercise in Multiple Sclerosis, *Therapeutic Exercise.* Sidney Licht, (ed.). New Haven, Conn., Elizabeth Licht, 1958, pp. 710–718.

CALIFORNIA RECREATION COMMISSION: *Recreation for Handicapped People in California.* Sacramento, California State Printing Office, 1955, 52 pp.

————: *Recreation for Older People in California.* Sacramento, California State Printing Office, 1951, 68 pp.

CANNON, WALTER B.: *The Wisdom of the Body.* New York, W. W. Norton and Co., Inc., 1939, 333 pp.

CARLSON, A. J., and JOHNSON, V.: *Machinery of the Body.* 4th ed. Chicago, University of Chicago Press, 1953, 663 pp.

Case studies from personal files of Dr. Charles LeRoy Lowman, and from the files of the Orthopedic Hospital, Los Angeles, California.

CASSIDY, ROSALIND: Democratic Leadership, *Developing Democratic Human Relations.* Washington, Amer. Ass'n. for Health, Physical Education and Recreation, 1951, pp. 101–115.

CHAPMAN, CARLETON B.: Exercise in Heart Disease, *Therapeutic Exercise.* Sidney Licht, (ed.). New Haven, Conn., Elizabeth Licht, 1958, pp. 762–769.

CLARKE, HENRY HARRISON: *Application of Measurement to Health and Physical Education.* 2nd ed. New York, Prentice-Hall, 1950, 493 pp.

CLARKE, HENRY HARRISON, and ELKINS, E. C.: Evaluation of Training of Physical Educationalists for Reconditioning and Rehabilitation, Arch. Phys. Med., *29*, 99–107, 1948.

COERS, CHRISTIAN: The Motor Unit, *Therapeutic Exercise.* Sidney Licht. (ed.). New Haven, Conn., Elizabeth Licht, 1958, pp. 1–19.

COGHILL, GEORGE ELLETT: *Anatomy and the Problem of Behavior.* New York, The Macmillan Co., 1929, 113 pp.

COLESTOCK, CLAIRE, and LOWMAN, CHARLES LEROY: *Fundamental Exercises for Physical Fitness.* New York, A. S. Barnes and Co., 1943, 314 pp.

COLSON, JOHN H. C.: *Postural and Relaxation Training in Physiotherapy and Physical Education.* Springfield, Charles C Thomas, 1956, 105 pp.

COMFORT, ALEXANDER: *The Biology of Senescence.* London, Rantledge and Paul, 1956, 257 pp.

COMMINS, W. D., and FAGIN, BARRY: *Principles of Educational Psychology.* 2nd ed. New York, Ronald Press Co., 1954, 795 pp.

CONANT, RICHARD D.: The Utilization of Photographic Techniques in Adapted Physical Education. Unpublished Master's thesis, The University of California, Los Angeles, 1956, 113 pp.

COOPER, L. F., BARBER, E. M., and MITCHELL, H. S.: *Nutrition in Health and Diseases.* 10th ed. Philadelphia, J. B. Lippincott Co., 1953, 790 pp.

COWELL, CHARLES C.: *Scientific Foundations of Physical Education.* New York, Harper Bros., 1953, 260 pp.

CRAIG, MARGARET B.: A Comparison of Five Methods Designed to Predict the Normal Weight of College Women, Res. Quart., *15*, 64–74, 1944.

CRAMPTON, C. WARD: Medical Services in Aging and De-Aging, J. Assoc. Phys. and Mental Rehabilitation, *9*, 39–43, 1955.

CROOK, BILLIE LOUISE: A Scale for Measuring the Antero-Posterior Posture of Pre-School Children, Res. Quart., 7, 96, 1936.

CROW, LESTER, and CROW, ALICE: *Adolescent Development and Adjustment.* New York, McGraw-Hill Book Co., Inc., 1956, 570 pp.

————: *Human Development and Learning.* New York, American Book Co., 1956, 578 pp.

CROWE, WALTER CAMPBELL: The Use of Audio-Visual Materials in Developmental (Corrective) Physical Education. Unpublished Master's thesis, The University of California, Los Angeles, 1950, 219 pp.

CUNNINGHAM, DANIEL JOHN: *Textbook of Anatomy.* 9th ed. J. C. Brash, (ed.). London, Oxford University Press, 1951, 1604 pp.

CURETON, T. K.: Bodily Posture as an Indicator of Fitness, Suppl. Res. Quart., *12*, 348–367, 1941.

————: *Physical Fitness, Appraisal and Guidance.* St. Louis, C. V. Mosby Co., 1947. 566 pp.

————: Weight and Tissue Symmetry Analysis, Suppl. Res. Quart., *2*, 331–347, 1941.

CURETON, T. K. and WICKENS, J. S.: The Center of Gravity of the Human Body in the Antero-Posterior Plane and Its Relation to Posture, Physical Fitness and Athletic Ability, Suppl. Res. Quart., *6*, 93–105, 1935.

CYRIAX, EDGAR F.: On the Anterior-Posterior Tilt of the Pelvis, Its Variations, and Their Clinical Significance in Children, British Journal of Children's Diseases, *24*, 279–283, 1924.

DACAO, MICHAEL M.: Rehabilitation of the Aged—Promise or Reality, *Age is No Barrier.* New York, New York State Joint Legislative Committee on Problems of the Aging, 1952, pp. 136–139.

DANIELS, ARTHUR S.: *Adapted Physical Education.* New York, Harper Bros., 1954, 538 pp.

DANIELS, L., WILLIAMS, M., and WORTHINGHAM, CATHERINE: *Muscle Testing.* Philadelphia, W. B. Saunders Co., 1956, 176 pp.

DARLING, ROBERT C.: Physiology of Exercise and Fatigue, *Therapeutic Exercise.* Sidney Licht, (ed.), New Haven, Conn., Elizabeth Licht, 1958, pp. 20–43.

DAVIS, ELWOOD C., and LAWTHER, JOHN D.: *Successful Teaching in Physical Education.* New York, Prentice-Hall, Inc., 1948, 617 pp.

DAVIS, G. G.: *Applied Anatomy.* Philadelphia, J. P. Lippincott Co., 1910, 630 pp.

DAVIS, JOHN EISELE: Exercise in Mental Disease, *Therapeutic Exercise.* Sidney Licht, (ed.), New Haven, Conn., Elizabeth Licht, 1958, pp. 719–736.

————: *Rehabilitation, Its Principles and Practice.* Rev. ed. New York, A. S. Barnes and Co., 1946, 264 pp.

DEARBORN, WALTER, and ROTHNEY, JOHN W. M.: *Predicting the Child's Development.* Cambridge, Mass, Science Art Publishers, 1941, 360 pp.

DE LONG, EVERETT W.: Contrasenescence, J. Appl. Nutrit., *9*, 415–421, 1956.

DICKSON, FRANK D., and DIVELEY, REX L.: *Fundamental Disorders of the Foot.* Philadelphia, J. B. Lippincott Co., 1953, 345 pp.

DOING, RUTH: Exercises for Senior Citizens, *Growing With The Years.* New York, New York State Joint Legislative Committee on Problems of the Aging, 1954, pp. 133–134.

DONAHUE, WILMA: The Human Machine at Middle Life, *Aging in the Modern World.* Clark Tibbitts and Wilma Donahue, (eds.). Ann Arbor, University of Michigan, 1957, pp. 47–66.

DREW, L. C.: *Individual Gymnastics.* 5th ed. Rev. and ed. by Hazel Kinzley, Philadelphia, Lea & Febiger, 1949, 222 pp.

DUVALL, ELLEN NEALL: *Kinesiology*. Englewood Cliffs, N. J., Prentice-Hall, Inc., 1959, 292 pp.

EBEL, ALFRED: Exercise in Vascular Diseases, *Therapeutic Exercise*. Sidney Licht, (ed.). New Haven, Conn., Elizabeth Licht, 1958, pp 770–785.

EDWARDS, LINDEN FOREST: *Concise Anatomy*. 2nd ed. New York, McGraw-Hill Book Co., Inc., 1956, 502 pp.

EWERHARDT, F. H., and RIDDLE, GERTRUDE F.: *Therapeutic Exercise*. Philadelphia, Lea & Febiger, 1947, 152 pp.

FINK, DAVID HAROLD: *Release from Nervous Tension*. New York, Simon and Schuster, Inc., 1943, 232 pp.

FISK, GUY H.: Motions of the Shoulder and Hip, *Therapeutic Exercise*. Sidney Licht, (ed.). New Haven, Conn., Elizabeth Licht, 1958, pp. 88–98.

FITZHUGH, M. L.: Some Effects of Early Sitting on Body Mechanics of Infancy and Childhood, Physiotherapy Rev., *23*, 8–13, 1943.

FLETCHER, W. D.: Exercise in Obstetrics, *Therapeutic Exercise*. Sidney Licht, (ed.). New Haven, Conn., Elizabeth Licht, 1958. pp. 786–795.

FLOYD, W. F., and SILVER, P. H. S.: Patterns of Muscle Activity in Posture and Movement, Science News, No. 22, November, 1951.

FORD, ADELBERT: *Foundations of Bioelectronics for Human Engineering*. Navy Electronics Laboratory Report 761. San Diego, California, U. S. Navy Electronics Laboratory, 4 April, 1957, 119 pp.

FOREST, ILSE: *Child Development*. New York, McGraw-Hill Book Co. Inc., 1954, 291 pp.

FOX, MARGARET G., and YOUNG, OLIVE G.: Placement of the Gravital Line in Antero-Posterior Standing Posture, Res. Quart., *25*, 277–285, 1954.

FRANCIS, ANDREW J.: Bases for Selection of Activities for Senior Citizens. Unpublished Research project, The University of California, Los Angeles, 1957, 73 pp.

GARDINER, M. DENA: *The Principles of Exercise Therapy*. London, G. Bell & Sons Ltd., 1954, 260 pp.

GARRISON, KARL C., and GRAY, J. STANLEY: *Educational Psychology*. New York, Appleton-Century-Crofts, Inc., 1955, 505 pp.

GESELL, ARNOLD LUCIUS: *Youth, the Years from Ten to Sixteen*. New York, Harper Bros., 1956, 542 pp.

GESELL, ARNOLD, and ILG, FRANCES L.: *Child Development: An Introduction to the Study of Human Growth*. New York, Harper and Bros., 1949, 475 pp.

————: *Infant and Child in the Culture of Today*. New York, Harper and Bros., 1943, 403 pp.

GESELL, ARNOLD, et al.: *The Child from Five to Ten*. New York, Harper and Bros., 1946, 475 pp.

GILLETTE, HARRIET E.: Exercises for Cerebral Palsy, *Therapeutic Exercise*. Sidney Licht, (ed.). New Haven, Conn., Elizabeth Licht, 1958, pp. 692–709.

GLUECK, SHELDON, and GLUECK, ELEANOR: *Physique and Delinquency*. New York, Harper Bors., 1956, 339 pp.

GOFF, C. W.: Mean Posture Patterns with New Postural Values, Am. J. Phys. Anthrop., *9*, 335–346, 1951.

————: Orthograms of Posture, J. Bone and Joint Surg., *34-A*, 115–122, 1952.

————: Posture in Children, Clin. Orthop., *1*, 66–79, 1953.

GOLDTHWAITE, J. E., SWAIN, L. T., and KUHNS, J. G.: *Essentials of Body Mechanics*. 5th ed. Philadelphia, J. B. Lippincott Co., 1952, 356 pp.

GOODHART, ROBERT S.: Nutrition and the Aging, *New Channels for the Golden Years*. New York, New York State Joint Legislative Com. on Problems of the Aging, 1956, pp. 81–82.

GORDON, I.: The Healthy Child: Its Many Disguises, Brit. Med. J., *1*, 611–622, 1951.

GRAY, HENRY: *Anatomy of the Human Body*. Ed. by Charles Mayo Goss. 27th ed. Philadelphia, Lea & Febiger, 1959, 1480 pp.

GREULICH, W. W., and PYLE, S. I.: *Radiographic Atlas of Skeletal Development of Hand and Wrist*. Stanford, Stanford University Press, 1950, 190 pp.

GUCKER, THOMAS: Exercise in Orthopedics, *Therapeutic Exercise*. Sidney Licht, (ed.). New Haven, Conn., Elizabeth Licht, 1958, pp. 581–608.

GULLICKSON, GLENN: Exercises for Amputees, *Therapeutic Exercise*. Sidney Licht, (ed.). New Haven, Conn., Elizabeth Licht, 1958, pp. 521–580.

GUTHRIE-SMITH, O.:   *Rehabilitation, Re-education and Remedial Exercise*. London, Bailliere, Tindall and Cox, 1949, 456 pp.

HALE, C. J.:   Changing Growth Patterns of the American Child, Education, *78*, 467–470, 1958.

HANSSON, K. G.:   Body Mechanics and Posture, J.A.M.A., *128*, 947–953, 1945.

HARRIS, DALE B.:   *The Concept of Development*. Minneapolis, University of Minn. Press, 1957, 287 pp.

HAWLEY, GERTRUDE: *The Kinesiology of Corrective Exercise*. 2nd ed. Philadelphia, Lea & Febiger, 1949, 192 pp.

HAYES, ASAHEL E.:   Determination of Bases for Developmental Physical Education in the Public Schools. Unpublished Master's thesis, The University of California, Los Angeles, 1950, 109 pp.

HAYES, SHIRLEY: The Use of Rhythmical Activities in Adapted Physical Education. Unpublished Master's thesis, The University of California, Los Angeles, 1957, 132 pp.

HELLEBRANDT, F. A., and FRANSEEN, E. B.:   Physiological Study of Vertical Stance of Man, Physiol. Rev., *23*, 220–255, 1943.

HINES, THOMAS F.:   Manual Muscle Examination, *Therapeutic Exercise*. Sidney Licht, (ed.). New Haven, Conn., Elizabeth Licht, 1958, pp. 159–251.

HOBERMAN, MORTON: Crutch and Cane Exercises and Use, *Therapeutic Exercise*. Sidney Licht, (ed.). New Haven, Conn., Elizabeth Licht, 1958, pp. 20–43.

HOBSON, WILLIAM, (ed.).:   *Modern Trends in Geriatrics*. London, Butterworth, 1956, 422 pp.

HOLLINSHEAD, W. Henry: *Functional Anatomy—Limbs and Back*. Philadelphia, W. B. Saunders Co., 1951, 341 pp.

Howarth, M. B.:   Dynamic Posture, Hygiea, *25*, 198, 1947.

HOWARTH, M. BECKETT, *et al.*:   *A Text-book of Orthopedics*. Philadelphia, W. B. Saunders Co., 1952, 1110 pp.

HUBBARD, A. W.:   Muscular Force in Reciprocal Movements, J. Gen. Psych., *20*, 315–325, 1939.

HUNT, VALERIE V.:   *Recreation for the Handicapped*. New York, Prentice-Hall, Inc., 1955, 340 pp.

HURLOCK, ELIZABETH B.:   *Adolescent Development*. Rev. ed. New York, McGraw-Hill Book Co., Inc., 1956, 703 pp.

————:   *Child Growth and Development*. New York, McGraw-Hill Book Co., Inc., 1956, 384 pp.

JACOBSON, EDMUND: *Progressive Relaxation*. 2nd ed. Chicago, University of Chicago Press, 1956, 493 pp.

————:   *You Must Relax*. 3rd ed. New York, McGraw-Hill Book Co., Inc., 1948, 282 pp.

JANSEN, MURK: *Feebleness of Growth*, London, Hodden and Stoughton, 1921, 82 pp.

JEFFREYS, R. J.:   *Life Will Begin at 100*. Columbus, Ohio, Capitol College Press, 1955, 239 pp.

JERSILD, ARTHUR T.:   *The Psychology of Adolescence*. New York, The Macmillan Co., 1957, 438 pp.

JOHNS, EDWARD B., SUTTON, WILFRED C., and WEBSTER, LLOYD E.:   *Health for Effective Living*. New York, McGraw-Hill Book Co., Inc., 1958, 507 pp.

JOHNSON, WINGATE M.:   *The Years after Fifty*. New York, McGraw-Hill Book Co., Inc., 1947, 153 pp.

JOINT COMMITTEE OF AMERICAN MEDICAL ASSOCIATION AND THE ASSOCIATION FOR HEALTH, PHYSICAL EDUCATION AND RECREATION.   Exercise and Fitness, J. Health, Phys. Educ., Recreation, *29*, 40–43, 1958.

JONES, EDWINA, MORGAN, EDNA, and STEVENS, GLADYS: *Methods and Materials in Elementary Physical Education*. New York, World Book Co., 1957, 432 pp.

JONES, H. E.:   *Motor Performance and Growth*. Berkeley, University of California Press, 1949, 181 pp.

————:   Those Physical Changes of Adolescence, Nat. Parent Teach., *52*, 8–10, Sept., 1957.

JONES, R. L.: The Human Foot. An Experimental Study of Its Mechanics, and the Role of Its Muscles and Ligaments in Support of the Arch, A. J. Anat., *68*, 1–40, 1941.

KABAT, HERMAN: Proprioceptive Facilitation in Therapeutic Exercise, *Therapeutic Exercise*. Sidney Licht, (ed.). New Haven, Conn., Elizabeth Licht, 1958, pp. 301–318.

KANSAS PUBLIC SCHOOLS: *Survey of Inter-School Tackle Football in Junior High School*. Kansas City, Board of Education, February 1958, 19 pp. (mimeographed.)

KELLY, ELLEN D.: A Comparative Study of Structure and Function of Normal, Pronated and Painful Feet Among Children, Res. Quart., *18*, 291–312, 1947.

KELLY, ELLEN D.: *Teaching Posture and Body Mechanics*. New York, A. S. Barnes and Co., 1949, 212 pp.

KELLOGG, JOHN HARVEY: Observations on the Relations of Posture to Health, and a New Method of Studying Posture and Development, Bull. Battle Creek Sanitarium-Hospital Clin., *22*, 1, 1927.

KENDALL, H. O., and KENDALL, F. P.: Normal Flexibility According to Age Groups, J. Bone & Joint Surg., *30-A*, 690, 1948.

————: The Role of Abdominal Exercises in a Program of Physical Fitness, J. Health and Phys. Educ., *14*, 480–481, 1943.

KENDALL, HENRY O., KENDALL, FLORENCE P., and BOYNTON, DOROTHY A.: *Posture and Pain*. Baltimore, Williams and Wilkins Co., 1952, 204 pp.

KENDALL, P. HUME: Exercises for Arthritis, *Therapeutic Exercise*. Sidney Licht, (ed.). New Haven, Conn., Elizabeth Licht, 1958, pp. 638–653.

KIERNANDER, BASIL: Physical Medicine in the Treatment of the Elderly, *Modern Trends in Geriatrics*. William Hobson, (ed.). London, Butterworth, 1956, pp. 344–345.

KIPHUTH, ROBERT: *How to be Fit*. New Haven, Yale University Press, 1956, 151 pp.

KITE, JOSEPH H.: Exercise in Foot Disabilities, *Therapeutic Exercise*. Sidney Licht, (ed.). New Haven, Conn., Elizabeth Licht, 1958, pp. 609–637.

KNAPP, MILAND E.: Exercises for Poliomyelitis, *Therapeutic Exercise*. Sidney Licht, (ed.). New Haven, Conn., Elizabeth Licht, 1958. pp. 494–520.

KNIGHT, R. A.: Developmental Deformities of Lower Extremities, J. Bone & Joint Surg., *36-A*, 521–527, 1954.

KNIPPING, H. W., and VALENTIN, H.: Sports in Medicine, *Therapeutic Exercise*. Sidney Licht, (ed.). New Haven, Conn., Elizabeth Licht, 1958, pp. 329–349.

KOZMAN, HILDA CLUTE, CASSIDY, ROSALIND, and JACKSON, CHESTER O.: *Methods in Physical Education*. Philadelphia, W. B. Saunders Co., 1952, 557 pp.

KOZMAN, HILDA CLUTE, (ed).: *Group Process in Physical Education*. New York, Harper Bros., 1951, 418 pp.

KRAUS, H.: *Principles and Practice of Therapeutic Exercise*. Springfield, Charles C Thomas, 1956, 309 pp.

KRAUS, RICHARD: *Play Activities for Boys and Girls*. New York, McGraw-Hill Book Co., Inc., 1957, 236 pp.

KROGMAN, W. M.: The Concept of Maturity from a Morphological Viewpoint, Child Development, *21*, 25–32, 1950.

KUHNS, J. G.: The Late Effects of Minor Degrees of Poor Posture, Phys. Therapy Rev., *29*, 165–168, 1949.

KUHNS, J. G., KLEIN, A., REGAN, E., WILLIAMS, P. C., and CROWE, H. E.: *Posture and Its Relationship to Orthopaedic Disabilities*. Report of the Posture Committee of the American Academy of Orthopedic Surgery, Chicago, Illinois, 1947.

LANE, JANET: *Your Carriage, Madam! A Guide to Good Posture*. 2nd ed. New York, John Wiley and Sons, Inc., 1947, 160 pp.

LA SALLE, DOROTHY: *Rhythms and Dances for Elementary Schools*. New York, A. S. Barnes and Co., 1951, 201 pp.

LEE, J. MURRAY, and LEE, DORRIS MAY: *The Child and His Development*. New York, Appleton-Century-Crofts, Inc., 1958, 624 pp.

LEE, MABEL, and WAGNER, MIRIAM M.: *Fundamentals of Body Mechanics and Conditioning*. Philadelphia, W. B. Saunders Co., 1949, 377 pp.

LE GRAND-LAMBLING, Y.: Exercises for Scoliosis, *Therapeutic Exercise*. Sidney Licht, (ed.). New Haven, Conn., Elizabeth Licht, 1958, pp. 449–493.

LERRIGO, CHARLES HENRY: *The Better Half of Your Life*. New York, J. Day Co., 1951, 270 pp.

LEWIN, PHILIP: *The Back and Its Disk Syndromes*. 2nd ed. Philadelphia, Lea & Febiger, 1955, 942 pp.

LICHT, SIDNEY, (ed.).: History, *Therapeutic Exercise*. New Haven, Conn., Elizabeth Licht, 1958. pp. 380–422.

————: Other Exercises, *Therapeutic Exercise*. New Haven, Conn., Elizabeth Licht, 1958, pp. 836–847.

————: *Therapeutic Exercise*. New Haven, Conn., Elizabeth Licht, 1958, 893 pp.

LIPOVITZ, FERDINAND JOHN: *Basic Kinesiology*. Minneapolis, Burgess Co., 1952, 105 pp.

————: *Medical Physical Education*. Minneapolis, Burgess Co., 1947, 417 pp.

LOGAN, GENE A., DUNKELBERG, JAMES G., GARDNER, GERALD W., and EGSTROM, GLEN H.: *Student Handbook for Adapted Physical Education*. Los Angeles, Adadon Press, 1956, 54 pp.

LOS ANGELES CITY SCHOOL DISTRICT: *Education of the Physically Handicapped*. School Publication, No. 215. Los Angeles, California, 1931, 38 pp.

LOS ANGELES CITY SCHOOLS: *Corrective Physical Education*. Los Angeles: Los Angeles Board of Education, 1958, 400 pp.

LOVETT, ROBERT W.: *Lateral Curvature of the Spine and Round Shoulders*. Philadelphia, P. Blakiston's Son and Co., 1931, 240 pp.

LOWEN, ALEXANDER: *Physical Dynamics of Character Structure, Bodily Form and Movement in Analytical Therapy*. New York, Grune and Stratton, 1958, 358 pp.

LOWMAN, CHARLES LEROY: A Contribution of Correctives to Child Welfare, J. Health and Phys. Educ., *12*, 10–11, 1941.

————: *Balance Skills in Physical Education*. Ann Arbor, Michigan, Edwards Brothers, 1935, 42 pp.

————: A Consideration of Teenage Athletics, J. Health and Phys. Educ., *12*, 398–399, 1941.

————: Education for the Handicapped, Los Angeles School J., *39*, 12, 1955.

————: Effect of Faulty Skeletal Alignment upon the Eyes, Am. J. Orthop. Surg., *16*, 459–492, 1918.

————: Feet and Body Mechanics, J. Health and Phys. Educ., *11*, 137, 1940.

————: Heavy Breasts as a Factor in Production of Faulty Posture, J.A.M.A., *78*, 173–175, 1922.

————: Importance of Stabilization, Phys. Therapy Rev., *29*, 253–255, 1949.

———— Orthopedic Problems: Responsibility of School Physicians, Health Educ. J. *14*, 3–4, 1951.

————: Posture in Early Childhood, California and Western Med., *41*, 382–385, 1934.

————: Faulty Posture in Relation to Performance, J. Health, Phys. Educ., Recreation, *29*, 14–15, 1958.

————: Sitting Position in Relation to Pelvis Stress, Physiotherapy Rev., *21*, 30–33, 1941.

————: Technical Use of Surgical Corsets and Girdles, Physiotherapy Rev., *27*, 156–158, 1947.

————: Therapeutic Indications for Pool Therapy, Phys. Therapy Rev., *37*, 224–225, 1957.

————: Therapeutic Use of Rocker Sole, Western J. Surg., *58*, 243–245, 1950.

————: The Relation of Postural States to Competitive Sports, Physical Educator, *9*, 67–68, 1952.

————: The Vulnerable Age, J. Health and Phys. Educ., *18*, 635, 1947.

————: Value of Pool Therapy, Physiotherapy Rev., *27*, 247–248, 1947.

LOWMAN, CHARLES LEROY, COLESTOCK, CLAIRE, and COOPER, HAZEL: *Corrective Physical Education for Groups*. New York, A. S. Barnes and Co., 1928, 521 pp.

LOWMAN, CHARLES LEROY, and ROEN, SUSAN G.: *Therapeutic Use of Pools and Tanks*. Philadelphia, W. B. Saunders Co., 1952, 90 pp.

McCLOY, C. H.: Anthropometry in the Service of the Individual, J. Health and Phys. Educ., *5*, 7–11, 1934.

————: *Philosophical Bases for Physical Education*. New York: Appleton-Century-Crofts, Inc., 1940, 311 pp.

————: *Tests and Measurements in Health and Physical Education*. New York: F. S. Crofts and Co., 1944, 412 pp.

————: X-ray Studies of Innate Differences in Straight and Curved Spines, Research Quarterly, *9*, 50–57, 1938.

McGRAW, M. B.: *Growth*: *A Study of Johnny and Jimmy*. New York, D. Appleton-Century Co., 1935, 319 pp.

————: Later Development of Children Specially Trained During Infancy: Johnny and Jimmy at School Age, Child Development, *10*, 1–19, 1939.

————: Neuromuscular Development of the Human Infant as Exemplified in the Achievement of Erect Locomotion, J. Pediat., *17*, 747–771, 1940.

————: *The Neuromuscular Maturation of the Human Infant*. New York, Columbia University Press, 1943, 140 pp.

McGRAW, MYRTLE B., and BREEZE, K. W.: Quantitative Studies in the Development of Erect Locomotion, Child Development, *12*, 267–303, 1941.

MacCARTHY, SHANE: Fitness and the Future, *Fitness of American Youth, Report of the Second Annual Meeting of the President's Council on Youth Fitness*. Washington, D.C.: United States Government Printing Office, 1958, pp. 27–33.

MacCONAILL, MICHAEL A.: Mechanical Anatomy of Motion and Posture, *Therapeutic Exercise*. Sidney Licht, (ed.). New Haven, Conn., Elizabeth Licht, 1958, pp. 44-87.

MARTIN, WILLIAM E., and STENDLER, CELIA BURNS: *Child Development: The Process of Growing Up in Society*. New York, Harcourt, Bruce & Co., 1953, 519 pp.

MASON, BERNARD, and MITCHELL, ELMER D.: *Social Games for Recreation*. New York, A. S. Barnes and Co., 1935, 421 pp.

MASSEY, WAYNE W.: A Critical Study of Objective Methods for Measuring Anterior Posterior Posture with a Simplified Technique, Res. Quart., *14*, 3–22, 1943.

MATTHIAS, EUGEN: *The Deeper Meaning of Physical Education*. New York, A. S. Barnes and Co., 1929, 88 pp.

MENSENDIECK, B. M.: *Look Better, Feel Better*. New York, Harper Bros., 1954, 276 pp.

MEREDITH, F., IRWIN, LESLIE W., and STATON, WESLEY M.: *Health and Fitness*. 3rd ed. Boston, D. C. Heath & Co., 1957, 450 pp.

MEREDITH, HOWARD V.: A Physical Growth Record for Use in Elementary and High Schools, Am. J. Publ. Health, *39*, 878, 1949.

MEREDITH, H. V., and KNOTT, V. B.: Changes in Body Proportions during Infancy and Preschool Years; Shelic Index, Child Development, *9*, 49–62, 1938.

METHENY, ELEANOR: *Body Dynamics*. New York, McGraw-Hill Book Co., Inc., 1952, 225 pp.

MICHAEL-SMITH, H. (ed.): *Management of the Handicapped Child*, New York, Grune & Stratton, 1957, 276 pp.

MILLARD, CECIL V.: *Child Growth and Development in the Elementary School Years*. Rev. ed. Boston, D. C. Heath and Co., 1958, 512 pp.

MITCHELL, ELMER D.: *Sports for Recreation*. New York, A. S. Barnes and Co., 1952, 522 pp.

MOREHOUSE, LAURENCE E.: A Conditioning Program for Sedentary Men, J. Ass'n Phys. and Ment. Rehabilitation, *7*, 39–43, 1953.

MOREHOUSE, LAURENCE E., and MILLER, AUGUSTUS T.: *Physiology of Exercise*. 5th ed. St. Louis, C. V. Mosby Co., 1959, 333 pp.

MORRISON, W. R., and CHENOWETH, LAURENCE B.: *Normal and Elementary Physical Diagnosis*. 5th ed. Philadelphia, Lea & Febiger, 1955, 412 pp.

MORTON, DUDLEY J.: *Human Locomotion and Body Form*. Baltimore, Williams and Wilkins Co., 1952, 285 pp.

————: *Oh Doctor, My Feet*. New York, D. Appleton-Century Co., 1939, 116 pp.

————: *The Human Foot*. New York, Columbia University Press, 1935, 244 pp.

MURPHY, GARDNER: *Personality*. New York, Harper Bros., 1947, 999 pp.

NAPIER, J. R.: The Foot and the Shoe, Physiotherapy, *43*, 65–74, 1957.

NASH, JAY B.: *Physical Education: Interpretations and Objectives*. New York, A. S. Barnes and Co., 1948, 288 pp

NATIONAL RESEARCH COUNCIL OF THE RESEARCH SECTION: *Measurement and Evaluation Materials*. Washington, Amer. Ass'n Health, Physical Education and Recreation, 1950, 138 pp.

NATIONAL SOCIETY FOR THE STUDY OF EDUCATION: *Adolescence, 43rd Yearbook Part I*. Chicago, University of Chicago Press, 1944, 358 pp.

NEILSON, N. P. and VAN HAGEN, WINIFRED: *Physical Education for Elementary Schools*. New York, A. S. Barnes and Co., 1954, 552 pp.

NELSON, W. E.: *Textbook of Pediatrics*. 7th ed. Philadelphia, W. B. Saunders Co., 1959, 1462 pp.

NORTHWAY, W. H.: Injuries to Joints, Arch. Phys. Therapy, *23*, 467–473, 1942.

OBERTEUFFER, DELBERT: *Physical Education*. Rev. ed. New York, Harper Bros., 956, 479 pp.

OLIVER, JEAN: Anatomic Changes of Normal Aging, *Geriatric Medicine*. Edward Stieglitz, (ed.). 3rd ed. Philadelphia, J. B. Lippincott Co., 1954, pp. 67–90.

OLSON, WILLARD C.: *Child Development*. Boston, D. C. Heath and Co., 1949, 417 pp.

OLSON, W. C., and HUGHES, B. O.: Growth of the Child as a Whole, *Child Behavior and Development*. R. G. Barker *et al.* (eds.). New York, McGraw-Hill Book Co., Inc., 1943, Ch. XII.

PESZCZYNSKI, MIECZYSLAW: Exercises for Hemiplegia, *Therapeutic Exercise*. Sidney Licht. (ed.). New Haven, Conn., Elizabeth Licht, 1958, pp. 654–673.

PHELPS, WINTHROP M., KIPHUTH, ROBERT J., and GOFF, CHARLES W.: *Diagnosis and Treatment of Postural Defects*. Springfield, Charles C Thomas, 1956, 190 pp.

PHYSICAL MEDICINE AND REHABILITATION SERVICE, CORRECTIVE THERAPY SECTION: *Guide to Proper Body Mechanics and Patient Self-Care*. Los Angeles, Veterans Adm. Center, 1959, 26 pp.

Physical Reconditioning. Dept. of the Army, Tech. Manual TM8-292; Dept. of the Air Force, Manual AFM 160-16, 1952, 219 pp.

Physical Training. War Department Field Manual, F.M. 21-22, January, 1946, 392 pp.

POLEY, M. S.: The Adapted Physical Education Program at the University of Oregon, J. Ass'n. Phys. and Ment. Rehabilitation, *11*, 81–84, 1957.

PRESCOTT, DANIEL ALFRED: *Emotion and the Educative Process*. Washington, American Council on Education, 1938, 323 pp.

PRESSEY, SIDNEY L., and KUHLEN, RAYMOND G.: *Psychological Development Through the Life Span*. New York, Harper Bros., 1957, 654 pp.

Proceedings of the Governor's Conference on the Problems of Aging. Div. F. Sec. 15, Mutual Health. Sacramento, California, 1951, 7 pp. (mimeo)

PRYOR, HELEN B.: *As the Child Grows*. New York, Silver Burdett Co., 1943, 400 pp.

————: *Width-Weight Tables*. Stanford, California, Stanford University Press, 1940, 15 pp.

QUIMBY, R. H.: What a Man Should Weigh., Res. Quart., *5*, 91–109, 1934.

QUINN, DON: Halls of Ivy Television Program, presented by Ronald Coleman, April, 1952.

RAND, WINIFRED, SWEENEY, MARY E. and VINCENT, E. LEE: *Growth and Development of the Young Child*. 6th ed. By Marian E. Breckenridge and Margaret Nesbit Murphy, Philadelphia, W. B. Saunders Co., 1958, 548 pp.

RASCH, PHILIP J. and BURKE, ROGER K.: *Kinesiology and Applied Anatomy*. Philadelphia, Lea & Febiger, 1959, 456 pp.

RASCH, PHILIP J., and MOREHOUSE, LAURENCE E.: Effect of Static and Dynamic Exercises on Muscular Strength and Hypertrophy, J. Appl. Physiol., *11*, 29–34, 1957.

RATHBONE, JOSEPHINE L.: *Corrective Physical Education*. 5th ed., Philadelphia, W. B. Saunders Co., 1959, 329 pp.

————: *Relaxation*. New York, Teachers College, Columbia University, 1943, 157 pp.

RESEARCH SECTION OF AMER. ASS'N FOR HEALTH, PHYSICAL EDUCATION AND RECREATION: *Research Methods Applied to Health, Physical Education, and Recreation*. Washington, Amer. Ass'n Health, Phys. Ed. & Rec., 1949, 535 pp.

RENFROW, LOUIS H.: News item in *Los Angeles* (California) *Times*, September, 1956.

RODGERS, MARTIN: *A Handbook of Stunts*. New York, The Macmillan Co., 1940, 515 pp.

ROGERS, JAMES FREDERICK: *What Every Teacher Should Know about the Physical Condition of Her Pupils*. Pamphlet No. 68 (revised) Washington, U. S. Office of Education, 1945.

ROYAL AIR FORCE: *Principles of Anatomy and Physiology for Physical Training Training Instructors*. London, His Majesty's Stationery Office, 1946, 180 pp.

RUSK, H. A., and TAYLOR, E. J.: Physical Disability: A National Problem, Am. J. Publ. Health, *38*, 1381–1386, 1948.

SALTER, NANCY: Muscle and Joint Measurement, *Therapeutic Exercise.* Sidney Licht. (ed.). New Haven, Conn., Elizabeth Licht, 1958, pp. 127–158.

SCHNEIDER, EDWARD C., and KARPOVICH, PETER V.: *Physiology of Muscular Activity.* 3rd ed., Philadelphia, W. B. Saunders Co., 1948, 346 pp.

SCHWARTZ, R. P.: Conservative Treatment of Functional Disorders of the Feet in the Adolescent and Adult, J. Bone and Joint Surg., *31-A*, 501–510, 1949.

SCOTT, M. GLADYS: *Analysis of Human Motion.* New York, F. S. Crofts and Co., 1942, 388 pp.

SELLWOOD, JOHN J.: Relationships of Growth and Developmental Patterns of Posture, J. School Health, *25*, 190–196, 1955.

————: The Integration of Physical Education with Physical Medicine and Rehabilitation Relative to the Preparation of Professional Personnel. Unpublished Doctor's dissertation, The University of California, Los Angeles, 1952, 282 pp.

SHELDON, WILLIAM H.: *Atlas of Men.* New York, Harper Bros., 1954, 357 pp.

SHELDON, WILLIAM H., STEVENS, S. S., and TUCKER, W. B.: *The Varieties of Human Physique.* New York, Harper Bros., 1940, 347 pp.

SHERMAN, H. C., and LANFORD, C. S.: *Essentials of Nutrition.* 4th ed., Philadelphia, W. B. Saunders Co., 1957, 505 pp.

SHERRINGTON, CHARLES SCOTT: *The Integrative Action of the Nervous System.* New Haven, Yale University Press, 1947, 433 pp.

SHOCK, NATHAN WETHERIL: *Trends in Gerontology.* Stanford, California, Stanford University Press, 1957, 214 pp.

SIMMONS, KATHERINE: *The Brush Foundation Study of Child Growth and Development II, Physical Growth and Development.* Monographs of the Society for Research in Child Development, Vol. 9, No. 1. Washington, National Research Council, 1944.

SINCLAIR, J. D.: Exercise in Pulmonary Disease, *Therapeutic Exercise.* Sidney Licht, (ed.), New Haven, Conn., Elizabeth Licht, 1958, pp. 737–761.

"Slippers," Senior Citizen, p. 48, November, 1956.

SMITH, ETHEL: *The Dynamics of Ageing.* New York, W. W. Norton, 1956, 191 pp.

SMOUT, C. F. V., and McDOWELL, R. J. S.: *Anatomy and Physiology for Students of Physiotherapy, Occupational Therapy and Gymnastics.* 2nd ed., Baltimore, William and Wilkins Co., 1947, 470 pp.

SNORRASON, EGILL: Exercise for Healthy Persons, *Therapeutic Exercise.* Sidney Licht, (ed.). New Haven, Conn., Elizabeth Licht, 1958, pp. 814–825.

SODEN, WILLIAM H.: *Rehabilitation of the Handicapped.* New York, Ronald Press Co., 1949, 399 pp.

SONTAG, L. W., and REYNOLDS, E. L.: The Fels Composite Sheet: I A Practical Method for Analyzing Growth Progress, II Variations in Growth Patterns in Health and Disease, J. Pediat., *5*, 194, 1934.

STAFFORD, GEORGE T.: *Exercise During Convalescence.* New York, A. S. Barnes and Co., 1947, 281 pp.

————: *Preventive and Corrective Physical Education.* New York, A. S. Barnes and Co., 1950, 312 pp.

————: *Sports for the Handicapped.* New York, Prentice-Hall, Inc., 1947, 334 pp.

STAFFORD, GEORGE T., and KELLY, ELLEN DAVIS: *Preventive and Corrective Physical Education.* 3rd ed., New York, Ronald Press Co., 1958, 395 pp.

STALEY, S. C.: *Calisthenics.* New York, A. S. Barnes and Co., 1936, 338 pp.

STEINDLER, ARTHUR: *Kinesiology of the Human Body.* Springfield, Charles C Thomas, 1955, 708 pp.

————: *Mechanics of Normal and Pathological Locomotion in Man.* Springfield, Charles C Thomas, 1935, 424 pp.

————: *Postgraduate Lectures on Orthopedic Diagnosis and Indications, Vol. I.* Springfield, Charles C Thomas, 1950, 289 pp.

STEINDLER, ARTHUR, and MARXER, JOHN LOUIS: *Traumatic Deformities and Disabilities of the Upper Extremity.* Springfield, Charles C Thomas, 1946, 494 pp.

STIEGLITZ, E. J.: The Personal Challenge of Aging: Biological Changes and Maintenance of Health, *Aging in the Modern World, Supplement I.* Clark Tibbitts. (comp.), Ann Arbor, University of Michigan, 1957, 246 pp.

STONE, ELEANOR, and DEYTON, JOHN M.: *Corrective Therapy for the Handicapped Child.* New York, Prentice-Hall, Inc., 1951, 315 pp.

STRONG, O. S., and ELWYN, A.: *Human Neuroanatomy*. 3rd ed., Baltimore, Williams and Wilkins Co., 1953, 442 pp.

STUART, H. C., and STEVENSON, S. S.: *Physical Growth and Development, Textbook of Pediatrics*. 7th ed., W. E. Nelson (ed.), Philadelphia, W. B. Saunders Co., 1959, 1462.

TANNER, J. M., *et al.*: Aberdeen Growth Study I. The Prediction of Adult Body Measurements from Measurements Taken Each Year from Birth to 5 Years, Arch. Dis. Childhood, *31*, 372–381, 1956.

TAYLOR, EUGENE J.: Rehabilitation in Community Programs for the Aged, *Age is No Barrier*. New York, New York State Joint Legislative Com. on Problems of the Aging, 1952, pp. 133–135.

THOMPSON, GEORGE G.: *Child Psychology, Growth Trends in Psychological Adjustment*. Boston, Houghton Mifflin Co., 1952. 667 pp.

THORPE, LOUIS P.: *Child Psychology and Development*. 2nd ed., New York, Ronald Press Co., 1955, 709 pp.

THORPE, LOUIS P., and CRUZE, W. W.: *Developmental Psychology*. New York, Ronald Press Co., 1956, 670 pp.

TIBBITTS, CLARK, and DONAHUE, WILMA, (eds.): *Aging in the Modern World*. Ann Arbor, University of Michigan, 1957, 175 pp.

TREANOR, WALTER J.: Motions of the Hand and Foot, *Therapeutic Exercise*. Sidney Licht, (ed.). New Haven, Conn,. Elizabeth Licht, 1958, pp. 99–115.

TRUSLOW, W.: Relationship of Foot Strains to Other Body Strains, Med. Times, *58*, 275, 1946.

V-5 ASSOCIATION OF AMERICA: *Conditioning Exercises, Games, Tests*. 3rd ed. by Karl C. H. Oermann and Carl Haven Young, *et. al.* Annapolis, Maryland, United States Naval Institute, 1960, 280 pp.

VAN DALEN, DEOBOLD B., and VAN DALEN, MARCELLA: *The Health, Physical Education, and Recreation Teacher*. New Jersey, Prentice-Hall, Inc., 1956, 436 pp.

VAN HAGEN, WINIFRED, DEXTER, GENEVIEVE, and WILLIAMS, JESSE FEIRING: *Physical Education in the Elementary Schools*. Sacramento, California State Dept. Educ., 1951, 1004 pp.

WAKIM, KHALIL G.: The Physiological Aspects of Therapeutic Physical Exercise, J.A.M.A., *142*, 100–108, 1950.

WASHBURN, A. H.: Appraisal of Healthy Growth and Development, *Practice of Pediatrics, Vol. I*. Hagerstown, Md., W. F. Prior Co., Inc., 1957, Chapter VIII.

WEIR, LEROY: Postwar Health and Physical Education, J. Health and Phys. Educ., *15*, 263–264, 1944.

WELLS, KATHERINE F.: *Kinesiology*. 2nd ed., Philadelphia, W. B. Saunders Co., 1955, 516 pp.

————: Practical Body Mechanics, J. Health and Phys. Educ., *19*, 591, 1948.

WESSEL, JANET A.: *Movement Fundamentals*. Englewood Cliffs, N.J., Prentice-Hall, Inc., 1957, 270 pp.

WETZEL, N. C.: Assessing Physical Condition of Children; Components of Physical Status and Physical Progress and Their Evaluation, J. Pediat., *22*, 329–361, 1943.

————: *Instruction Manual in the Use of the Grid for Evaluating Physical Fitness*. New York, N. E. A. Service, Inc., 1941, 11 pp.

————: Physical Fitness in Terms of Physique, Development, and Basal Metabolism, J.A.M.A., *116*, 1187–1195, 1941.

————: The Baby Grid, An Application of the Grid Techniques to Growth and Development in Infants, J. Pediat., *29*, 439–454, 1946.

WHEATLEY, GEORGE M., and HALLOCK, GRACE: *Health Observation of School Children*. New York, McGraw-Hill Book Co., Inc., 1956, 488 pp.

WHITE HOUSE CONFERENCE ON CHILD HEALTH AND PROTECTION: *Body Mechanics: Education and Practice*. New York, Century Co., 1932, 166 pp.

————: *Growth and Development*. New York, Century Co., 1932.

————: 1930 Committee on Special Classes. *Special Education: the Handicapped and the Gifted*. New York, Century Co., 1931–32, 604 pp.

WHITE, P. D.: The Role of Exercise in the Aging, J.A.M.A., *165*, 70, 1957.

WICKENS, J. S., and KIPHUTH, OSCAR: Body Mechanics Examination of Yale University Freshmen, Res. Quart., *13*, 102–108, 1942.

WILES, PHILIP: *Essentials of Orthopedics*. Boston, Little, Brown and Company, 1955, 538 pp.

WILLIAMS, JESSE FEIRING: *The Principles of Physical Education*. 5th ed., Philadelphia, W. B. Saunders Co., 1954, 366 pp.

WILLIAMS, M., and WORTHINGHAM, CATHERINE: *Therapeutic Exercise for Body Alignment and Function*. Philadelphia, W. B. Saunders Co., 1957, 127 pp.

WILLIAMS, ROGER JOHN: *Biochemical Individuality*. New York, John Wiley and Sons, Inc., 1956, 214 pp.

WOLFFE, JOSEPH B.: Future Basic Research Relating Physical Education to Sports Medicine, *College Physical Education Association, 59th Annual Proceedings*. 1956, pp. 115–125.

WRIGHT, W. G.: *Muscle Function*. New York, Paul B. Hoeber, Inc., 1928, 188 pp.

WYNN-PARRY, C. B.: Vicarious Motions, *Therapeutic Exercise*. Sidney Licht, (ed.). New Haven, Conn., Elizabeth Licht, 1958, pp. 116–126.

YALE UNIVERSITY CLINIC OF CHILD DEVELOPMENT: *The First Five Years of Life*. A Guide to the Study of the Pre-school Child, New York, Harper Bros., 1940, 393 pp.

YOUNG, CARL HAVEN: A Procedure in the Organizing of a Corrective Physical Education Program for High School Boys. Unpublished Master's thesis, The University of Southern California, Los Angeles, 1935, 150 pp.

————: A Research Design for the Acceleration of Professional Competence and Status, J. Ass'n Phys. and Men. Rehabilitation, *12*, 149–153, 1958.

————: Broadening the Corrective Program, California J. Second. Educ., *15*, 87–88, 1940.

————: Challenging Portals in the Profession, J. Health and Phys. Educ., *18*, 647–649, 1947.

————: *Directional Goals for Clinical Therapy Experiences*. New York: Ass'n Phys. and Men. Rehabilitation, 1958, 39 pp.

————: Integrative Field Work Experiences for Pre-Therapists, J. Ass'n Phys. and Men. Rehab., *11*, 11–16, 1957.

————: Meeting Needs of the Individual, J. Health and Phys. Educ., *11*, 71, 1940.

————: My Aching Back, *Kiwanis Club Bulletin of Westwood Village*, November 18, 1955, p. 1.

————: Operational Principles in Physical Education Administration: Organization and Staff, *College Physical Education Association, 58th Annual Proceedings*. 1955, pp. 180–182.

————: The Construction of a Manual for Use in The Physical Appraisal and Development of Cadets in the Naval Aviation Training Program. Unpublished Doctor's dissertation, Stanford University, Stanford, California, 1946, 81 pp. plus Manual of 235 pp.

————: What the Services Teach Us about Physical Education, California J. Second. Educ., *20*, 9–15, 1945.

YOUNG, CARL HAVEN, and CRAIG, ROBERT E.: Control Objectives in Adapted Physical Education, *College Physical Education Association, 61st Annual Proceedings*. 1958, pp. 244–250.

Appendixes

SINCE the exercise schedules presented in the former publication, *Corrective Physical Education for Groups* are no longer available, it has been suggested by many that because these schedules have stood the test of time, they should be included for those who wish to make use of them.

These former lesson plans have been closely scrutinized, reworked and revised. The programs have been shortened to 10 exercises for each day, and have been based on the need kinetically for antigravity value and progressive complexity.

For the growing individual, it is essential that the fundamental basis of all early exercises should strongly emphasize the antigravity values in order to improve the skeletal alignment in anticipation of later activities in athletic and recreational fields.

Such prescriptions are planned for the use of classroom teachers, with the vertical forms for daily use, while the horizontal forms are intended for specific application to individual needs on the basis of increasing complexity.

It will be found that through the use of such procedures, programs will take on new meaning, and that there may be some assurance that the exercise program will be beneficial rather than potentially harmful. Every effort has been made to include all necessary exercises for use in schools, however, it should be appreciated that they are adaptable for use in hospitals and in the home by individuals of all ages.

Wisely used, exercise becomes a means for development, prevention, habilitation, rehabilitation and maintenance of postural fitness. It may also contribute to other aspects of health which as yet are not clearly defined, but believed to be of considerable benefit to the welfare of mankind.

APPENDIX A.

ELEMENTARY SCHOOL

LESSON I

1. Feet.
    a. Lying on back, knees bent (hook lying), heels and outer borders fixed, press ball and toes to the floor—One! Relax—Two!

b. Keeping heels fixed, turn soles of feet toward each other—One!
Return to floor pressing toes and ball down—Two!
Relax—Three!

NOTE: Pressing big toe and ball to floor actuates peroneus longus, the depressor of the front foot and thus aids in maintaining the stability of the front abutment of the long arch.

2. Knee Alignment.
Lying on back, legs extended or sitting back to wall or braced with arms (long sitting)
Push heel down, right foot turned in—One!
Return and relax—Two!
Same, left.

NOTE: Exercise to stretch tight hamstrings and calf muscles when knees tend to flex.

3. Lower Back.
a. Lying on back
Contract abdominals and press back to floor—One!
Relax—Two!
b. Standing one or more feet from wall, toeing in. Let head, shoulders and back touch the wall, bend knees and lower to sitting position, take small steps backward with feet, gradually straightening knees, keeping back to wall, come to erect position (5 to 10 counts). Resume sitting against wall and repeat.

NOTE: Stout children with prominent buttocks may not be able to flatten back to wall so they may, when possible, stand in a doorway with back to the edge of door jamb so that the sacrum may touch and thus back can be flattened to eliminate the lumbar curve.

4. Abdomen.
Supine, knees bent (hook lying), soles together, knees apart (abducted).
Bend hips and knees (back flat, hips on floor)—One!
Gripping thighs back of knees, pull thighs to chest—Two!
Return—Three!
Position—Four! (Throat open by counting or exhaling).

NOTE: Thigh abduction before lifting relaxes the thigh adductors and doesn't allow them to assist an already tightened psoas (hip flexor).

5. Upper Back and Chest.
Supine, knees bent, hands to neck moving arms, palms up, to elbow bent position, flattening back, arm and wrist to floor—One!

17

Hold—Two!

Relax—Three!

Return hands to neck—Four!

NOTE: To increase force, imagine resistance to arms as arms are pulled down to bent position.

6. Head.

Sitting astride bench, feet forward (Check on correct back and head position).

Push head up, chin back (Stretch tall, tense abdomen)—One!

Relax—Two!

NOTE: Spinal push-up improves relation of head, trunk and pelvis.

7. Trunk.

   a. Same position astride bench. Cross feet under bench—One!

Bend forward (hands on hips)—Two!

Up—Three!

Position—Four!

   b. Or side bend, right then left.

8. Balance—Feet.

   a. Standing on tilted balance board, posture board on head, walk by file—One!

Two! Three! Four!

NOTE: If tilted balance board is not available, tilt feet to outer border.

   b. Same with hands on head holding boards or hands on hips, four steps forward, then four back.

9. Spinal Stretch (Suspension).

   a. Face stall bars, right foot on lower bar, right hand grasp one bar above horizontal—One!

Left hand, left foot next bar up—Two!

Continue—Three! and Four!

   b. Hanging, face out, hands wide apart, slowly allow stretch to 8 counts.

Return feet to bar and relax. Repeat.

NOTE: Hanging face out, hands wide, puts arms in external rotation and abduction and stretches pectorals without flaring scapulæ and stretching scapular adductors (rhomboids and lower trapezius).

10. Standing.

Feet parallel, push up spine—One!

Rotate thighs outward—Two!

Rotate arms out—Three!

Position—Four!

LESSON II

1. Feet.
   a. and b. as in Lesson I.
   c. Lying prone, legs extended, heels apart, toes touching.
      Pinch buttocks, rotate thighs outward till heels touch—One!
      Relax—Two!
2. Knee Alignment (To stretch hamstrings and tendo achillis).
      Sitting, legs extended.
      Cross right foot over left, turn foot in, push heel down—
      One!
      Raise leg—Two!
      Lower—Three!
      Relax—Four!
      Repeat, left.
3. Lower Back.
      Lying on back, knees bent (hook lying), hands on neck,
      elbows on floor. Contract abdomen and raise head forward
      —One! (Keep low back flat and arms on floor)
      Relax—Two!
      Note: Actuates abdominals to raise head and flexes
   low spine and corrects lordosis and forward pelvic tilt.
4. Abdomen.
      Same as 3, arms at "T" position, palms down.
      Put soles of feet together and separate knees—One!
      Raise legs in that position to chest—Two!
      Return slowly—Three!
      Position—Four!
      Note: Arms "T" stretches pectorals while abdominals
   are shortened and back flattened.
5. Upper Back and Chest.
      Same as 4, arms diagonal.
      Bring arms to elbow-bent position against imaginary resist-
      ance. (Keep back flat and elbows on floor)—One!
      Hold—Two!
      Return arms up to diagonal informally—Three!
      Repeat.
6. Head.
      Sitting astride bench or cross sitting on floor, feet forward,
      hands on hips (Check correct sitting position).
      Cross feet, drop head forward on chest, push head back,
      chin in against imaginary resistance—One! (Keep abdom-
      inals tense and back flat).
      Hold—Two!
      Relax—Three!
      Repeat.

7. Trunk.
>Astride bench or sitting on floor, knees bent, feet crossed, arms horizontal.
>
>Bend right until right hand touches floor—One! (Keep head in line with trunk).
>
>Return—Two!
>
>Repeat, left.

8. Balance and Feet.
>Standing on tilted balance board.
>
>Raise right leg, turn foot toward body—One!
>
>Replace—Two!
>
>Repeat with opposite foot and progress along board.
>
>NOTE: Arms may be placed in varying positions or if no balance board, from plain stand and rotate thighs outward, hold and raise foot across knee, sole up and replace one foot forward and repeat for progression.

9. Suspension.
>Climb from rungs up as in previous lesson, turn, reverse grasp, hands wide, hang 4 counts and lower right hand and left foot, left hand and right foot to starting 4 counts.

10. Standing.
>As in 9, in front of stall bars.
>
>Hands to neck, head and spine push up, rotate thighs out till weight is on outer border of feet and march out maintaining position.

LESSON III

1. Feet.
>Lying, knees bent, feet straight.
>
>Press toes to floor and separate knees slightly—One!
>
>Relax—Two!
>
>NOTE: As the weight of legs goes outward there is a tendency for the feet to invert and supinate and in resisting this effect by pressing down on the ball, the peroneus longus and plantar flexors are actuated and tend to raise the arch.

2. Knees. (Leg alignment)
>Lying on back, legs extended.
>
>Point the heels and push down as though making the legs longer—One!
>
>Hold and relax—Two!
>
>Exercise should be hard enough to feel the tension on posterior leg and thigh muscles.

3. Lower Back.
>Lying on back, knees bent (Hook lying), hands on head.

Bend trunk right—One!

Return—Two!

Repeat, left. (Keep shoulders and elbows on floor).

4. Abdomen.

Back lying, knees bent (hook lying), arms "T" position, soles of feet together, knees separated.

Raise knees to chest—One!

Raise head, exhaling—Two!

Return head—Three!

Position—Four!

NOTE: Various arm positions may be used, also in lowering head keep back of neck flat.

5. Upper Back and Chest.

Prone lying, hands clasped in rear.

With head and arms relaxed, pinch shoulder blades together —One!

Hold—Two! Three!

Relax—Four!

NOTE: With arms back and head relaxed, it is easier to localize on the shoulder blades.

6. Head.

Sitting, legs crossed, knees bent, hands clasped in rear.

Bend head to right shoulder, keeping back of neck flat— One!

Return—Two!

Repeat, left.

NOTE: Hands clasped behind back fixes shoulders so that they do not raise shoulder when bending to opposite side.

7. Trunk.

Same position as 6, or astride a bench, arms side horizontal.

Twist trunk right and clap right hand with left one—One!

Return—Two!

Same, left.

8. Balance—Feet.

Standing on balance board.

Raise right leg forward, turn foot toward body—One!

Raise right leg backward—Two!

Forward again turning foot in—Three!

Step forward—Four!

Same left and repeat across board.

9. Suspension.

Climb up, starting right hand and right foot—four counts.

Hang back to bars, hands wide apart, palms forward, contract abdominals and flatten back—One!

Rotate thighs outward—Two!
Return—Three!
Turn and maintain abdominal tension while going down
four steps.

LESSON IV

1. Feet.
   Back lying, knees bent.
   Place right heel on left knee—One!
   Bend ankle up—Two!
   Turn foot up till bottom can be seen—Three!
   Replace to floor—Four!
   Same, left.

2. Knee (To stretch hamstrings).
   Backward lying, thighs to chest, knees separated.
   Extend both legs upward forcibly pointing heels—One!
   Hold—Two! Three!
   Position—Four!
     NOTE: (Hands may steady the legs.) This is a further
   stretch for tight Achilles.

3. Lower Back.
   Back lying, knees bent, arms to the diagonal.
   Roll trunk to right, carry left arm over body to floor,
   opposite side—One!
   Keeping right shoulder stationary, return—Two!
   Same to left.

4. Abdomen.
   Same as 3, arms diagonal.
   Separate knees and raise knees to chest—One!
   Roll knees to right to floor—Two!
   Return—Three!
   Position—Four!
   Same, left.

5. Upper Back and Chest.
   Prone lying position, arms straight, palms down at side
   horizontal, head on floor.
   Raise head 2 inches from floor—One!
   Palms up—Two!
   Return—Three!
   Position—Four!
     NOTE: Neck should be kept flat.

6. Head.
   Sitting legs crossed, knees bent, or astride bench.
   Head circling forward to right and backward to left and
   forward again—One!

Two! Three! Four!
Same, left!

7. Trunk.
    Same position as 6, hands on neck (wing position).
    Twist trunk right—One!
    Bend forward over right knee—Two!
    Return—Three!
    Position—Four!
    Same, left.

8. Balance—Feet.
    Standing on tilted balance board.
    Bend knee upward and turn outward—One!
    Back—Two!
    Down—Three! (Stepping one step forward).
    Same, left. Walk across the board.

9. Suspension.
    Standing facing stall bars.
    Step up, right foot on first bar, hand grasp forward—One!
    Left up one step—Two! And continue four bars.
    Then change and hang back to bars, hands wide.
    Tense abdominal muscles—One!
    Raise right leg outward—Two!
    Return—Three!
    Position—Four!
    Same, left, then step down 4 bars to floor.

10. Dismissal.
    Line up in file, hands on hips. Two steps forward, twist
    left—One!
    Same, twist right—Two!
    Repeat to door. NOTE: Step high like a majorette, keep-
    ing low back flat and placing feet with weight on outer
    border.

LESSON V

1. Feet.
    Back lying, knees bent.
    a. Press down ball and toes to floor, keep heel and outer
       border stationary—One!
       Relax—Two!
    b. Or Touch soles of feet together, bend ankles up—One!
       Return—Two!

2. Knee Alignment.
    Lying on the right side, lower under knee bent for support.
    Bend left ankle upward, raise left leg forward as far as
    possible—One!

Return—Two!
Repeat on left side.

3. Lower Back.
Prone lying, forearms under abdomen.
Separate legs (leg abduction)—One!
Return—Two!
Repeat as desired.

4. Abdomen.
Same as 2, lying on right side, right knee bent.
Left leg circumduction—One! Two! Three! Four!
Repeat opposite side.
NOTE: To get fixation the pelvis is stabilized by the supporting leg and trunk muscles (quadratus lumborum and abdominal obliques) act as fixators.

5. Upper Back and Chest.
Sitting knees bent, legs crossed, arms side horizontal, palms up.
Describe small arm circles backward (Keep upper back flat) One! Two! Three! Four!
Repeat as many times as desired making circles a little larger.
NOTE: Keeping upper back and scapulæ flat and putting emphasis on the backward circling actuates the external rotators which are synergists or helpers of the scapular adductors.

6. Head.
Same position, hands on hips (Check for good sitting position).
Push head up to stretch the spine making supporting pressure with the hands to hold the shoulders down. Push up —One!
Relax—Two!
Repeat as desired.

7. Trunk.
Same position as 6, either astride bench or on the floor.
Bend forward—One!
Twist right—Two!
Return—Three!
Position—Four!
Same, left!
Repeat as desired.

8. Balance—Feet.
Standing on tilted balance board, hands on hips or shoulders or head.
Touch right heel forward—One!

Step—Two! (Swinging weight forward on ball of foot).
Same, left, and alternate across board.

NOTE: When one foot is raised, the supporting leg must contract all supporting muscles and because of the tilt the foot muscles must come into balance, *i.e.*, tight abductors must elongate but remain in a holding position, while the weakened muscles of the inner border and arch must take up the slack.

9. Suspension.

Face stall bars and climb 4 bars, alternating feet and hands to count, then turn and hang face out, hands wide apart.
Abduct or spread legs—One!
Touch heels together (knees bent)—Two!
Repeat and return, 4 counts.

10. Dismissal.

   a. Some progressive marching or dance movement toward exit or substitute (*b*).
   b. Face the bars, feet straight and weight on outer borders, one foot in front of bars or wall and one foot apart, hands grasp bar at shoulder height, wide apart, keeping neck and back flat, slowly let body sag forward 4 counts and return. Repeat as desired.

   NOTE: Good to stretch tight pectorals and tight hamstrings and Achilles (gastrocnemius).

LESSON VI

1. Feet.

   Sitting, feet on floor, legs crossed, knees bent.
   Press toes, right, to floor, feet toeing in—One!
   Turn right foot toward left (Keep outer border on floor—Two!
   Hold—Three! Four! (Hold strongly enough so that the foot cannot be pulled straight by the teacher.)
   Same, left.

2. Knee Alignment.

   Sitting, legs straight.
   Bend trunk forward, twist to left and touch left foot with right hand—One!
   Return—Two!
   Same, left.
   Repeat as desired.

4. Abdomen.

   Side lying, lying on right side, both knees slightly bent, right leg back, left leg forward.
   Separate knees widely and straighten left leg—One!

Feet together—Two! (Like scissors kick.)

Same other side.

Repeat as desired.

NOTE: Pelvis is balanced by position of legs and lateral leg raising and straightening actuates lateral abdominals and hip abductors.

5. Upper Back and Chest.

Sitting on bench or floor, legs crossed as before, arms diagonal.

Bend elbows against imagined resistance—One!

Elbows back to side horizontal—Two!

Return—Three!

Position—Four! (Keep back flat).

6. Head.

Same sitting position, hands on head.

Push hands upward stretching spine, tensing abdominals and flattening low back—One!

Twist head right—Two!

Return—Three!

Position—Four!

Same, left.

Repeat as desired.

7. Trunk.

Same position as 6, hands on abdomen.

Bend trunk forward—One!

Bend to right—Two!

Press hands to abdomen to keep the forward bent position —Three!

Return—Four!

Same, left, and repeat as desired.

NOTE: Pressure on abdomen good to stimulate intestinal tract, increase by exhaling on the forward bend.

8. Balance—Feet.

Standing on tilted balance board, hands on head, hips, or extended.

Touch right heel forward—One!

Extend leg backward, touch toe—Two!

Right heel forward again—Three!

Step—Four!

Same, left, and on across board.

9. Suspension.

Face stall bars.

Climbing, right foot and left hand to bar—One!

Each one placed one bar higher—Two! Three! Four!

Change and face out, arms wide, both feet on the bars.

Release right foot and let it hang free—One!
Same, left—Two!
Hip raising, right, and replace foot—Three!
Same, left—Four!
Repeat as desired.

NOTE: Hip raising actuates external abdominal obliques and quadratus.

10. Dismissal.

Line up in file in correct standing position, hands to head, elbows back, abdomen tense (but not pulled in), march out or around the room and back to seats, if used in classroom.

LESSON VII

1. Feet.

Sitting on bench facing sideward, pupils side by side, properly spaced, feet on floor 2 inches apart. (In classroom sitting sideways feet in aisle).
Bring right foot to left knee—One!
Turn heel in—Two!
Return—Three!
Position—Four!
Same, left.
Repeat four to eight times.

NOTE: Combination outward thigh rotation and foot inversion with low back flat.

2. Knee Alignment.

Position as above, hands at sides on bench, feet 6 inches apart.
Lift arches keeping toes flat—One!
Rotate feet inward—Two!
Return—Three!
Relax—Four!

3. Lower Back.

Right side lying, lower knee bent.
Raise left leg sideward upward—One!
Hold—Two! Three!
Return slowly—Four!
Repeat twice.
Turn to opposite side and repeat, right.

NOTE: This actuates the abductors of the right thigh for stabilizing the pelvis by pressure downward on the floor.

4. Abdomen.

Kneeling on right knee, right foot in moderate inversion.
Fold arms across lower abdomen, bend trunk forward—One!
Twist left—Two!

Return—Three!

Position—Four!

Reverse and do same, twisting right.

Repeat as desired.

NOTE: Good for constipation as the bend with twist alternately presses and relaxes the abdominal cavity.

5. Upper Back and Chest.

Astride bench toeing in, hands on hips or cross sitting on floor.

Bend trunk forward, upper back flat—One!

Drop head to chest—Two!

Return head, chin back strongly—Three!

Position—Four!

6. Head.

Position as in 5, trunk forward, shoulder blades flat. Drop head foward slightly, rotate left to right and return, 6 or 8 times, forcefully but not with a jerk.

7. Trunk.

Position as in 6, hands to neck, elbows back.

Twist left—One!

Bend right and touch right elbow to right knee—Two!

Return—Three!

Position—Four!

Reverse and repeat as desired.

8. Balance—Feet.

Standing on balance board or on floor with feet inverted, arms side horizontal.

Bend right knee upward, turned out—One!

Extend leg forward turning foot in—Two!

Bend knee—Three! (Bring leg back to forward position).

Step forward—Four!

Repeat, left, and go across board.

9. Suspension.

Back to stall bars.

Left foot to bottom bar, left hand grasping as high as possible, step up—One!

Repeat, right foot and hand—Two!

Repeat again, opposite side—Three!

Repeat, right foot and hand—Four!

Shift hands, wide apart and hang, tensing abdomen, flattening low back, touch soles together—One!

Hold soles together and raise knees—Two!

Return—Three!

Position—Four! (Feet on bars)

Step down four counts to floor.

10. Dismissal Exercise.

Correct standing position, hands to neck, march out with alternate trunk twists right elbow with left leg and reverse.

LESSON VIII

1. Feet.

Sitting on bench facing sideward, feet properly spaced.
Raise right foot to left knee, heel in front of knee joint—One!
Grasp right forefoot with left hand and pull toward the body—Two!
Release—Three!
Position—Four!
Same, left foot, grasping with right hand.
Repeat as desired.

NOTE: In cases of pronated ankles and flat, everted feet this will stretch the tightened or short abductors (peroneals).

2. Knee Alignment.

Bear position on all fours, legs straight, toes in.
Sag forward stretching Achilles—One!
Return—Two!
Repeat as desired.

CAUTION: Not to be done by those who have backknees or relaxed knees.

3. Lower Back.

Lying on back, arms at sides.
Soles together, draw feet toward body, knees back as far as possible and draw hands along sides to the armpits—One!
Extend arms sidewards, thumbs up, extend legs to the diagonal—Two!
Arms to sides and soles together—Three!
Position—Four!

4. Abdomen.

Lying on back, arms "T" position, soles of feet together.
Raise head keeping arms on the floor—One!
Raise legs, knees apart, feet pressed together—Two!
Return legs—Three!
Position—Four!

NOTE: Make more difficult by having student exhale when raising head and legs.

5. Upper Back.

Sitting, crossed feet, knees separated, arms side horizontal.
Pinch shoulder blades together—One! (Do not raise or pull back on arms or shoulders. Limit movements to scapulæ only.)
Turn palms upward—Two!

Return, holding shoulder blades firm—Three! Four!
Relax and repeat as desired.

6. Head.

Stand before wall, arm's length away, place hands on wall shoulder height, bend elbows slightly leaning a little forward.

Drop head forward—One!

Raise head, chin in, pinch shoulder blades together—Two!

Straighten elbows, hold scapulæ firm—Three!

Position—Four!

Repeat.

7. Trunk.

Standing, arms side horizontal.

Place right foot forward, foot slight toe-in—One!

Twist trunk right, turn palms upward—Two!

Return—Three!

Position—Four!

Same, opposite.

NOTE: Twisting trunk right with right foot forward gives maximum torsion to spine and renders balance more difficult, actuates abdominal obliques, latissimus dorsi, serrati, and quadrati lumborum.

8. Balance—Feet.

Standing on tilted balance board, arms side horizontal.

Bend knee upward outward—One!

Stretch right leg backward—Two!

Return to knee forward position—Three!

Step—Four!

Same, left, across the board.

NOTE: Be careful to tense abdomen on the leg extension backward in order to avoid increasing hollow in back (lordosis).

9. Suspension.

Standing facing bars.

Climbing one bar at a time with opposite hand and foot, 4 counts.

Reverse to hanging position, hand grasp wide.

Hang, place soles together, draw feet toward body—One!

Extend legs diagonally outward—Two!

Feet together—Three!

Back to bars—Four!

NOTE: Raising legs abducted with abdominal wall tight minimizes the pull on the thigh flexors (mainly psoas), thereby preventing assumption of hollow back.

Return to floor, 4 counts.

Repeat cautiously in accordance with muscle strength and tone.

10. Dismissal Exercise.

Standing in file, 2 to 3 feet apart, hands on head, good spinal position.

Raise right knee to right angle, knee and hip flexion, replace with force on extension as body shifts forward. Repeat, left, and march out in good snappy tempo.

NOTE: Any type of marching calisthenics can be used for dismissal exercises.

LESSON IX

1. Feet—General Posture.

   a. Sitting in seats, back supported, soles of feet together, arm bend position.

   Stretch left arm upward, right arm downward, flatten back against seat—One!

   Reverse arm position, right arm sideward downward, left arm sideward upward, press low back against back—Two!

   Return—Three!

   Position—Four!

   NOTE: Sitting in this position and pressing knees to floor stretches foot abductors and tight outer thigh fascia.

2. Lower Back.

   Sitting on top of desks, legs hanging free, grasp edge of desk. Raise legs alternately with small movements from hips, knees straight (as in flutter kick in swimming)—One! Two! Three! Four!

3. Abdomen.

   Sitting astride bench, feet on floor toeing forward, hands on abdomen.

   Trunk rotation, right, bend right—One!

   Forward—Two!

   Left—Three!

   Position—Four!

   NOTE: Backward bending eliminated to prevent assumption of hollow back position.

4. Upper Back.

   Sitting, hands in lap.

   Push head up, chin in, stretch spine (up as tall as possible) —One!

   Relax—Two!

   Repeat.

   NOTE: Spinal push up, chin in brings about correct

Describe small arm circles backward—One! Two! Three! Four!

Repeat making larger circles.

NOTE: Keep upper back flat and shoulder blades together.

6. Head.

Sitting in seat or on benches, back supported, feet on floor toeing forward, arms side horizontal.

Drop head forward—One!

Hands to back of head—Two!

Push head back to vertical, chin in—Three!

Position—Four!

7. Trunk—Big Muscle Mimetic, Back Stroke Swimming using One Leg at a Time.

Standing, turn right knee out, raise right foot to left knee, sole of foot on knee.

Draw hands along sides to arm pits—One!

Extend arms sidewards, palms down, extend right leg to diagonal outward—Two!

Arms to sides, feet together—Three!

Hold—Four!

Same, left.

Repeat.

8. Balance—Feet.

Standing in aisle or on gym floor, feet on outer borders, hands at sides.

Raise arms to side horizontal and raise right knee to horizontal, right toe pointing down and in—One!

Hands to hips—Two!

Extend right leg—Three!

Position—Four!

Same, left.

Repeat.

9. Suspension.

   a. If in gym, repeat Exercise 9, Lesson IX.

   b. Or in classroom, standing in aisles, hands on seat backs. Elbows straighten to push shoulders up—One!

   Let knees bend to lower body against the push up of arms —Two!

   Hold—Three!

   Position—Four!

   NOTE: Watch to prevent pointing the shoulders forward. Emphasize keeping shoulder blades back. This will hold shoulder in balance between front and back depressors.

10. Dismissal.

Marching, skipping steps, various arm positions: Extended and hands flapping as a bird for small children; arms horizontal, elbows bent to imitate airplane wings for older ones, forward and back, toeing in slightly to prevent flattening lowered arches. Continue around the room to exit. May be adapted to classroom, up and down the aisles.

LESSON XI

1. Feet and General Posture.

   a. Sitting in seats, feet on floor, soles together, arms forward, elbows bent.

   Extend right arm sidewards, left hand to right shoulder, arm at horizontal, flatten back against seat—One!

   Sweep both arms upward to left bringing left arm to side horizontal, right hand to left shoulder as in One, back pressed to seat—Two!

   Return—Three!

   Position—Four!

   Same, starting left.

   Repeat.

   b. Same seated on benches without back support, feet on the ground toeing in.

   NOTE: To get full foot value hold soles together throughout exercise in (a) and in (b) keep outer border and big toes firmly on the floor.

2. Knee Alignment.

   Sitting as in (a) or (b), hands at sides, feet on floor toeing forward, weight on the outer borders.

   Extend arms forward—One!

   Extend right leg strongly forward and push forward on arms—Two!

   Return—Three!

   Position—Four!

   Same, start left leg.

   Repeat.

   NOTE: Pushing arms forward tenses abdominals, keeps low back flat, thereby fixing the pelvis so that the extension of the leg stretches the hamstrings.

3. Lower Back.

   Seated on desks facing to side of room, legs hanging, hands grasping edge of desk.

   Straighten legs—One!

Place soles of feet together, separate and bend knees
slightly—Two!
Return—Three!
Position—Four!
  NOTE: In case aisle is too narrow for full leg extension,
push feet against opposite desk on count One.

4. Abdomen.

Sitting astride benches or stools, feet on ground or floor,
toeing forward, hands on top of head.
Trunk rotation, right bend—One!
Bending forward—Two!
Bending left—Three!
Position, pushing hands up with head—Four!
Same, starting left.
Repeat.

5. Upper back.

Sitting in seats or on benches or stools, hands on head,
palms together, arms forward, elbows bent.
Arms to horizontal, keep elbows bent, hands open, fingers
touching—One!
Roll hands on head to palms up and press elbows back—
Two!
Return—Three!
Position—Four!
Repeat.
  NOTE: Rolling forearms from neutral to supination
while elbows are carried back, strongly activates anti-
gravity muscles of shoulder blade area.

6. Head.

Sitting as in No. 5, hands on head, palms up.
Press head up, chin in—One!
Bend right—Two!
Bend left—Three!
Position—Four!

7. Trunk—Big Muscle Mimetic, Basket Ball Throw for Distance.

Standing, feet in stride position, left shoulder forward.
Hold imaginary ball in right hand, right arm extended back-
ward, weight on right foot, knee slightly bent, left arm
forward for balance—One!
Swing right arm forward upward discharging the ball while
left arm swings backward outward to counter balance—
Two!
Return arms—Three!
Feet to position—Four!
Repeat.

NOTE: Any left handed students to execute exercise in their natural way.

8. Balance—Feet.

Standing in the aisle facing side wall, or on gym floor.

Hands to hips, arms to side horizontal—One!

Raise right leg sideward slowly but strongly, balance with arms but do not bend trunk—Two!

Slow return of leg—Three!

Position—Four!

Same, left.

Repeat.

NOTE: This is also a good exercise on the tilted balance board if you have it. The side leg raising not only actuates the thigh abductor (gluteus medius) of the moving side but staticly provokes the opposite gluteus to firm, steady holding action to maintain balance.

9. Suspension.

Climb stall bars, 4 counts.

Hang facing sidewards by one hand, placing opposite hand to the back to grasp bar—One!

Extend leg sideward—Two!

Return—Three!

Position—Four!

Same, opposite way, and then climb down.

NOTE: For older age group may be repeated.

10. Dismissal.

Line up in file, arms length apart.

Extend left arm forward, hand ready to grasp—One!

Lean forward as if reaching—Two!

Right arm and right leg back—Three!

Position—Four!

Repeat, advancing one step, starting opposite sides.

Progress to exit.

LESSON XII

1. Feet.

Sitting in seats facing aisle, or if in gym on benches, feet forward, hands in lap.

Cross feet, outer borders firmly placed on floor—One!

Lean slightly forward and rise to standing position. feet remaining crossed—Two!

Resume sitting position—Three!

Uncross feet—Four!

Repeat.

NOTE: Hands in lap keeps student from using them in rising, necessitating use of extensors of legs and trunk, strong holding action of foot muscles, concentrical contraction of adductors (anterior and posterior tibials) and excentric contraction while elongated on the part of the lateral stabilizers or adductors (peroneus longus and brevis).

2. Knee Alignment.

Seated on desk, legs hanging in aisle, hands grasping edge of desk.

Cross right knee over left—One!

Extend right leg—Two!

Point heel, pushing down—Three!

Return to position—Four!

Same, left.

Repeat.

NOTE: Stretches calf, hamstrings and fascia lata (the tight flat tendon of the auxiliary abductor, the tensor fascia femoris). In knock knees and tibial torsions this band may become contractured and tends to perpetuate the deviation.

3. Lower Back.

Sitting in seats, facing the aisle, feet on floor, 2 inches apart, toeing forward, hands at sides.

Tighten abdominal muscles and flatten back—One!

Rise to standing position holding pelvis and low back firm —Two!

Sit—Three!

Relax—Four!

Repeat.

4. Abdomen.

Seated on desks, feet hanging in aisle, hands grasping edge of desk.

Raise and lower legs with short quick strokes keeping knees stiff but feet relaxed (as in treading water)—One! Two! Three! Four!

Relax and repeat.

5. Upper Back.

Sitting in seats back supported (or on benches, sitting astride), feet on floor toeing forward, hands on neck (wing position).

Bend slightly forward, upper back flat—One!

Twist head slowly right—Two! Do not move hands.

Same, left—Three!

Position—Four!

Repeat.

6. Head.

Sitting as in No. 5, hands on head, palms up.

Pivot head right—One!

Front—Two!

Left—Three!

Position—Four!

Repeat.

NOTE: Keep chin in, neck flat and twist on a central axis with the pivot centered on the hands. To execute well will require a straight spine and neck.

7. Trunk—Big Muscle Mimetic, Crawl Stroke Swimming.

Standing position, left arm to vertical.

Head relaxed forward—One!

Pull left arm down strongly, right arm up to vertical turning head to right lifting chin for breath—Two!

Repeat as desired.

NOTE: May adapt various arm movements to different strokes.

8. Balance—Feet.

Standing in aisle facing wall or on gym floor, right hand on abdomen, left hand behind, feet 6 inches apart toeing forward.

Twist to left—One!

Bow from hips—Two!

Return—Three!

Position—Four!

Same reversed.

Repeat.

NOTE: Twisting trunk and pelvis far to one side rotates the standing leg, strongly activating foot and leg muscles for stabilization, while the opposite leg and foot only maintain a steadying action, *i.e.*, rotating far to the left may even lift the right heel and only slight pressure on right forefoot maintains balance.

9. Suspension.

Repeat Exercises No. 9, Lesson XI.

NOTE: As this is rather difficult it may appeal to elementary age group as a stunt, therefore rather intriguing, but if there are any students with scoliosis, they should do the side hanging with the arm on the concave side uppermost and the opposite arm grasping downward.

10. Dismissal of Period.

Can be used in classroom or gym.

Marching, facing two march steps backward combined with facing.

Two steps forward, four step hops.
Same backward if remaining in room or continuously forward if progressing to exit.

LESSON XIII

1. Feet and General Posture.
   Standing, feet 6 inches apart, arms side horizontal.
   Place right foot sideward—One!
   Arm rotation outward, palms up with outward thigh rotation—Two!
   Return—Three!
   Position—Four!
   Same left.
   Repeat.

2. Knee Alignment.
   Sitting on desk, legs hanging in aisle (or on bench in gym).
   Raise right leg passing right foot over left knee, grasping foot with left hand—One!
   Extend left knee—Two!
   Return left to position—Three!
   Return right to position—Four!
   NOTE: Grasping foot stretches tight abductors of foot as well as tight fascia of thigh, while it goes into external rotation.

3. Lower Back.
   Sitting feet in the aisle, or on benches facing sideward, hands in lap.
   Cross feet placing them firmly on outer borders—One!
   Tense abdomen flattening lower back and rise to standing position—Two!
   Arms to vertical—Three!
   Position sitting—Four!
   NOTE: Do not drop into seat suddenly but let arms down easily and gracefully, while low back is held in same position as when rising.

4. Abdomen.
   Standing feet in stride position, hands on abdomen.
   Trunk rotation to right, pressing hands to abdomen—One!
   Forward bend, press—Two!
   Bend to left, press—Three!
   Position, pushing head up, chin in—Four!
   Same, left.
   Repeat.
   NOTE: Hand pressure acts to improve local circulation and has massaging effect on muscles and bowel.

5. Upper Back.

Sitting in seats, feet in aisle or on benches sitting astride feet on floor toeing forward, hands on hips. Push up with head, chin in, neck flat—One!

Keeping head fixed, rotate trunk to right—Two!

To left—Three!

Position—Four!

6. Head.

Standing, stride position, arms to side horizontal, chin in, neck flattened—One!

Turn left and bend left—Two!

Up—Three!

Position—Four!

Same, turning right.

Repeat.

7. Trunk—Big Muscle Mimetic, Chest Throw for Basket.

Standing position.

Hold imaginary ball with both hands in front of chest, elbows bent and close to body, place left foot forward, knees slightly bent, weight on balls of feet—One!

Extending and jump as in shooting a basket—Two!

Repeat as desired.

8. Balance—Feet.

Standing in aisle facing wall, elbows bent, hands touching in front of chest.

Raise right leg outward—One!

Bend slightly forward—Two! (Keeping weight on outer border of supporting foot).

Return—Three!

Position—Four!

Same, left.

Repeat.

NOTE: May be done on tilted balance board.

9. Suspension.

Class in twos, fours or sixes as apparatus permits, hanging from ladder or stall bars, hands three feet apart.

Contract abdomen and flatten back—One!

Raise legs, knees separated—Two!

Return—Three!

Position—Four!

10. Dismissal.

Marching, facing, step sideward crossing left foot over right.

Step right crossing left foot behind right.

Repeat four counts, on last coming to position of attention.

Repeat, hands at any desired position. May be adapted to classroom, gym or playground.

LESSON XIV

1. Feet and General Posture.
   Standing, arms side horizontal.
   Placing right foot forward toeing in—One!
   Arms folded over top of head, push up against arms—Two!
   Return—Three!
   Position—Four!

2. Knee Alignment.
   Standing in aisle, facing forward, hands on hips, feet toeing in
   Step back with right foot—One!
   Bend left knee slightly and bend forward—Two!
   Keep back flat and right knee straight with heel held down and foot inverted—Three!
   Position—Four!

3. Lower Back.
   Standing back to wall, feet 4 inches away from it, arms at sides.
   Drop body back against wall, shoulders relaxed, tighten abdominal muscles and flatten low back against wall—One!
   Push head back to wall, chin in—Two!
   Keep abdomen tight and push forward with hands—Three!
   Relax—Four!
   Repeat as desired.
       NOTE: If no flat wall in classroom, use the doors and take turns.

4. Abdomen.
   Standing, feet 1 foot apart, arms over head, hands clasped.
   Flatten low back—One!
   Hold and push arms up—Two!
   Relax arms—Three!
   Position—Four!

5. Upper Back.
   Sitting, feet in the aisle and toeing forward. (In gym or out of doors use benches, in classroom as below).
   Drop head forward—One!
   Hands on head—Two!
   Push up and back, chin in, elbows back to flatten neck and bring shoulder blades together—Three!
   Position—Four!

6. Head.
   Standing in aisle, facing side wall, legs in moderate stride, arms side horizontal, palms up trunk flat.
   Bend forward about 20 to 30 degrees, describe small arm circles backward—One!

Two!—Three!—Four!

NOTE: Emphasis on the over and back part of the stroke. The outward rotators of the scapula require posterior fixation when circling.

7. Trunk—Big Muscle Mimetic, Soccer, Free Kick.

Standing position.

Run forward, four steps, right, left, right, left—One!—Two! —Three!—Four!

Kick with right, swing leg through forward and upward, point toe and use instep for the kick—Five!

Right foot to position—Six!

Repeat.

8. Balance and Feet.

Standing in aisle, facing forward, arms in "T", elbows bent.

Airplane in flight—One!

Bend body forward with right leg back—Two!

Return—Three!

Position—Four!

Same, left leg, and repeat.

NOTE: If aisle is narrow and pupils are lower grade level, they may at first lightly touch desks on either side to help balance while pushing the leg backward and upward. The supporting foot must be kept toe-in and inverted. This is especially good on the tilted balance board.

9. Suspension.

Same as Exercise 9 in Lesson XIII.

10. Dismissal—General Marching and Facing.

Single or double march steps combined with facing.

Run four steps sideward crossing right foot in front of left and alternate step behind left.

About face and repeat, left foot.

Continue for required count or arrange progress toward exit.

LESSON XV

1. Feet and General Posture.

Standing, hands on neck.

Place right foot sideward—One!

Arms stretch sideward to diagonal with heel raising and turning toes in—Two!

Return—Three!

Position—Four!

Same, left.

2. Knee Alignment.

Standing in the aisle facing forward, hands on hips.

Lunge forward a short step, right, with right arm straight

forward, left arm back, keeping left knee very straight—
One!
Bring left foot to right—Two!
Return hands—Three!
Position—Four!
Same, left.
Repeat the reverse, stepping back.

3. Lower Back.
Standing as in No. 3, Lesson XIV.
Drop back against wall, flatten low back—One!
Chin in, head to wall—Two!
Push away from wall and take two steps forward—Three!
Two steps back to position—Four!
Repeat.

4. Abdomen.
Stand facing wall, bent arms's length away, body slightly
inclined forward, back flat, hands on wall, shoulder high
and shoulder width apart, elbows slightly bent, feet toeing
forward. Tighten abdominal muscles, flattening low back,
let body fall toward wall until chest touches—One!
Return—Two!
Repeat.

NOTE: The distance from the wall should be determined
by the strength of student's abdominal muscles. Keep
body straight throughout exercise. In case low back tends
to sag into lordosis, stand closer to wall.

5. Upper Back.
Sitting on benches or in classroom, feet in aisle.
Relax head forward, hands on neck, elbows forward, pinch
shoulder blades together—One!
Bring elbows back—Two!
Head back, chin in, flatten neck—Three!
Position—Four!

6. Head.
Stand in aisle, stride position, arms horizontal, hands grasp-
ing those of students on each side.
All drop heads—One!
Lean forward to bow—Two!
Raise head, chin in, shoulders back—Three!
Position—Four!

7. Trunk—Big Muscle Group, Mimetic, Tennis Serve.
Stride standing, left shoulder forward.
Place weight on right foot, head back and facing forward,
right hand grasps imaginary racquet, right arm shoulder

high, elbow bent, left arm extended forward holding ball
—One!

Swing right arm overhead and down finishing across the
body with weight on left foot—Two!

Repeat.

NOTE: For left handers, use opposite stance and action.

8. Balance and Feet.

Standing facing forward, hands on neck, feet on outer
border, big toe held down firmly.

Raise right knee, right foot pointing down and in—One!

Turn body to left slowly—Two!

Return—Three!

Position—Four!

9. Suspension.

Passive hang, ladder or bars, hands grasp wide, soles of
feet together.

Draw feet toward body, knees apart—One!

Straighten legs to diagonal—Two!

Return—Three!

Position—Four!

Repeat.

NOTE: Estimate students laxity of muscles or strength,
also excess weight, and reduce repetitions accordingly.

Watch for straining when extending legs and keep throat
open.

10. Dismissal.

Marching and facing, four running steps forward (hands
on hips).

Point toe forward—One!

Extend backward and point—Two!

Swing forward—Three!

Position—Four!

Same, left, and progress to exit or to end of desired count
if in classroom.

LESSON XVI

1. Feet and General Posture.

Standing, arms bent.

Place right foot forward—One!

Stretch arms to "tall walk" with heel raising and turning
toes in—Two!

Return—Three!

Position—Four!

2. Knee Alignment.

Standing, hands at sides, feet toeing in.

Raise right foot and place it across opposite knee—One!
Turn to left—Two!
Return—Three!
Position—Four!
Same, left.
Repeat.

NOTE: Supporting foot should be held firm. The trunk rotation raises the arch of the standing foot. Students with high arches should be cautioned about twisting too far for fear of tipping the foot over and getting a strained ankle.

3. Lower Back.

Stand in aisle, opposite the back of the seat, bend forward with hands grasping the front of seat edge on each side of the aisle (for some use desk edges).
Relax body and then tighten abdomen and hump the back up—One!
Raise the head, chin in—Two!
Return—Three!
Position—Four!

4. Abdomen.

Standing in aisle facing wall, legs at stride position.
Lean forward, hands on opposite desk—One! (If in gym or on playground, use benches).
Tense abdominal muscles to keep low back flat and lower the trunk till elbows are at a right angle bend—Two!
Return—Three!
Position—Four!

NOTE: Not good for severe round shoulders, too much pectoral and serratus action.

5. Upper Back.

Seated, feet in aisle, or sidewards on bench, feet toeing forward.
Hands on head, palms upward—One!
Elbows strongly back—Two!
Turn right—Three!
Position—Four!
Same, left.
Repeat.

6. Head.

Standing in aisle, leaning forward with hands on desks or bench.
Drop head forward pointing chin forward, lifting face—One!
Drop forehead down and draw chin in and back and up strongly—Two!
Return—Three!

Position—Four!

Repeat.

NOTE: This can be modified to swing relaxed head and neck from side to side or twisting back and forth, facing first left, then right, or doing a complete circumduction.

7. Trunk—Big Muscle Group Mimetic, Breast Stroke Swimming.

Standing, arms vertical, palms forward forefingers touching (head between arms as though in a straight line in water.)

Arms sideward, palms back—One!

Draw elbows in, hands touching in front of chest—Two!

Arms vertical—Three!

Repeat.

8. Balance and Feet.

Standing in aisle facing forward, feet parallel, toeing forward, four inches apart.

Extend left arm forward—One!

Lean slightly, raise right leg back and carry right arm back —Two! (Position of pursuit and light).

Return slowly—Three!

Position—Four!

Same, left.

Repeat.

NOTE: In case students are small or rather incoordinate, let them touch the toe in rear rather than raise the leg with knee straight.

9. Suspension.

Same as in Exercise 9, Lesson XV. As this is rather hard, it can well be repeated both as a test of form as well as strength.

10. Dismissal.

Standing in file, canoeing movement.

Hold paddles, right arm high, left arm forward grasping imaginary paddle, bend left—One!

Dip left—Two!

Long step forward, right—Three!

Position—Four!

Same, left, progressing thus to exit.

NOTE: This may be done to music or waltz rhythm and made graceful as a movement in a dance.

APPENDIX B.

JUNIOR HIGH SCHOOLS AND
SENIOR HIGH SCHOOLS

LESSON I

1. Feet.
   > Sitting, legs extended.
   > Turn balls of feet toward each other until toes touch—One!
   > Bend ankles up—Two!
   > Down—Three!
   > Position—Four!
   >
   > NOTE: Do not use in very flexible flatfeet in which anterior tibials are strong and tend to supinate the forefeet strongly, because such action relaxes the peroneus longus which is essential to depression of the first metatarsal.

2. Knee Alignment-Stretching Tendo Achillis and Hamstrings.
   > Sitting as in No. 1 above, back to wall or hands back on floor for support.
   > Push heels down—One!
   > Hold while trunk is bent forward with low back flat—Two!
   > Straighten—Three!
   > Position—Four!
   > Repeat as desired.

3. Lower Back.
   > Lying on back, knees bent (hook lying).
   > Raise head slightly forward—One!
   > Press lower back to floor—Two!
   > Return head—Three!
   > Position—Four!
   > Repeat desired number of times.

4. Abdomen.
   > Backward lying, legs extended.
   > Soles of feet together, separate knees, bring thighs to chest, back flat—One!
   > Grasp thighs back of knees and pull down to chest—Two!
   > Return to knee bent hook lying position—Three!
   >
   > NOTE: Separating knees before raising actuates outward rotators of thighs and abductors, thus throwing out the adductors which help to tilt pelvis forward and hollow the back.

5. Upper Back.
   > Lying, knees bent.
   > Press neck to floor—One!
   > Relax—Two!
   > Repeat as desired.

NOTE: Good for forward head and round shoulders, cervical lordosis and round back (kyphosis).

6. Head and Upper Back.

> Sitting, knees bent, feet crossed (cross sit).
> Arms side horizontal, turn palms upward forcibly—One!
> Hands to neck, elbows back—Two!
> Return—Three!
> Position—Four!
> Repeat.

7. Trunk.

> Sitting, knees bent, feet crossed, hands on floor.
> Hands to neck, head up, elbows back—One!
> Return—Three!
> Position—Four!
> Same, left.
> Repeat.

8. Balance—Feet.

> Standing, hands on hips, on tilted balance board.
> Bend trunk forward, touch board if possible—One!
> Return—Two!
> Right hand against pelvis behind, palm out, left hand palm down on lower abdomen (over symphysis), push up on left hand, down on right, gripping buttocks together—Three!
> Hands to hips—Four!
> Same, hands reversed.
> Repeat.

9. Suspension.

> Standing facing stall bars.
> Right hand to bars, shoulder high, right foot to lower bar —One!
> Climb up one bar—Two!—Three!—Four!
> Reverse position, hand grasp wide, hang flattening back— One!—Two!—Three!—Four!
> Feet to bar, relax, climb down alternating hands and feet.
> Repeat as desired.

10. In file, hands on hips, stepping in place for four counts and then skipping, toes in, to exit.

LESSON II

1. Feet.

> Standing, arms at sides.
> Turn arms strongly outward, turn knees out, grip buttocks together, keep big toes pressed to floor—One!
> Relax—Two!
> Repeat.

19

NOTE: Attention to tensing the buttocks adds to thigh rotation and results in lifting the arches and correcting pronation.

2. Knee Alignment.

Standing facing the wall or stall bars at arm's length, feet toeing in.

Lean forward, elbows to half bend, knees straight—One!—Two!—Three!

Return—Four!

3. Lower Back.

Lying on back, knees bent, arms in reversed "T" position, palms down.

Raise head forward, chin in, press palms to floor—One!

Return—Two!

Repeat.

NOTE: Arms reversed "T" stretches adductors and depressors (the pectorals major and minor). It affords a broad fixation base for trunk flexors (longus colli) and abdominals which correspondingly flatten low back and decrease pelvic tilt.

4. Abdomen.

Same as No. 3.

Knee raising, separated, grasp thighs behind knees and pull to chest—One!

Return against resistance of hands holding—Two!

Prolong the count to accentuate the action.

NOTE: Arm resistance produces trunk fixation by spinal extensors and thus decreases the tendency for psoas to pull lumbar spine forward, also reduces the tendency for the diaphragm to force downward.

5. Upper Back.

Lying on the face, hands under abdomen, palms up.

Raise head, chin in, face three inches from floor—One!

Return to floor, right cheek down—Two!

Alternate, returning to left cheek.

Repeat.

NOTE: Hands fixed by body weight tends to localize action to the shoulder and guards against arching the low back.

6. Head and Upper Back.

Sitting, knees apart and feet crossed.

Arms side horizontal, pinch shoulder blades together (do not raise or pull the shoulders back)—One!

Turn palms up—Two!

Return (holding shoulder blade tight)—Three!
Position—Four!
  NOTE: This exercise allows localized action of the scapular adductors (rhomboids and lower trapezius), throws out the arm adductors which, when contracted, are scapular abductors (teres and latissimus dorsi).

7. Trunk—For Big Muscle Action.
  Kneeling on right knee, hands on hips, right foot inverted, toeing in.
  Bend trunk forward—One!
  Return—Two!
  Repeat 3 times.
    NOTE: Given for constipation; pressure over right knee compresses ascending colon and over the left thigh the descending colon.

8. Balance—Feet.
  Standing on tilted balance board.
  Hands to neck, turn trunk to left and bend left—One!
  Position—Two!
  Alternate to right and repeat.
    NOTE: Standing on the tilt is of benefit to feet in holding them in a correct position while the balance muscles act.

9. Suspension.
  Stand one foot away from stall bars.
  Place right hand and left foot on the bar, foot on the first bar, hand grasping the bar that can be conveniently reached by standing on tip toe—One!
  Climb—Two!—Three!—Four! Alternate hand and foot.
  Hands wide grasp, hang four counts.
  Descend four counts to position.
    NOTE: Upward backward reach brings scapulæ back. Hanging stretches tight pectorals, keeping back flat actuates abdominals.

10. Dismissal.
  Standing in file, arm's length apart, arms side horizontal, rotate trunk forward on right, alignment of shoulder and arm fixed, step forward with left foot a good stride.
  Alternate, progressing to door.

LESSON III

1. Feet.
  Lying on back, knees bent (hook lying).
  Balls of feet together—One!
  Bend ankles up—Two!
  Hold and extend legs—Three!

Position—Four!
Repeat.
2. Knee Alignment.
Backward lying, legs diagonal.
Raise knees to chest, legs abducted—One!
Extend upward forcibly—Two!
Return—Three!
Position—Four!
Repeat.
3. Lower Back.
Lying, knees bent (hook lying), arms side horizontal, palms up.
Press back of hand to floor and raise head—One!
Return slowly—Two!
Repeat.
NOTE: Actuates posterior shoulder blade muscles and front abdominals. Good for relaxed wall and dependent abdomen or visceroptosis.
4. Abdomen.
Position as in No. 3, hands on neck, soles together.
Separate knees and raise keeping pelvis still and knees bent, at the same time raise the head—One!
Return—Two!
Repeat.
NOTE: Strong actuation of neck flexors, holding shoulder girdle fixators firm, while the abdominals fix pelvis on thorax as a base in order to allow legs to be raised by thigh flexors without arching low back.
5. Upper Back.
Prone lying, hands under abdomen, back of hands to floor and making fists.
Raise head three inches from floor, chin in—One!
Press elbows to sides—Two!
Return elbows—Three!
Return head—Four!
Repeat.
NOTE: Also good for constipation, for bowel falls forward off the spinal ridge and pressure of fists is increased by action of abdominal muscles tensing for the fixation needed for head action.
6. Head.
Sitting, feet crossed, knees apart.
Drop chin to chest—One!
Pull back slowly and firmly to neck flat position—Two!
Relax.

Repeat as desired, adding arms horizontal making outward circles, palms upward.

Repeat as desired.

NOTE: Elongates pectorals and subscapularis, actuating posterior scapular muscles and external arm rotators.

7. Trunk—Big Muscle Action.

Kneeling on right knee, right foot inverted, left knee forward, at right angles, left foot toe in.

Fold arms across lower abdomen, bend forward—One!

Twist trunk right—Two!

Return—Three!

Position—Four!

Repeat twisting to left.

Shift to left knee, kneel and repeat.

NOTE: Greater pressure on relaxed abdomen and reduced balance stress.

8. Balance and Feet.

Standing on tilted balance board or on floor with feet inverted, hands on neck, elbows back.

Lift right foot keeping it inverted, cross and touch outer border to opposite tread (if on floor, touch floor in front of left foot)—One!

Return to one foot ahead—Two!

Shift weight forward—Three!

Repeat with left progressing forward as many steps as desired.

9. Suspension.

Hanging on stall bars or horizontal ladder, hands wide apart.

Swing body to right and left—Eight counts.

10. Dismissal.

Facing in rank, march column left by twos and fours with cross-foot gait (pigeon toe walk).

NOTE: Any students with high arches or who have a toe-in gait should be excused.

LESSON IV

1. Feet and General Posture.

Standing, heels apart, toes in.

Grip buttocks—One!

Slide heels together against floor resistance—Two!

Step forward to toe-in position—Three!

Return, left same—Four!

Repeat as desired.

NOTE: Gripping buttocks aids external thigh rotators and helps flatten the low back.

2. Knee Alignment.
> Lying on back, legs extended.
> Invert right heel—One!
> Press right knee to floor—Two!
> Relax foot—Three!
> Relax knee—Four!
> Same, left.
> Repeat as desired.
> NOTE: Pressing knee to floor actuates external thigh rotators and relaxes inner rotators and adductors.

3. Lower Back.
> Lying, knees bent and feet and knees wide apart, arms "T".
> Arms vertical, hands clasped above—One!
> Roll trunk to right—Two!
> Return—Three!
> Position—Four!
> Repeat.
> NOTE: Knees and feet wide apart gives a more stable base from which trunk rotators may act.

4. Abdomen.
> Same as No. 3, arms reverse "T".
> Soles of feet together, separate knees—One!
> Raise legs to chest, still separated—Two!
> Head raise forward—Three!
> Position—Four!
> NOTE: Student to count aloud or exhale on leg raising to keep throat open.

5. Upper Back.
> Sitting, knees bent, feet crossed.
> Pinch shoulder blades together—One!
> Hold, arms raising sideward, palms down—Two!
> Palms up—Three!
> Position—Four!

6. Head and Upper Back.
> Same position as No. 5.
> Drop head forward, pull chin in—One!
> Twist to right strongly—Two!
> To left—Three!
> Position—Four!

7. Trunk and Big Muscle Action.
> Kneeling on right knee, toes in, left leg forward, knee at right angle, foot moderately inverted, hands on abdomen, fingers clasped.
> Squeeze elbows to sides—One!
> Bend trunk to right—Two!

To left—Three!
Position—Four!
Repeat and then shift to left knee down.

8. Balance and Feet.
Same position as in Lesson III.
Hands on hips—One!
Raise right foot inverted and place it in left hand—Two!
Hand pulls foot more inward—Three!
Position—Four!
One foot forward.
Same, left.
Repeat across board or number of steps desired.
NOTE: Hand grasp on forefoot pulling in and up stretches tight (peroneals), foot abductors.

9. Suspension.
As in Lesson III.
Hang, contract abdominal wall—One!
Bend ankles up, pushing down on heels—Two!
Turn thighs outward tensing buttocks—Three!
Position—Four!
Repeat as desired.

10. Dismissal.
In file, pigeon toe, running around the room and out.

LESSON V

1. Feet—General Posture.
Standing, feet parallel, three-quarter inches apart.
Rotate thighs outward enough to raise arches, keep big toe down flat—One!
Bend knees slightly holding foot position—Two!
Return—Three!
Position—Four!

2. Knee Alignment.
Standing, hands on hips.
Step forward, left, a half step, knees slightly bent—One!
Straighten right knee forcibly—Two!
Bend left knee a little more holding right fixed to stretch hamstrings—Three!
Position—Four!
Repeat as desired.

3. Lower Back.
Lying on back, knees bent, right hand on abdomen, palm down, left hand in small of back, palm down.
Press abdomen down to flatten back enough to pinch rear hand—One!

Relax—Two!

Repeat.

4. Abdomen.

Same as No. 3, arms reverse "T", feet apart, knees resting against each other.

Press down on feet flattening low back—One!

Hold and press hands to floor—Two!

Relax hands—Three!

Position—Four!

Repeat.

5. Upper Back.

Lying prone, heels apart, toes touching, hands under abdomen.

Raise head, face three inches from floor—One!

Press elbows to sides—Two!

Grip buttocks—Three!

Position—Four!

6. Head and Upper Back.

Sitting, knees bent, feet crossed (cross sit).

Hands on knees, press knees toward floor, helping with hands—One!

Forward lean, back flat—Two!

Up—Three!

Position—Four!

7. Trunk—Big Muscle Action.

Standing, archery position, in file, legs astride, students two steps apart.

Hands as in grasping bow—One!

Raise to left—Two!

Pull right fingers to chin, neck flat—Three!

Position—Four!

Repeat.

8. Balance and Feet.

As in previous lesson, head board in left hand.

Raise board and place on head—One!

Raise right knee—Two!

Take board—Three!

Position—Four! Returning foot, 1 foot ahead.

Same, left.

Repeat across the board or 8 steps forward on the floor.

9. Suspension.

Stall bars or horizontal ladder as in previous lesson.

Hang, abduct legs—One!

Rotate thighs outward—Two!

Return—Three!

Position—Four!

Rest with feet on appropriate bar.

Repeat as desired.

10. Dismissal.

Facing forward, hands on hips, toes in.

Side-step to right maintaining toe-in—One!

Cross over with left and place toe-in—Two!

Right foot to right —Three!

Left foot to position—Four!

Same, right foot crossing over to left.

Run to door, feet crossed in exaggerated pigeon toe.

NOTE: Excuse any student with high arches or who has varus or adductus of forefeet (pigeon-toed).

LESSON VI

1. Feet—General Posture.

Stand in stride position, hands on head with head board or bean bag.

Push up, flatten neck—One!

Maintain head and shoulder position, shift trunk to left —Two!

To right—Three!

Position—Four!

NOTE: Center of gravity shifted from one foot to the other, altering tension on lateral balance muscles.

2. Knee Alignment.

Standing in front of wall, feet 4 inches away, moderate toe-in.

Lean against wall and flatten back—One!

Slide down to quarter knee bend—Two!

Slide up to starting position—Three!

Relax—Four!

Repeat.

NOTE: Actuates gluteals and quadriceps. (Buttocks and front thigh muscles).

3. Lower Back.

Same position as No. 2.

Drop body forward—One!

Tighten abdomen—Two!

Hold and push up to erect position, chin back—Three!

Position—Four!

Repeat.

4. Abdomen.

Lying, knees bent.

Place soles together, raise legs keeping feet together—One!

Hips to left—Two!
Straight—Three!
Down—Four!
Same to right.
Repeat as desired.

NOTE: Soles together, knees apart brings external thigh rotators into action.

5. Upper Back.

Sitting, knees bent, soles touching, arms folded behind back.
Drop head and trunk forward—One!
Return to position against resistance of arms—Two!
Repeat.

NOTE: Obtains passive stretch of foot abductors (peroneals) and allows resistance to trunk extensors without arching the back.

6. Head and Upper Back.

Same position as in No. 5, hands on hips, good shoulder alignment.
Head circling first to right four counts.
Then to left four counts.

7. Trunk.

Sitting knees bent.
Extend arms forward a little wide as in grasping bars while leaning forward—One!
Extend legs against imaginary resistance as in rowing and pull back bringing body slightly beyond the right angle and elbows to a half-bend position—Two!
Repeat as desired.

NOTE: This may be modified by having pupils sit opposite each other, knees bent and have soles braced against those of an opponent while they grasp a wand, alternating the pull back and thus getting some resistance. Note also teacher might pass around the group and observe any lateral tilting of the pelvis during the exercises.

8. Balance and Feet.

Standing on floor, feet on outer borders or on tilted boards, head board in right hand.
Correct standing push up, arms side horizontal—One!
Raise right knee—Two!
Pass the board to opposite hand behind the knee—Three!
Arms horizontal—Four!
Step—Five!
Repeat, opposite knee.

9. Suspension.

Standing, right side to stall bars.

Left arm up and grasp bars above with left hand and below
with right hand, abduct left leg—One!

Down—Two!

Position—Three!

Turn around—Four!

Same, opposite arm and leg.

Repeat as desired.

10. Dismissal.

Standing in file, arms over head.

Clap hands and advance right foot.

Arms down as weight is transferred to right foot.

Same, left.

Repeat to door.

LESSON VII

1. Feet and General Posture.

Standing, arms to side horizontal.

Jump to a stride position, feet toeing in—One!

Hands to top of head, push head up, chin in, stretch tall
tensing abdominal muscles, flatten back—Two!

Return—Three!

Position—Four!

Repeat.

2. Knee Alignment.

Stand 4 inches away from wall.

Drop back against wall, flatten low back to wall, head back
to wall, hands to wall, tense abdomen—One!

Press hard to wall and push body away from wall with the
fingers—Two!

Step forward—Three!

Step back—Four!

Drop back to wall and see whether back position has been
retained.

3. Lower Back.

Sitting, knees bent, feet crossed.

Place hands on top of head—One!

Bend trunk right (Keeping elbows well back)—Two!

Return—Three! (Elbows kept back)

Position—Four!

Same, left.

Repeat.

4. Abdomen.

Lying on back, knees bent, arms "T", soles of feet together.

Raise legs to chest, keeping hips down—One!

Raise head—Two! (Keep hands on floor)

Return head—Three!

Position—Four!

Repeat.

5. Upper Back.

Lying prone, hands under abdomen, heels apart, toes touching.

Tense buttocks, rotating thighs outward until heels touch, raise head, chin in, face 3 inches from floor—One!

Hold—Two!—Three!

Relax—Four!

NOTE: Powerful antigravity movement; the difficulty is increased by holding the head and thigh rotators throughout the exercise.

6. Head and Upper Back.

Sitting, knees bent, feet crossed; by twos facing each other. Grasp partner's hands, No. 1 drops head and trunk forward —One!

Return to position against partner's resistance—Two!

Reverse and repeat.

7. Trunk—Mimetic. Batting Ball.

Standing, feet 14 to 18 inches apart, hands together in front, elbows slightly bent as in grasping a bat.

Turn trunk, to right—One!

Swing forward and follow through to trunk twist to left —Two!

Return—Three!

Position—Four!

Repeat.

8. Balance and Feet.

Standing on tilted boards or on floor, feet on outer borders.

Arms to side horizontal—One!

Carry right leg back in full extension, body slight bend forward—Two!

Hands to hips and right leg forward—Three!

To the floor in position—Four!

Same, left.

Repeat across board or for 8 steps on floor.

9. Suspension.

Standing, right side to stall bars, 18 inches away, grasp bars left hand over head, right hand 2 feet lower.

Rotate body half turn forward—One!

Return—Two!

Backward—Three!

Position—Four!

Same, left.

Repeat.

10. Dismissal.

Line up in file, arm's length apart, hands on shoulders of pupil next ahead.

Stepping high, abdominal muscles tensed as knee is raised —One!

Down forcibly—Two! (Feet toeing in)

Continue to exit.

LESSON VIII

1. Feet and General Posture.

Standing, hands on hips.

Thigh rotation outward—One!

Charge forward, right, toeing forward (keep body in line with rear leg), stretch Achilles' tendon and hamstrings— Two!

Return—Three!

Position—Four!

Repeat.

2. Knee Alignment.

Back lying, legs extended, arms as desired.

Place right foot on left thigh just above knee—One!

Press right knee down—Two!

Turn right foot up—Three!

Return—Four!

Same, left.

Repeat as desired.

NOTE: Adduction and inversion of foot should actuate the posterior tibial; weight of one leg on the other tends to stretch hamstrings.

3. Lower Back.

Sitting, knees bent, feet crossed, hands on head.

Twist trunk right (keep elbows back)—One!

Bend trunk left—(keep elbows back), left elbow to left knee—Two!

Return—Three!

Position—Four!

Same, left.

Repeat.

4. Abdomen.

Lying on back, arms "T" position, soles of feet together.

Raise legs, knees apart, soles pressed together—One!

(Pupils count aloud to keep throat open).

Raise head (keep arms on floor)—Two!

Return—Three!
Position—Four!

5. Upper Back.

Lying on face, hands under abdomen, heels apart, toes touching.

Tense buttocks, rotate thighs outward till heels touch, press elbows to sides hard—One!

Raise head, chin in, about 3 inches from floor—Two!

Return—Three!

Position—Four!

Repeat.

NOTE: Raising head slightly flattens neck and actuates spinal extensors but not enough to provoke lordosis below, and elbows to sides moderately actuates scapular adductors.

6. Head and Upper Back.

Sitting, knees bent, feet crossed, hands on hips.

Hands to neck, twist trunk right, elbows back—One!

Bend trunk forward over right knee, elbows back—Two!

Return—Three!

Position—Four!

Same, left.

Repeat.

7. Trunk—Bicycling.

Lying on back, knees bent, arms to diagonal.

Raise right knee to chest—One!

Extend right leg up while left knee is raised to chest—Two!

Alternate pushing up forcefully and pointing heels—16 counts.

8. Balance and Feet.

Standing on tilted boards or (on floor, feet slightly inverted).

Arms to side horizontal, palms forward—One!

Hands to neck, bend knees slightly keeping heels down —Two!

Return—Three!

Position—Four!

Repeat.

9. Suspension.

Hanging, back to stall bars, both hands grasp high.

Release right foot and let it hang close to bars—One!

Same, left—Two!

Hip raising, right, and replace right foot—Three!

Same, left—Four!

Repeat three times.

NOTE: Hip raising actuates quadratus lumborum and side abdominals.

10. Dismissal.
    Marching in file, hands on heads, trunk push up.
    Side step, right—One!
    Step forward, left—Two!
    Position—Three!
    Same, left.
    Repeat, progressing to exit.

LESSON IX

1. Feet and General Posture.
    Standing position, arms at sides.
    Arms straight over head—One!
    Push up, right foot to the side—Two!
    Return (continue pushing up tall)—Three!
    Position—Four!
    Same, left.
    Repeat.
        NOTE: Caution, do not carry arm push up back of the
    line of the face because there are so many with tight pec-
    torals that the rib cage will be lifted forward and there is a
    tendency to produce compensatory lordosis in low back.

2. Knee Alignment.
    Standing, weight on outer border of feet, elbows bent, finger
    tips touching in front of chest.
    Pull left shoulder back and twist trunk left—One!
    Return—Two!
    Same, left.
    Repeat.
        NOTE: The twist of trunk and pelvis further increases
    the inversion effect on foot passively stretching hamstrings,
    gastrocnemius and peroneals.

3. Lower Back.
    Sitting, knees bent, feet crossed, arms vertical, hands
    clasped.
    Twist trunk right—One!
    Bend trunk to right knee (keeping head in line with body)
    —Two!
    Return—Three!
    Position—Four!
    Same, left.
    Repeat.

4. Abdomen.
    Lying on back, arms "T" position, soles of feet together.
    Raise head (keep arms to floor)—One!
    Raise legs, knees apart, soles pressed together (keep hips

Position—Four!

Repeat same, left.

   NOTE: If any pupil has an undue pelvic tilt or twist, he may not be able to sit this way or his hips may be different on the two sides, in which case observe class closely and investigate any such condition.

4. Abdomen.

Sitting, knees bent, feet with soles together, hands on hips.

Trunk circling, bend trunk to right—One!

Forward—Two!

To left—Three!

Return—Four!

Same to left and repeat.

5. Upper Back.

Position as in No. 4, hands on hips.

Hands to neck, bend forward trunk, head and elbows—One!

Chin in, elbows strongly back—Two!

Return—Three!

Position—Four!

6. Head and Upper Back.

Same as in No. 3 and No. 4, hands on neck.

Pinch shoulder blades together (do not pull shoulders back or up)—One!

Elbows forward—Two!

Arms extend forward—Three!

Position—Four!

   NOTE: Arms forward only in case scapular pinch can be held.

7. Trunk, Mimetic Back Stroke Swimming Movement.

Lying on back, soles of feet together, arms at sides.

Simultaneously draw legs up to body, draw hands up the sides to the armpits—One! (Hold knees outward and as near to floor as possible.)

Extend arms sidewards, a little above side horizontal, and legs outward to diagonal—Two!

Return feet together, arms to sides—Three!—Four!

Repeat.

8. Balance and Feet.

Standing on boards or on floor as previously explained, hands on top of head.

Bend body left—One!

Bend right knee—Two! (If on the boards, try to touch right foot to floor right while holding trunk bend.)

Return—Three!

Position—Four!

Same, left.

Repeat.

NOTE: Bending trunk to side increases load on the standing leg and increases balance stress, while lifting the relaxed leg actuates loin muscles on that side, and when right foot reaches down to floor from the board, the opposite loin muscles must tense to keep balance.

9. Suspension.

Hanging on stall bars or ladder.

Release right foot, pass it across in front of left—One!

Return—Two!

Left over right—Three!

Return—Four!

Repeat.

NOTE: Trunk twist in reverse with shoulder girdle fixed.

10. Dismissal.

In file, arms length apart, arms side horizontal.

Right arm and right leg forward—One!

Left arm and left leg forward a full step—Two!

Repeat to exit.

LESSON XI

1. Feet and General Posture.

Standing, arms at side.

Bend elbows, place right foot sideward—One!

Fling arms sidewards, palms upward, thigh rotation outward—Two!

Return—Three!

Position—Four!

Same, left.

Repeat.

2. Knee Alignment.

Sitting, legs extended, hands on floor.

Place right foot across left knee, invert feet, push left heel down—One!

Return—Two!

Same, left—Three!

Position—Four!

Repeat.

3. Lower Back.

Lying on side, lower leg bent, upper arm on hip, lower arm bent under head for support.

Extend upper leg forward—One!

Backward—Two!

Return—Three!

Position—Four!

Repeat.

Same, left.

Repeat.

NOTE: Gravity load falls on abductors and side trunk fixators and not on thigh flexors.

4. Abdomen.

Sitting, soles of feet together, hands on knees.

Bend trunk forward—One!

Push to upright position as against resistance, chin in, shoulder blades together—Two!

Repeat.

5. Upper Back.

Lying prone, fists under abdomen, legs separated.

Raise head, chin in, face 3 inches from floor—One!

Bend knees, heels to buttocks—Two!

Return—Three!

Position—Four!

Repeat.

6. Head and Upper Back.

Sitting, knees bent, feet crossed, hands on hips.

Bend trunk forward extending arms forward and strongly outward, turning head to right—One!

Return head and arms forward—Two!

Body up—Three!

Arms position—Four!

Same, head turn left.

Repeat.

7. Trunk, Mimetic, Shoot for Basket.

Standing, elbows fully flexed in front of chest, left foot slightly forward.

Knees quarter bend, weight on balls of feet—One!

Jump and thrust arms forward and upward as in basketball throw—Two!

Repeat.

8. Balance and Feet.

Standing on boards or floor as previously indicated, elbows bent.

Stretch right arm upward, palm in, left arm to side horizontal, palm forward—One!

Reverse arm position—Two!

Reverse again—Three!

Position—Four!

Same, left.

Repeat.

9. Suspension.

> Stall bars, face forward, four bars up.

> *a.* Grasp high, feet on lower bar, shift pelvis to right—One!
> To left—Two!—Three!
> Position—Four!
> Repeat, each time one bar lower to floor.

> *b.* When using a hanging ladder, raise right foot to inside of
> left knee—One!
> Extend out to diagonal—Two!
> Return—Three!
> Position—Four!
> Repeat opposite.

10. Dismissal.

> Stand back to bars or wall, shoulders and head touching
> wall, back flattened, hands on hips.
> Sway forward keeping pelvis fixed and abdomen tight—
> One!
> Step forward, left—Two!
> Step forward, right—Three!
> Heels together—Four!
> Continue to exit or as many steps as desired.

LESSON XII

1. Feet and General Posture.

> Standing.
> Arms sideward upward to diagonal, right foot sideward—
> One!
> Rotate arms and thighs outward (keeping toes and ball
> of foot down)—Two!
> Return—Three!
> Position—Four!
> Same, left.
> Repeat.

2. Knee Alignment.

> Lying on back, knees bent.
> Extend right leg, forcefully pointing heel—One!
> Same, left, returning right to position—Two!
> Repeat, alternating, eight counts.
> NOTE: Pupils with high arched feet should be told to
> eliminate pointing heels.

3. Lower Back.

> Lying on side, right knee bent under left leg, right arm bent
> under head.
> Raise left leg upward—One!
> Hold—Two!—Three!

Position—Four!
Repeat.
Change sides and repeat reversed.

4. Abdomen.
   Sitting, knees bent 45 degrees.
   Separate knees, raise trunk forward—One!
   Arms to vertical, clasp hands over head—Two!
   Trunk erect—Three!
   Position—Four!
   Repeat.

   NOTE: Bending trunk forward between knees actuates abdominals, and the hip flexors only minimally. Keeping head and arms in line of the body prevents rounding of back and shoulders.

5. Upper Back.
   Lying on face, bend knees, heels to buttocks.
   Grasping ankles pull heels down strongly—One!
   Raise head, chin in, face 3 inches from floor—Two!
   Return—Three!
   Position—Four!
   Repeat.

6. Head and Upper Back.
   Sitting, knees bent, feet crossed, hands on hips.
   Bend trunk forward, bring arms to arm bent position—One
   Arm stretch sidewards, palms up—Two!
   Return to arm bent—Three!
   Position—Four!
   Repeat.

7. Trunk, Big Muscle Mimetic, Golf Drive.
   Standing at stride, hands grasping club, right little finger locked with left forefinger, arms hanging.
   Drop head and shoulders forward, eyes on the ball, swing arms to right and up letting elbows bend, twist trunk right —One!
   Swing forward, down and up to left—Two!
   Hold and look for ball to land—Three!
   Position—Four!

8. Balance and Feet.
   Standing on boards or floor.
   Hands to neck—One!
   Press elbows back, neck firm, lean slowly forward—Two (Keep back flat.)
   Raise left leg backward—Three!
   Position—Four!
   Repeat.

Same, right leg.

Repeat.

9. Suspension.

Facing bars climb upward alternating hand and foot, four counts.

Turning back to bars and hang.

Rotate thighs out—One!

Flatten abdomen—Two!

Hold—Three!

Position—Four!

Repeat.

10. Dismissal.

Standing in file, arm's length apart, hands on hips.

Right leg forward diagonal, touch pointed toe to floor, lean slightly forward and bow—One!

Straighten body—Two!

Swing left leg through and touch toe bowing—Three!

Alternate, progressing to exit. Keep body position but make all movements smooth and graceful.

LESSON XIII

1. Feet and General Posture.

Standing, heels apart, toes together.

Grip buttocks—One!

Slide heels together against resistance of floor—Two!

Jump to stride, feet straight ahead—Three!

Jump to starting position, heels apart, toes together—Four!

Repeat.

2. Knee Alignment.

Standing, hands on hips.

Lean forward—One!

Arms side horizontal—Two!

Kick right leg back with heel pointed (forcefully to straighten knee and stretch Achilles)—Three!

Position—Four!

Repeat.

3. Lower Back.

Lying on side, right, supporting knee bent under left leg, right elbow bent under head, left arm lying on left side.

Raise left leg to diagonal and left arm to vertical—One!

Position—Two!

Repeat.

Same, left.

Repeat.

4. Abdomen.
   Lying, legs extended.
   Press down on heels and raise body to vertical, bringing knees to chest, grasp knees and pull to chest strongly—One! Position—Two!
   Repeat.
   NOTE: Keep back and shoulder girdle flat. Changing to arm pull of knees relaxes abdominals and makes passive pressure; good for constipation.

5. Upper Back.
   Lying on face, arms "T" position.
   Raise head, chin in, face 3 inches from floor—One!
   Raise elbows keeping forearms in line (airplane position) —Two!
   Return—Three!
   Position—Four!
   Repeat.

6. Head and Upper Back.
   Sitting, knees bent, feet crossed, hands on hips.
   Bring trunk forward and arms to bent position, palms down —One!
   Arms up, out and back, palms up—Two!
   Return—Three!
   Position—Four!
   Repeat.

7. Trunk, Big Muscle Mimetic, Breast Stroke as in Swimming.
   Standing, arms vertical, palms forward, forefingers touching forehead.
   Arms sideward, palms upward, knees slightly bent—One!
   Jump to stride stand, draw elbows to side, forefingers to chest—Two!
   Feet together—Three!
   Position—Four!
   Repeat.

8. Balance and Feet.
   Standing on floor, weight on outer borders of feet, two arms' length apart, enough to grasp hand of next student.
   Raise arms to side horizontal, grasp other student's hand, bend right knee—One!
   Hold knee up and drop head forward—Two!
   Chin in, head up—Three!
   Position—Four!
   Same, left.
   Repeat.

9. Suspension.

Standing, back to bars, climb up alternate hand, opposite foot.

Reach right hand up and grasp bar—One!

Raise left knee tensing abdomen—Two!

Place left foot on first bar higher—Three!

Reach and grasp opposite hand one bar higher and thus repeat up four bars and down four bars.

10. Dismissal.

Stand in file, arms length apart.

Charge forward outward to diagonal with right leg—One!

Twist toward right and forcefully extend arms in line with right leg—Two!

Bring left foot up to right—Three!

Position—Four!

Repeat, left, and continue to exit or as many steps as desired.

LESSON XIV

1. Feet and General Posture.

Standing, arms side horizontal.

Lunge sideward, right foot toeing forward and landing on outer border—One!

Hands to neck, bend trunk sideward to right—Two!

Straight—Three!

Position—Four!

Same, left.

2. Knee Alignment.

Standing, stride position.

Arms over head—One!

Bend to the left foot—Two!

Return—Three!

To the right—Four!

Position—Five!

Repeat.

3. Lower Back.

Right side lying, right knee bent.

Raise left leg and head—One! (Sliding left hand down left thigh)

Position—Two!

Repeat same, right.

4. Abdomen.

Lying on back, knees bent, arms reverse "T", leg circling.

Knees bent and separated to chest—One!

Circling to right—Two!

Down but feet do not touch floor—Three!
Same, reverse direction.
> NOTE: Powerful movement involving trunk and pelvic stabilizers. Caution, should not be done by any student complaining of low back pain, or girls near or during menstrual period.

5. Upper Back.
Lying on face, arms reverse "T".
Raise head and arms from floor, head to right—One!
Bend trunk right keeping face 3 inches from floor—Two!
Return—Three!
Position—Four!
Same, to left.
Repeat.

6. Head and Upper Back.
Sitting, knees bent, feet crossed, hands on hips.
Trunk bend forward, arms to side horizontal—One!
Chin in, neck flat, turn palms up, rotating arms—Two!
Return—Three!
Position—Four!
Repeat.

7. Trunk, Big Muscles, Mimetic, Crawl Stroke.
Standing position.
Left arm to vertical, head relaxed forward—One!
Pull left arm down strongly, right arm to vertical, turning head to left, lifting chin to breathe—Two!
Repeat.
> NOTE: For variety adapt arm detail as desired.

8. Balance—Feet.
Standing in rank, legs at stride, outer borders of feet against those of students on each side.
Grasp hands or wrists, all sway to left—One!
Return—Two!
To right—Three!
Position—Four!
Repeat.
> NOTE: Should be done slowly and feet should be kept on the floor, firmly and toeing straight ahead. This will stretch tight foot evertors (peroneals).

9. Suspension.
Standing, facing bars.
Climb upward, alternate hand and foot—Four counts on right side of bars.
Release right hand and foot and twist to left until hand and foot can be placed.

Change to left hand and foot and hang—Four counts.
Climb down—Four counts.

10. Dismissal.
Line up in column of twos.
Turn and face each other, arm's length apart, hands on
each other's shoulders, side step right—One!
Carry left foot through and place toes in.
Repeat to exit.

LESSON XV

1. Feet and General Posture.
Standing.
Raise right foot, grasp front foot with left hand—One!
Bend left knee slightly, pull right foot up—Two!
Return—Three!
Position—Four!
Same, left.
Repeat.

2. Knee Alignment.
Line up in rank, arm's length apart, hands on back of next
student in rank.
All step forward with left foot keeping right heel down—
One!
Bend left knee slowly—Two! (Keeping right heel down)
Return—Three!
Position—Four!
Same, reversed.
Repeat.
NOTE: All keep backs flat and abdominals tight to main-
tain fixed pelvic position for stretch of tight hamstrings
and Achilles.

3. Lower Back.
Lying on right side, supporting leg bent at hip and knee.
Left leg extended strongly—One! (Left hand sliding down
thigh)
Bend trunk upward raising right arm to horizontal—Two!
Return—Three!
Position—Four!

4. Abdomen.
Lying on back, legs extended, arms at side horizontal
Bring hands to forehead—One!
Raise head forward against weight of hand—Two!
Return—Three!
Position—Four!

5. Upper Back.
> Lying on the face.
> Clasp hands in rear, pinch shoulder blades together keeping head on floor—One! (Arms remain relaxed)
> Hold—Two!—Three!
> Position—Four!
>
>   NOTE: Teacher should feel arm muscles to see that they remain relaxed.

6. Head and Upper Back.
> Standing, stride position.
> Relax trunk and head forward, arms hanging—One!
> Tense abdominals and raise trunk and head, hands to neck, chin in—Two!
> Keep back flat!
> Return—Three!
> Position— Four!

7. Trunk, Big Muscles, Mimetic, Bowling.
> Standing position.
> Step forward, left—One! (Holding ball in right hand, left arm forward sideward to balance)
> Step forward, right—Two!
> Charge forward, left, right arm stroke forward, left arm back—Three!
> Position—Four!
> Reverse.
> Continue for sixteen counts.

8. Balance and Feet.
> Standing on tilted boards or on floor, weight on outer borders.
> Touch right foot to floor—One!
> Raise right foot and place against left leg just above knee, hands to head—Two!
> Hold—Three!
> Position—Four!

9. Suspension.
> Standing facing stall bars.
> Climb upward, alternate hand and foot for four counts.
> Active hanging, back to bars, hands 3 feet apart—Eight counts.
> Return to passive hang slowly—Four counts.
>
>   NOTE: After shoulder depressors, notably pectorals and teres have been sufficiently stretched, there should be strong activation of scapular adductors (rhomboids and trapezius). As the arm adductors act also as scapular abductors, it is essential to disassociate the synergistic action of these

groups, *i.e.*, obtaining scapular adduction while the arms are fixed in abduction.

10. Dismissal.

Columns of twos, hands on hips.

Step right, swing left forward, step left, swing right forward, three running steps, 1–2–3–hop.

Right swing, left forward and repeat to exit.

LESSON XVI

1. Feet and General Posture.

Standing, arms side horizontal.

Charge forward, right, toeing in a little, keep body in line with rear leg—One!

Bend forward, touch hands to floor—Two!

Return—Three!

Position—Four!

Same, left.

Repeat.

2. Knee Alignment.

Sitting, legs extended, hands a little to rear supporting.

Push left heel down to lengthen leg—One!

Cross right foot over left leg and place on floor, foot turned in—Two!

Return—Three!

Position—Four!

Same, reversed.

Repeat.

3. Lower Back.

Lying on right side, supporting knee bent, right elbow bent, supporting head.

Raise left leg and circle it four times one way.

Reverse, four counts.

Repeat, left side.

4. Abdomen.

Lying on back, legs extended at diagonal, hands on forehead.

Raise head and shoulders—One!

Turn shoulders right—Two!

Left—Three!

Position—Four!

Repeat.

5. Upper Back.

Lying on face, arms at side horizontal.

Raise head and arms, face 3 inches from floor—One!

Turn palms up—Two!

Return—Three!

Position—Four!
6. Head and Upper Back.
    Standing, stride position.
    Hands to neck, pinch shoulder blades together—One!
    Bend trunk forward, keep elbows well back, chin in, back flat—Two!
    Return—Three!
    Position—Four!
7. Trunk, Big Muscle, Mimetic, Soccer Free Kick.
    Run forward two steps, right, left—One!
    Kick right, swing leg forcefully forward upward and leave the ground from the left foot, arms sideward upward for balance—Two!
    Land on left, foot comes to ground directly, weight forward on right—Three!
    Repeat.
8. Balance and Feet.
    Standing on tilted balance board or on floor, feet inverted slightly, hands on hips.
    Bend forward touching board or floor if possible—One!
    Return pushing head up with chin in—Two!
    Place right hand on lower abdomen (over symphysis pubis), left hand to small of back, push the right hand upward with the pubic bone, grip buttocks—Three!
    Hands to hips—Four!
    Repeat, changing hands.
9. Suspension.
    Standing facing stall bars.
    Climb upward, alternate hand and foot—Four counts!
    Passive hanging back to the bars, hand grasp wide.
    Place soles of feet together and draw them up to the body, knees wide apart—One! (Beginning of leg movement for frog kick in back stroke swimming.)
    Extend legs diagonally outward—Two!
    Together—Three!
    Hold—Four!
    Repeat on one bar lower each time to floor.
10. Dismissal.
    Line marching, hands on head, push up tall.
    Stepping forward, left—1, 2, 3, 4,—on four point outside, foot forward.
    Repeat, start right—1, 2, 3, 4, point. Continue to exit.
      NOTE: This can be modified to slide 2, 3, hop on 4, or in column of two's, holding hands and swinging them with stepping, one, two, three, change hands, and so forth.

Index